Minimally Invasive Foregut Surgery for Malignancy

Steven N. Hochwald
Editor
Moshim Kukar
Associate Editor

Minimally Invasive Foregut Surgery for Malignancy

Principles and Practice

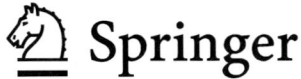
Springer

Editor
Steven N. Hochwald, MD, FACS
Department of Surgical Oncology
Roswell Park Cancer Institute
Buffalo, NY
USA

Associate Editor
Moshim Kukar, MD
Department of Surgical Oncology
Roswell Park Cancer Institute
Buffalo, NY
USA

Videos to this book can be accessed at
http://www.springerimages.com/videos/978-3-319-09341-3.

ISBN 978-3-319-09341-3 ISBN 978-3-319-09342-0 (eBook)

DOI 10.1007/978-3-319-09342-0
Springer Cham Heidelberg New York Dordrecht London

Library of Congress Control Number: 2014957156

Printed on acid-free paper

Springer is part of Springer Science+Business Media (www.springer.com)

Foreword

It has taken several decades for physicians and surgeons to accept that the management of the cancer patient is no longer discipline based but disease based.

The majority of advances that have come about have been the result of increased knowledge and understanding of pathogenesis, molecular diagnosis, natural history, and prognostic factors for progression and survival. This knowledge, accompanied by controlled trials, has allowed the integration of meaningful treatment. No longer can the oncologist expect patient management to be solely driven by his or her own discipline.

With such knowledge-based care, traditional views of surgical approaches can now be maximized, balancing morbidity against outcome. The rapid evolution of minimal access techniques has quickly demonstrated that morbidity can be minimized over and above more radical classical approaches. The perioperative advantages of such approaches were easy to define. Initially, these were confined to the benefits of solely ablative procedures such as hysterectomy or cholecystectomy done through minimal incisions with low risk and low morbidity. In situations where cancer care involved more extensive procedures, particularly those requiring reconstruction, progress was slower but is clearly being made. Once it was established that a minimal access approach could provide adequate oncological resection with similar lymph node yield where appropriate, then those advantages were confirmed. Internal reconstruction techniques were defined, and the benefits of minimal access surgery seen in the perioperative period could then be examined in the context of long-term outcome. This has now been established such that the perioperative benefits are associated, when done well, with equivalent long-term outcome. The ability of surgeons to utilize the technical improvements in vision and robotic instruments is expanding exponentially.

The present text by Drs. Kukar and Hochwald brings together this combination of knowledge-based treatment with minimal access techniques as they apply to foregut surgery for malignancy. The authors have assembled an international cast, many of whom have been leaders in bringing such techniques to the fore.

For any physicians involved in the surgical management of foregut malignancy, this text will be required reading

NY, USA   Murray F. Brennan, MD

Preface

Malignancies of the stomach and esophagus remain devastating for the patient and challenging for the treating physician. Worldwide, these cancers remain a major health concern, and due to varied presentation on different continents, surgical practice and expertise varies considerably. The aggressive biology of these tumors coupled with the advanced stage at presentation in many patients mandates multidisciplinary care. Such care is frequently associated with the careful integration of radiotherapy and chemotherapy either before or after surgery. No matter what the approach, esophagectomy or gastrectomy is associated with measurable deficits for the patient and the need for physical as well as functional rehabilitation.

Minimally invasive surgical treatment of these malignancies allows for more rapid return of preillness physical strength due to a reduced physiological insult resulting from smaller incisions, more rapid mobilization of the patient, decreased narcotic use, and shorter hospital time. Up until recently, minimally invasive surgery for esophageal or gastric malignancy was not considered mainstream due to fear of inadequacy of oncological resection in the face of advanced disease at presentation. Technological advancements and the published results of surgical pioneers in these areas have allowed for rapid progress in minimally invasive esophagogastric surgical approaches that closely emulate and potentially improve upon the traditional open approaches. Furthermore, the development of robotic surgery platforms offers great promise for refinements of techniques and outcomes in the near future.

This global, comprehensive work captures the brilliant progress made in the minimally invasive surgical care of gastric and esophageal cancer patients. There is much to learn from our physician colleagues as patterns of disease presentation have led to the development of distinct and regional experts in minimally invasive treatment approaches. No existing book on this topic has assembled essential background chapters discussing tumor biology and treatment approaches as well as comprehensive technique chapters complemented extensively by high-definition videos illustrating salient surgical points. To accomplish this, we have assembled an international group of experts that discuss and demonstrate every major minimally invasive surgical and endoscopic treatment modality including the use of endoscopic submucosal dissection and robotic surgery for stomach and esophageal cancer. In order to give the reader an opportunity to visualize several different approaches for one operation, minimally invasive esophagectomy with cervical anastomosis is described utilizing both laparoscopic and robotic approaches. In addition, minimally invasive esophagectomy with intrathoracic anastomosis is described utilizing both an EEA circular stapler in an end-to-side fashion as well as the use of a linear stapler to create a side-to-side anastomosis. Both robotic and laparoscopic approaches to gastric cancer surgery are extensively reviewed and described.

The work is divided into background chapters useful for current treatment recommendations, while technique chapters enriched with multiple figures demonstrate the various minimally invasive surgical approaches. Finally, as visual demonstrations of techniques are essential for more widespread adaptation, each technique chapter is accompanied by at least one video demonstrating the critical portion of the procedure.

We have learned much during our assembly of the outstanding contributions and from watching superb videos available through an online link. We are confident that you will look to this book as an integrated state-of-the-art invaluable resource.

Buffalo, NY, USA   Moshim Kukar, MD
Buffalo, NY, USA   Steven N. Hochwald, MD

Internet Access to Video Clips: The owner of this text will be able to access these video clips through Springer with the following Internet link: http://www.springerimages.com/videos/978-3-319-09341-3.

Contents

Contributors

Sang-Hoon Ahn, MD Department of Surgery, Seoul National University Bundang Hospital, Seongnam, Gyeonggi, Republic of Korea

Yuji Akiyama, MD, PhD Department of Surgery, Iwate Medical University School of Medicine, Morioka, Iwate Prefecture, Japan

Christopher Armstrong, MD, FRCSC Department of General Surgery, Rockyview General Hospital and South Health Campus, University of Calgary, Calgary, AB, Canada

Kfir Ben-David, MD Department of Surgery, University of Florida Health, Gainesville, FL, USA

George Bouras, BMBS, BMedSci, FRCS Department of Surgery and Cancer, Imperial College London, London, UK

Fátima Carneiro, MD, PhD Department of Pathology, IPATIMUP and Medical Faculty, Centro Hospitalar de São João, Porto, Portugal

Todd L. Demmy, MD Department of Thoracic Surgery, Roswell Park Cancer Institute, Buffalo, NY, USA

Yuichiro Doki, MD Department of Gastroenterological Surgery, Osaka University Graduate School of Medicine, Suita, Osaka, Japan

Joshua Ellenhorn, MD Department of Surgery, Cedars-Sinai Medical Center, Los Angeles, CA, USA

Fumitaka Endo, MD, PhD Department of Surgery, Iwate Medical University School of Medicine, Morioka, Iwate Prefecture, Japan

Mei Ka Fong, PharmD Department of Pharmacy, Roswell Park Cancer Institute, Buffalo, NY, USA

Dido Franceschi, MD Department of Surgery, University of Miami Hospital and Jackson Memorial Hospital, Miami, FL, USA

Heike I. Grabsch, MD, PhD, FRCPath Department of Pathology, Maastricht University Medical Center, AZ Maastricht, The Netherlands

Steven N. Hochwald, MD, FACS Department of Surgical Oncology, Roswell Park Cancer Institute, Buffalo NY, USA

Toshitaka Hoppo, MD, PhD Department of Surgery, Institute for the
Treatment of Esophageal and Thoracic Disease, The Western Pennsylvania
Hospital, Pittsburgh, PA, USA

Harohiro Inoue, MD, PhD Digestive Disease Center,
Showa University, Northern Yokohama Hospital, Yokohama, Japan

Takeshi Iwaya, MD, PhD Department of Surgery, Iwate Medical
University School of Medicine, Morioka, Iwate Prefecture, Japan

Blair A. Jobe, MD, FACS Department of Surgery, Institute for the
Treatment of Esophageal and Thoracic Disease, The Western Pennsylvania
Hospital, Pittsburgh, PA, USA

Kaitlyn J. Kelly, MD Department of Surgery, University of California,
San Diego, La Jolla, CA, USA

Hyung-Ho Kim, MD, PhD Department of Surgery, Seoul National
University Bundang Hospital, Seongnam, Gyeonggi, Republic of Korea

Yusuke Kimura, MD, PhD Department of Surgery, Iwate Medical
University School of Medicine, Morioka, Iwate Prefecture, Japan

Keisuke Koeda, MD, PhD Department of Surgery, Iwate Medical
University School of Medicine, Morioka, Iwate Prefecture, Japan

Masafumi Konosu, MD Department of Surgery, Iwate Medical
University School of Medicine, Morioka, Iwate Prefecture, Japan

A. Christiaan Kroese, MD Division of Anesthesiology,
Intensive Care and Emergency Medicine, University Medical Center
Utrecht, Utrecht, The Netherlands

Moshim Kukar, MD Department of Surgical Oncology,
Roswell Park Cancer Institute, Buffalo, NY, USA

Yukinori Kurokawa, MD Department of Gastroenterological Surgery,
Osaka University Graduate School of Medicine, Suita, Osaka, Japan

Sang-Woong Lee, MD, PhD Department of General
and Gastroenterological Surgery, Osaka Medical College,
Takatsuki, Osaka, Japan

Charles LeVea, MD, PhD Department of Pathology and Laboratory
Medicine, Roswell Park Cancer Institute, Buffalo, NY, USA

Donald E. Low, FACS, FRCS(c) Department of General, Thoracic,
and Vascular Surgery, Virginia Mason Medical Center, Seattle, WA, USA

James D. Luketich, MD Department of Cardiothoracic Surgery,
University of Pittsburgh Medical Center, UPMC Presbyterian,
Pittsburgh, PA, USA

Usha Malhotra, MD Department of Medicine, Roswell Park
Cancer Institute, Buffalo, NY, USA

Sheraz R. Markar, MRCS(Eng), MA, MSc Department of Thoracic Surgery, Virginia Mason Medical Center, Seattle, WA, USA

Robert C.G. Martin II , MD, PhD, FACS Division of Surgical Oncology, University of Louisville, Louisville, KY, USA

Isaac P. Motamarry, MD Department of General Surgery, University of Florida Shands, Gainesville, FL, USA

Didier Mutter, MD, PhD, FACS Department of Digestive and Endocrine Surgery, IRCAD, IHU, University Hospital of Strasbourg, Nouvel Hôpital Civil – Pôle Hépato-Digestif, Hôpitaux Universitaires de Strasbourg, Strasbourg, Alsace, France

Marius Nedelcu, MD Department of Digestive and Endocrine Surgery, University Hospital of Strasbourg, Nouvel Hôpital Civil – Pôle Hépato-Digestif, Hôpitaux Universitaires de Strasbourg, Strasbourg, Alsace, France

Nihn T. Nguyen, MD Department of Surgery, University of California Irvine Medical Center, Orange, CA, USA

Hiroyuki Nitta, MD, PhD Department of Surgery, Iwate Medical University School of Medicine, Morioka, Iwate Prefecture, Japan

Toru Obuchi, MD, PhD Department of Surgery, Iwate Medical University School of Medicine, Morioka, Iwate Prefecture, Japan

David D. Odell, MD, MMSc Department of Cardiothoracic Surgery, University of Pittsburgh Medical Center, UPMC Presbyterian, Pittsburgh, PA, USA

Koki Otsuka, MD, PhD Department of Surgery, Iwate Medical University School of Medicine, Morioka, Iwate Prefecture, Japan

C. Palanivelu, MS, MCh, FRCS, FACS Division of Oesophagastric Surgery, GEM Hospital and Research Centre, Coimbatore, TN, India

Wesley A. Papenfuss, MD Department of Surgical Oncology, Roswell Park Cancer Institute, Buffalo, NY, USA

R. Parthasarathi, MS, FMAS Division of Advanced Minimally Invasive and GI Surgery, GEM Hospital and Research Centre, Coimbatore, TN, India

Elizabeth Paulus, MD Division of Surgical Oncology, University of Miami – Miller School of Medicine/Jackson Memorial Hospital, Miami, FL, USA

Palanivelu Praveen Raj, MS, DNB(GI), DNB(SGI), FALS, FMAS Department of Surgical Gastroenterology GEM Hospital and Research Centre, Coimbatore, TN, India

R. Taylor Ripley, MD Division of Thoracic Surgery, Memorial Sloan-Kettering Cancer Center, New York, NY, USA

Georgios Rossidis, MD Department of Surgery, University of Florida, Gainesville, FL, USA

Jelle P.H. Ruurda, MD, PhD Department of Surgery, University Medical Center Utrecht, Utrecht, The Netherlands

Akira Sasaki, MD, PhD Department of Surgery, Iwate Medical University School of Medicine, Morioka, Iwate Prefecture, Japan

Hiroki Sato, MD Digestive Disease Center, Showa University, Northern Yokohama Hospital, Yokohoma, Japan

Erin Schumer, MS, MD Department of General Surgery, University of Louisville, Louisville, KY, USA

Roderich E. Schwarz, MD, PhD, FACS Department of Surgical Oncology, Indiana University Health Goshen Center for Cancer Care, Goshen, IN, USA

Palanisami Senthilnathan, MS, DNBGen, MRCSEd, DNB GISurg, FACS Department of Surgical Gastroenterology, GEM Hospital and Research Centre, Coimbatore, TN, India

J. Shapiro, MD Department of Surgery, Erasmus Medical Center, Rotterdam, CA, The Netherlands

Vivian E. Strong, MD Department of Surgery, Memorial Sloan-Kettering Cancer Center, New York, NY, USA

Shuji Takiguchi, MD Department of Gastroenterological Surgery, Osaka University Graduate School of Medicine, Suita, Osaka, Japan

A. Koen Talsma, MD, MSc Department of Surgery, Erasmus Medical Center, Rotterdam, CA, The Netherlands

Nobuhiko Tanigawa, MD, FACS Department of Surgery, Tanigawa Memorial Hospital, Ibaraki, Osaka, Japan

Richard van Hillegersberg, MD, PhD Department of Surgery, University Medical Center Utrecht, Utrecht, The Netherlands

J. Jan B. Van Lanschot, MD, PhD Department of Surgery, Erasmus Medical Center, Rotterdam, CA, The Netherlands

Pieter C. van der Sluis, MD, MSc Department of Surgery, University Medical Center Utrecht, Utrecht, The Netherlands

Roy J.J. Verhage, MD, PhD Department of Surgery, University Medical Center Utrecht, Utrecht, The Netherlands

Noriko Wada, MD Department of Gastroenterological Surgery, Osaka University Graduate School of Medicine, Suita, Osaka, Japan

Go Wakabayashi, MD, PhD Department of Surgery, Iwate Medical University School of Medicine, Morioka, Iwate Prefecture, Japan

Bas P.L. Wijnhoven, MD, PhD Department of Surgery, Erasmus Medical Center, Rotterdam, CA, The Netherlands

Danny Yakoub, MD, PhD Division of Surgical Oncology, University of Miami – Miller School of Medicine/Jackson Memorial Hospital, Miami, FL, USA

Monica T. Young, MD Department of General Surgery, University of California Irvine Medical Center, Orange, CA, USA

Pathogenesis of Esophageal Cancer

Charles LeVea

Introduction

Worldwide, esophageal cancer is most common in Asia, primarily Northern Iran, Central Asia, and Northern China. The majority of esophageal cancers in Asia, histologically, are squamous cell carcinoma. In Western countries only a third of carcinomas represent squamous cell carcinoma, where the majority of cancers, histologically, are adenocarcinoma. The differences in pathogenesis of esophageal cancer in Asia versus Western countries may be due to differences in environmental and lifestyle habits. Genetic differences may also come into play as China becomes more westernized but, even with the westernization, Barrett's esophagus and adenocarcinoma remain uncommon [1, 2].

Approximately 18,000 Americans will develop esophageal carcinoma in 2013 [3]. Esophageal carcinoma encompasses a variety of histological subtypes. Worldwide, the predominant subtype is squamous cell carcinoma. However, in the United States, it is estimated that only one-third of patients will develop squamous cell carcinoma. The majority of the remainder of the patients will develop adenocarcinoma. However, rarer

subtypes, such as undifferentiated carcinoma, adenosquamous carcinoma, adenoid cystic carcinoma, neuroendocrine carcinomas, and small cell carcinoma, also occur. This chapter will focus on the pathogenesis of squamous cell carcinoma and adenocarcinoma, the two most common cancers of the esophagus (Table 1.1).

Table 1.1 Risk factors for esophageal cancer [4–11]

Risk factor	Risk
Tobacco	4–8×
Alcohol	1.3–8×
Alcohol dehydrogenase	4×
Fruits and vegetables	0.53–0.56×
Poverty	8×
Gastroesophageal reflux	7.7×
Obesity	3.1×
Helicobacter pylori infection	0.56–1.1×

Squamous Cell Carcinoma

Worldwide squamous cell carcinoma is the most common cancer of the esophagus. Tobacco use, alcohol consumption, genetic abnormalities in the enzymes that metabolize alcohol, caustic injury to the esophagus, infrequent consumption of fruits and vegetables, and poverty have been implicated in the pathogenesis of squamous cell carcinoma (Table 1.2). Each of these risk factors for the development of squamous cell carcinoma of the esophagus will be discussed below.

C. LeVea, MD, PhD
Department of Pathology and Laboratory Medicine,
Roswell Park Cancer Institute,
Elm & Carlton Streets, Buffalo, NY 14263, USA
e-mail: charles.levea@roswellpark.org

S.N. Hochwald, M. Kukar (eds.), *Minimally Invasive Foregut Surgery for Malignancy: Principles and Practice*,
DOI 10.1007/978-3-319-09342-0_1, © Springer International Publishing Switzerland 2015

Table 1.2 Factors involved in the pathogenesis of squamous cell carcinoma of the esophagus

Tobacco smoke –> polycyclic aromatic hydrocarbons and N-nitrosamines –> DNA adducts, methylation, and chromosomal translocations
Alcohol –> metabolized in liver and oral bacteria –> acetaldehyde –> covalent DNA bonds
Alcohol –> squamous mucosa cytochrome P450 induction –> reactive oxygen species –> lipid peroxidation and oxidative cell injury –> DNA adducts
Alcohol dehydrogenase mutation –> inefficient metabolism of alcohol –> increased acetaldehyde in blood stream –> covalent DNA bonds
Genes affected –> p53, p14[ARF], p16[INK4a], cyclin D1, EGFR, COX-2, retinoic acid, retinoic acid receptor beta 2, and the fragile histidine triad
Other factors –> caustic injury due to lye, infrequent consumption of raw fruits and vegetables, poverty

Tobacco Use and Squamous Cell Carcinoma of the Esophagus

Cigarette smoke contains polycyclic aromatic hydrocarbons and N-nitrosamines, which have been shown to be carcinogenic [12, 13]. Cigarette smoke has a number of other carcinogens, but polycyclic aromatic hydrocarbons and N-nitrosamines are the most important in regard to esophageal squamous cell carcinoma development. The mechanisms of carcinogenesis by tobacco smoke may include formation of DNA adducts, silencing of genes by methylation, and chromosomal translocations [14].

Tobacco smoke causes cancer through the formation of covalent bonds between the carcinogen and cellular DNA, producing DNA adducts. The more DNA adducts formed, the more likely permanent mutations, in genes in cellular division regulating pathways, occur. When DNA adducts are bypassed incorrectly by DNA polymerases, permanent mutation in genes that deregulate cellular division is formed [15, 16].

Hypermethylation of promoters and intragenic hypermethylation can silence the transcription of genes, and DNA translocations can lead to mutational activation or to silencing of growth-regulating genes [17, 18].

A number of genes regulating cellular division have been implicated in the pathogenesis of squamous cell carcinoma of the esophagus. These include p53, p14[ARF], p16[INK4a], cyclin D1, epidermal growth factor receptors, COX-2, retinoic acid, retinoic acid receptor beta2, and the fragile histidine triad.

P53 is a cellular stress sensor, a tumor suppressor, which normally functions to maintain the integrity of cellular DNA. Loss of function of p53 in esophageal squamous cell carcinoma occurs in approximately 50–60 % of Japanese patients [19–21] making the tumor cells unable to enter into apoptosis or senescence. The tumor cells cannot repair the tobacco-mediated DNA damage, and the result is dysregulated cellular division [22, 23]. P14 [ARF] blocks MDM2-mediated degradation of p53, leading to increased expression of p53. Tobacco smoke causes the p14[ARF] promoter to be methylated, silencing expression of p14[ARF], which results in decreased p53 expression in about 60 % of patients with esophageal squamous cell carcinoma [24].

Loss of protein expression of the cyclin-dependent kinase inhibitor, p16[INK4a], has been observed early in the development of squamous cell carcinoma of the esophagus. This occurs predominantly through loss of heterozygosity of the p16[INK4a] gene or through silencing of the p16[INK4a] promoter by methylation [25]. P16[INK4a] proteins normally function to inhibit cyclin-dependent kinase 4 and cyclin-dependent kinase 6, preventing cellular division. Loss of p16[INK4a] allows cellular division of squamous cell tumors by allowing the cells to progress unchecked through G1 to S phase of the cell cycle [17].

While p16[INK4a] normally inhibits cyclin-dependent kinase 4 and cyclin-dependent kinase 6, cyclin D1 activates cyclin-dependent kinase 4/cyclin-dependent kinase 6 leading to progression through the cell cycle. Tobacco has been shown to increase levels of cyclin D1 in vitro [26], thus, facilitating cell cycle progression.

Other signaling molecules that have been linked to the development of squamous cell carcinoma include overexpression of epidermal growth factor receptors and associated overexpression of COX-2 and Her2/neu overexpression [27–29]. Retinoic acid and retinoic acid receptor beta2 induction can downregulate epidermal growth factor receptor expression. Tobacco smoke can suppress retinoic acid receptor beta2 by methylating the retinoic acid receptor beta2 gene promoters [30]. This may be a tobacco-mediated mechanism contributing to overexpression of epidermal growth factor receptor and, possibly, COX-2 and Her2/neu in squamous cell carcinoma.

The fragile histidine triad gene, encoding a tumor suppressor, has been shown to be inactivated in squamous cell carcinoma of the esophagus [31, 32]. The mechanism of inactivation occurs through silencing of the gene, by promoter methylation, or silencing through genome instability/chromosome translocations [33, 34].

Alcohol Consumption and Squamous Cell Carcinoma of the Esophagus

In the liver, ethanol is metabolized by alcohol dehydrogenase. The acetaldehyde generated by alcohol dehydrogenase has been shown to be carcinogenic in squamous cell carcinoma of the esophagus [35]. Additionally, oral bacteria metabolize ethanol to acetaldehyde resulting in a 10–100 times higher concentration of acetaldehyde in the oral cavity [36, 37]. The acetaldehyde in the saliva comes into direct contact with the squamous mucosa of the esophagus upon swallowing, directly adding to the amount of acetaldehyde that the squamous mucosa is already being exposed to via the blood during alcohol consumption.

Acetaldehyde forms covalent bonds with DNA, and the resulting DNA adducts can escape cellular DNA repair mechanisms causing detrimental mutations in growth-regulating genes [38]. In addition to directly causing mutations in DNA, acetaldehyde indirectly causes DNA mutations by binding to enzymes involved in DNA repair and DNA methylation. Alterations in these enzymes lead to mutations and aberrant regulation of genes [37].

Esophageal squamous mucosa from patients with chronic alcohol consumption demonstrated induction of cytochrome P450 2E1 (CYP2E1) when compared to the squamous mucosa from a teetotaler control group [39]. The cytochrome P450 system generates reactive oxygen species,

primarily hydrogen peroxide and superoxide anions. The reactive oxygen species cause lipid peroxidation and other forms of oxidative injury to the cell, which leads to DNA adducts [37, 40]. The resulting DNA adducts can cause permanent mutations.

Chronic alcohol consumption also results in aberrant gene regulation through ineffective promoter methylation (hypomethylation). Alcohol inhibits the synthesis of S-adenosyl-L-methionine, the donor group used for the methylation of promoter regions [41, 42]. Hypomethylated genes can be aberrantly transcribed, dysregulating cellular division [37].

Patients with squamous cell carcinoma of the esophagus, who consumed alcohol more than four times a week, demonstrated decreased levels of retinoic acid receptor gamma in their nonneoplastic squamous mucosa when compared to control patients, who consumed one drink a week or less [43]. Retinoic acid through its receptor's activation leads to decreased expression of epidermal growth factor receptors. By decreasing retinoic acid receptor expression, alcohol may dysregulate growth by increasing expression and activation of epidermal growth factor receptor signaling pathways.

Alcohol Dehydrogenase Mutation and Squamous Cell Carcinoma of the Esophagus

Ethanol is metabolized into acetaldehyde by alcohol dehydrogenase, and acetaldehyde is further metabolized to acetate by aldehyde dehydrogenase. Prevalent in East Asians are the ADH2*1/2*1 alleles of alcohol dehydrogenase and the ALDH2*2 alleles of aldehyde dehydrogenase [35]. The concentration of acetaldehyde in the bloodstream is increased by both of these enzymes. The ADH2*1/2*1 allele encodes a superactive form of alcohol dehydrogenase producing acetaldehyde quicker. The ALDH2*2 allele of aldehyde dehydrogenase produces an inactive enzyme slowing the removal of acetaldehyde from the blood. The formation of acetaldehyde DNA adducts is mutagenic.

Caustic Injury and Squamous Cell Carcinoma of the Esophagus

The first association of a lye burn and squamous cell carcinoma of the esophagus was reported in 1904 by Telesky [44]. The average interval between a caustic burn to the esophagus and the development of squamous cell carcinoma is approximately 40 years [44]. Chemical injury from a caustic chemical, such as lye, leads to fibrosis with stricture of the esophagus in the area of injury. The narrowed lumen causes an obstruction during swallowing, and the constant irritation leads to repeated injury, inflammation, and repair, which, over time, leads to carcinogenesis. For similar reasons, achalasia is a risk factor for developing squamous cell carcinoma. Why lye injury leads to squamous cell carcinoma and why the caustic injury from acid reflux (to be discussed more below) leads to adenocarcinoma of the esophagus is unclear.

Infrequent Consumption of Raw Fruits and Vegetables and Squamous Cell Carcinoma of the Esophagus

A number of studies [45, 46] have shown an inverse relationship between raw fruit and vegetable consumption and the risk of squamous cell carcinoma of the esophagus. Lower consumption of vegetables and fruits is associated with a higher risk of squamous cell carcinoma. Odds ratios were adjusted for alcohol consumption, tobacco use, and gender. The mechanism of the protective effect of fruit and vegetables is unclear, but it may be related to the vitamins and minerals contained in the foods.

Poverty and Squamous Cell Carcinoma of the Esophagus

The development of squamous cell carcinoma of the esophagus is strongly associated with low income. While the majority of the risk of developing squamous cell carcinoma of the esophagus can be explained by alcohol, tobacco, and low fruit and vegetable intake, low socioeconomic status has an independent effect [47]. Whether this independent effect can be explained by poor dental care or other nutritional or environmental factors needs to be further investigated.

Adenocarcinoma

The incidence of adenocarcinoma of the esophagus has been increasing in Western countries over the last few decades [48]. Environmental factors are most likely to have caused the increase in adenocarcinoma incidence, as it is unlikely that genetic risk/predisposition to adenocarcinoma has changed so abruptly. There is a gender influence on the development of adenocarcinoma of the esophagus, as, in the United States, men are six times more likely to develop esophageal adenocarcinoma than women [48]. Up to 13 % of adenocarcinomas of the esophagus may be due to patients inheriting a genetic predisposition. Genetic predisposition as well as the environmental influences of gastroesophageal reflux disease, obesity, and *Helicobacter pylori* infection on the development of adenocarcinoma of the esophagus will be discussed.

Genetic Factors and Adenocarcinoma of the Esophagus

Three candidate genes containing germline mutations were identified in patients with esophageal adenocarcinoma: MSR1, ASCC1, and CTHRC1 [49]. MSR1 encodes the class A macrophage scavenger receptor, whose protein function becomes disrupted by the germline mutation. The MSR1 mutation suggests a link between esophageal adenocarcinoma and inflammation. ASCC1 encodes activating signal cointegrator 1, which activates NF kappa B, serum response factor, and activating protein 1 [50]. Therefore, ASCC1 is another signaling molecule putatively linking inflammation to growth signal transduction pathways. Another germline mutation was found in CTHRC1, a protein expressed during tissue repair processes, called collagen triple helix repeat containing 1 protein [51]. CTHRC1 signaling regulates TGF beta pathways, thus, is an additional protein linking inflammation/repair processes to control of cellular proliferation [52].

Patients with a single gene polymorphism in the matrix metalloproteinase gene family, specifically MMP1 1G/2G, have a higher risk of developing esophageal adenocarcinoma [53]. Matrix metalloproteinase proteins are involved in extracellular matrix and basement membrane degradation. A synergistic effect of gastroesophageal reflux disease combined with the MMP1 1G/2G polymorphism increases the risk of developing esophageal adenocarcinoma [53].

A decreased local secretion of epidermal growth factor (EGF) has been associated with the development of esophageal adenocarcinoma [54]. The EGF 5′ UTR G/G genotype confers an increased risk of developing adenocarcinoma and is associated with low EGF levels. Interestingly, epidermal growth factor receptor levels in these patients are overexpressed, possibly caused by lack of an inhibitory effect on EGF receptor expression due to the low circulating EGF hormone levels.

Vascular endothelial growth factor is involved in the regulation of angiogenesis. The variant T allele of the VEGF gene in the +936CT/TT polymorphism is associated with increased risk of esophageal adenocarcinoma, especially in smokers [55]. Carriers of the T allele of VEGF have higher levels of VEGF. VEGF-induced angiogenesis has been shown to be an early event in esophageal adenocarcinoma development [55].

Interleukin-18 is a cytokine, whose inflammatory responses have been linked to antitumor immunity [56]. The single-nucleotide polymorphism, IL-18-607 C/A in its promoter, is associated with the development of Barrett's esophagus and esophageal adenocarcinoma. Alternatively, the IL-18RAP rs917997C allele is associated with a protective effect on Barrett's esophagus from developing into adenocarcinoma. The DNA repair protein O(6)-methylguanine-DNA methyltransferase, which repairs DNA adducts, has a variant single-nucleotide polymorphism – rs12268840, when homozygous, which is associated with an increased risk for esophageal adenocarcinoma [57].

Gender Influence and Adenocarcinoma of the Esophagus

Worldwide, there is a male predominance for developing adenocarcinoma. In the United States, the association is even stronger with a 3:1 (Native American) to 9:1 (Caucasian) ratio between men and women [58]. Thus, female sex hormones may have a protective effect. This is supported by the delayed development of adenocarcinoma on average by 17 years in women when compared to men [59]. Another interesting observation is the protective effect of breastfeeding on esophageal adenocarcinoma. Increased duration of breastfeeding is correlated with a reduced risk of developing esophageal adenocarcinoma [60]. More research is required to determine the hormonal mechanisms involved.

Gastroesophageal Reflux Disease and Adenocarcinoma of the Esophagus

Gastroesophageal reflux is an important risk factor for the development of esophageal adenocarcinoma. When compared to the risk of people without reflux symptoms developing adenocarcinoma, an individual experiencing reflux symptoms on a weekly basis has a lower risk of developing adenocarcinoma (5-fold risk) than someone experiencing daily reflux symptoms (7-fold risk) [61]. Reflux of the acid contents of the stomach into the esophagus causes caustic damage to the esophageal squamous mucosa. This leads to injury of the squamous mucosa and acute and chronic inflammation. Repair does not involve scarring as seen with lye but, rather, involves glandular metaplasia (Barrett's metaplasia) of the esophagus. Barrett's esophagus is when the squamous mucosa is replaced by intestinal-type glandular epithelium containing goblet cells. Further reflux damage results in further injury with subsequent chronic inflammation and repair. The resulting increased cellular turnover makes the mucosa susceptible to mutations in growth-regulating genes, which leads to glandular dysplasia. Low-grade glandular dysplasia may lead to high-grade glandular dysplasia and esophageal adenocarcinoma [62, 63].

The majority of people with Barrett's esophagus do not progress to esophageal adenocarcinoma. Neoplastic transformation of Barrett's esophagus can be difficult to identify, as dysplasia can be focal. Thus, a number of biopsies are required to prevent sampling errors and false-negative results [63, 64]. Low-grade glandular dysplasia has a low rate of progression to esophageal adenocarcinoma [65]. Even high-grade glandular dysplasia progresses to esophageal adenocarcinoma only 10–60 % of the time [66, 67].

The future of predicting which patients with Barrett's esophagus are at higher risk of progressing to esophageal adenocarcinoma and which have a low risk of progression may be with molecular and chromosomal markers. Chromosome instability, demonstrated by a combined panel of abnormalities encompassing 9p loss of heterozygosity (LOH), 17p LOH, and DNA aneuploidy or DNA tetraploidy in Barrett's esophagus, predicted subsequent development of esophageal adenocarcinoma, relative risk = 38.7, and a 5-year cumulative risk of developing adenocarcinoma of 79.1 %. Those patients without any demonstrable chromosome instability in their Barrett's esophagus had 0 % cumulative incidence of adenocarcinoma at 8 years [68]. Molecular markers of chromosome instability in Barrett's esophagus would be useful to determine patients that would benefit from close clinical surveillance.

Obesity and Adenocarcinoma of the Esophagus

Obesity is a strong risk factor for developing esophageal adenocarcinoma [69]. The risk is even greater for people with central and intraabdominal obesity [70, 71]. Various mechanisms for obesity-related cancer have been proposed, including increased levels of endogenous sex hormones, leptin, plasminogen activator inhibitor-1, and IGF-1, and decreased adiponectin, and chronic inflammation. This metabolic syndrome

caused by obesity has been correlated with length of Barrett's esophagus [72–74].

Alternatively, instead of being caused by this obesity-related metabolic syndrome, Barrett's esophagus may be a response to increased acid reflux caused by the increased intra-abdominal pressure due to intra-abdominal obesity. There is a direct correlation between increased body mass index and increased esophageal reflux [75]. The increased esophageal reflux or a combination of risk factors associated with reflux and the metabolic syndrome of obesity may lead to the development of esophageal adenocarcinoma.

Helicobacter Pylori Infection and Adenocarcinoma of the Esophagus

Helicobacter pylori infection occurs in 50 % of the worldwide population and commonly colonizes the stomach of children [76]. Up to a 50 % decrease in esophageal adenocarcinoma risk has been attributed to *Helicobacter pylori* infection [77]. One possible mechanism includes *Helicobacter pylori* infection leading to gastric atrophy. The reduction in the acidity and volume of gastric contents leads to an associated decrease in esophageal reflux disease.

Acute and Chronic Inflammation and Esophageal Carcinoma

Acute and chronic inflammation may provide the mechanisms common to the development of esophageal carcinoma. In both squamous cell carcinoma and adenocarcinoma, reactive oxygen species generated by acute and chronic inflammation can be mutagenic. An esophageal inflammatory reaction is seen in response to smoking, alcohol consumption, lye injury, chronic reflux, and obesity.

Acute and chronic esophageal inflammation causes intracellular oxidative stress [78, 79]. Increased serum levels of inflammatory cytokines, such as Il-6, TNF-alpha, C-reactive protein, and leptin, have been observed in patients with chronic reflux and obesity [80, 81]. When the inflammatory reaction is localized to the esophageal mucosa, the oxidative stress can lead to DNA damage and mutagenesis. Further genomic alterations can lead to DNA and chromosomal instability and the development of esophageal adenocarcinoma or squamous cell carcinoma [82, 83].

References

1. Chai J, Jamal MM. Esophageal malignancy: a growing concern. World J Gastroenterol. 2012;18(45):6521–6.
2. Huang Q, Fang DC, Zhang J, et al. Barrett's esophagus-related diseases remain uncommon in China. J Dig Dis. 2011;12(6):420–7.
3. National Cancer Institute at the National Institutes of Health USA. 2013. http://www.cancer.gov/cancertopics/types/esophageal. Accessed 7 Oct 2013.
4. Bosman FT, Carneiro F, Hruban RH, Theise ND. WHO Classification of Tumours, IARC. WHO Classification of Tumours. 2010;3:18.
5. Bagnardi V, Rota M, Botteri E, et al. Light alcohol drinking and cancer: a meta-analysis. Ann Oncol. 2013; 24:301–8.
6. IARC Monographs on the Evaluation of Carcinogenic Risks to Humans IARC Monographs, WHO Press. 2012;100:381.
7. Zhang GH, Mai RQ, Huang B. Meta-analysis of ADH1B and ALDH2 polymorphisms and esophageal cancer risk in China. World J Gastroenterol. 2010; 16(47):6020–5.
8. Morris Brown L, Hoover R, Silverman D, et al. Excess incidence of squamous cell esophageal cancer among Black Men: role of social class and other risk factors. Am J Epidemiol. 2001;53(2):114–22.
9. Lagergren J, Bergstrom R, Lindgren A, et al. Symptomatic gastroesophageal reflux as a risk factor for esophageal adenocarcinoma. N Engl J Med. 1999; 340(11):825–31.
10. Morris Brown L, Swanson CA, Gridley G, et al. Adenocarcinoma of the esophagus: role of obesity and diet. J Natl Cancer Inst. 1995;87(2):104–9.
11. Islami F, Kamangar F. Helicobacter pylori and esophageal cancer risk – a meta-analysis. Cancer Prev Res (Phila). 2008;1(5):329–38.
12. Boffetta P, Jourenkova N, Gustavsson P. Cancer risk from occupational and environmental exposure to polycyclic aromatic hydrocarbons. Cancer Causes Control. 1997;8:444–72.
13. Kamangar F, Strickland PT, Pourshams A, et al. High exposure to polycyclic aromatic hydrocarbons may contribute to high risk of esophageal cancer in Northeastern Iran. Anticancer Res. 2005;25:425–8.
14. Xu XC. Risk factors and gene expression in esophageal cancer. Methods Mol Biol. 2009;471:335–60.
15. Hoeijmakers JH. Genome maintenance mechanisms for preventing cancer. Nature. 2001;411:366–74.
16. Mangerich A, Dedon PC, Fox JG, et al. Chemistry meets biology in colitis-associated carcinogenesis. Free Radic Res. 2013;47(11):958–86. doi: 10.3109/10715762.2013.832239. Epub 2013 Oct 4.
17. Belinsky SA. Silencing of genes by promoter hypermethylation: key event in rodent and human lung cancer. Carcinogenesis. 2005;26:1481–7.
18. Ehrlich M, Lacey M. DNA methylation and differentiation: silencing, upregulation and modulation of gene expression. Epigenomics. 2013;5(5):553–68.
19. Egashira A, Morita M, Kakeji Y, et al. p53 gene mutations in esophageal squamous cell carcinoma and their relevance to etiology and pathogenesis: results in Japan and comparisons with other countries. Cancer Sci. 2007;98:1152–6.
20. Oki E, Zhao Y, Yoshida R, et al. The difference in p53 mutations between cancers of the upper and lower gastrointestinal tract. Digestion. 2009;79 Suppl 1:33–9.
21. Egashira A, Morita M, Yoshida R, et al. Loss of p53 in esophageal squamous cell carcinoma and the correlation with survival: analyses of gene mutations, protein expression and loss of heterozygosity in Japanese patients. J Surg Oncol. 2011;104(2):169–75.
22. Efeyan A, Serrano M. P53: guardian of the genome and policeman of the oncogenes. Cell Cycle. 2007; 6(9):1006–10.
23. Jackson SF, Bartek J. The DNA-damage response in human biology and disease. Nature. 2009;461(22): 1071–8.
24. Ito S, Ohga T, Saeki H, et al. Promoter hypermethylation and quantitative expression analysis of CDKN2A (p14ARF and p16INK4a) gene in esophageal squamous cell carcinoma. Anticancer Res. 2007; 27:3345–53.
25. Tokugawa T, Sugihara H, Tani T, et al. Modes of silencing of p16 in development of esophageal squamous cell carcinoma. Cancer Res. 2002;62: 4938–44.
26. Hu H, Zhang S, Zhu S. Influence of aspirin and cigarette smoke extract on the expression of cyclin D1 and effects of cell cycle in esophageal squamous cell carcinoma cell line. Dis Esophagus. 2009;22:310–6.
27. Kuwano H, Kato H, Miyazaki T, et al. Genetic alterations in esophageal cancer. Surg Today. 2005;35:7–18.
28. Moraitis D, Du B, De Lorenzo MS, et al. Levels of cyclooxygerase-2 are increased in the oral mucosa of smokers: evidence for the role of epidermal growth factor receptor and its ligands. Cancer Res. 2005;65: 664–70.
29. da Costa NM, Soares Lima SC, de Almeida Simao T, et al. The potential of molecular markers to improve interventions through the natural history of oesophageal squamous cell carcinoma. Biosci Rep. 2013; 33(4):art e00057.
30. Wang XD, Liu C, Bronson RT, et al. Retinoid signaling and activator protein-1 expression in ferrets given beta-carotene supplements and exposed to tobacco smoke. J Natl Cancer Inst. 1999;91:60–6.

31. Mori M, Mimori K, Shiraishi T, et al. Altered expression of Fhit in carcinoma and precarcinomatous lesions of the esophagus. Cancer Res. 2000;60:1177–82.

32. Chava S, Mohan V, Shetty PJ, et al. Immunohistochemical evaluation of p53, FHIT, and IGF2 gene expression in esophageal cancer. Dis Esophagus. 2012;25(1):81–7.

33. Zochbauer-Muller S, Fong KM, Maitra A, et al. 5′ CpG island methylation of the FHIT gene is correlated with loss of gene expression in lung and breast cancer. Cancer Res. 2001;61:3581–5.

34. Jeong YJ, Jeong HY, Lee SM, et al. Promoter methylation status of the FHIT gene and Fhit expression: association with HER2/neu status in breast cancer patients. Oncol Rep. 2013;30(5):2270–8.

35. Yokoyama A, Kato H, Yokoyama T, et al. Genetic polymorphisms of alcohol and aldehyde dehydrogenases and glutathione S-transferase M1 and drinking, smoking, and diet in Japanese men with esophageal squamous cell carcinoma. Carcinogenesis. 2002;23:1851–9.

36. Homann N, Tillonen J, Meurman JH, et al. Increased salivary acetaldehyde levels in heavy drinkers and smokers: a microbiological approach to oral cavity cancer. Carcinogenesis. 2000;21:663–8.

37. Seitz HK, Stickel F. Molecular mechanisms of alcohol mediated carcinogenesis. Nat Rev Cancer. 2007;7: 599–612.

38. Bartsch H. DNA adducts in human carcinogenesis: etiological relevance and structure – activity relationship. Mutat Res. 1996;340:67–79.

39. Millonig G, Wang Y, Homann N, et al. Ethanol-induced carcinogenesis in the human esophagus implicates CYP2E1 induction and generation of carcinogenic DNA-lesions. Int J Cancer. 2011;128:533–40.

40. Homann N, Seitz HK, Wang XD, et al. Mechanisms in alcohol-associated carcinogenesis. Alcohol Clin Exp Res. 2005;29:1317–20.

41. Baylin SB. DNA methylation and gene silencing in cancer. Nat Clin Pract Oncol. 2005;2 Suppl 1:S4–11.

42. Obeid R. The metabolic burden of methyl donor deficiency with focus on the betaine homocysteine methyltransferase pathway. Nutrients. 2013;5:3481–95.

43. Bergheim I, Wolfgarten E, Bollschweiler E, et al. Role of retinoic acid receptors in squamous-cell carcinoma in human esophagus. J Carcinog. 2005;8:4–20.

44. Hopkins RA, Postlethwait RW. Caustic burns and carcinoma of the esophagus. Ann Surg. 1981;194(2):146–8.

45. Link LB, Potter JD. Raw versus cooked vegetables and cancer risk. Cancer Epidemiol Biomarkers Prev. 2004;13(9):1422–35.

46. Chen YK, Lee CH, Wu IC, et al. Food intake and the occurrence of squamous cell carcinoma in different sections of the esophagus in Taiwanese men. Nutrition. 2009;25(7–8):753–61.

47. Brown LM, Hoover R, Silverman D, et al. Excess incidence of squamous cell esophageal cancer among US Black men: role of social class and other risk factors. Am J Epidemiol. 2001;153(2):114–22.

48. Edgren G, Adami HO, Weiderp E, et al. A global assessment of the oesophageal adenocarcinoma epidemic. Gut. 2013;62:1406–14.

49. Orloff M, Peterson C, He X, et al. Germline mutations in MSR1, ASCC1, and CTHRC1 in patients with Barrett esophagus and esophageal adenocarcinoma. JAMA. 2011;306:410–9.

50. Jung DJ, Sung HS, Goo YW, et al. Novel transcription coactivator complex containing activating signal cointegrator 1. Mol Cell Biol. 2002;22(14):5203–11.

51. Durmus T, LeClair RJ, Park KS, et al. Expression analysis of the novel gene collagen triple helix repeat containing-1 (Cthrc1). Gene Expr Patterns. 2006;6(8):935–40.

52. LeClair R, Lindner V. The role of collagen triple helix repeat containing 1 in injured arteries, collagen expression, and transforming growth factor beta signaling. Trends Cardiovasc Med. 2007;17(6):202–5.

53. Cheung WY, Zhai R, Bradbury P, et al. Single nucleotide polymorphisms in the matrix metalloproteinase gene family and the frequency and duration of gastroesophageal reflux disease influence the risk of esophageal adenocarcinoma. Int J Cancer. 2012;131:2478–86.

54. Menke V, Pot RG, Moons LM, et al. Functional single-nucleotide polymorphism of epidermal growth factor is associated with the development of Barrett's esophagus and esophageal adenocarcinoma. J Hum Genet. 2012;57:26–32.

55. Zhai R, Liu G, Asomaning K, et al. Genetic polymorphisms of VEGF, interactions with cigarette smoking exposure and esophageal adenocarcinoma risk. Carcinogenesis. 2008;29:2330–4.

56. Babar M, Ryan AW, Anderson LA, et al. Genes of the interleukin-18 pathway are associated with susceptibility to Barrett's esophagus and esophageal adenocarcinoma. Am J Gastroenterol. 2012;107:1331–41.

57. Doecke J, Zhao ZZ, Pandeya N, et al. Australian Cancer Study. Polymorphisms in MGMT and DNA repair genes and the risk of esophageal adenocarcinoma. Int J Cancer. 2008;123:174–80.

58. Cook MB, Chow WH, Devesa SS. Oesophageal cancer incidence in the United States by race, sex, and histologic type, 1977–2005. Br J Cancer. 2009;101:855–9.

59. Derakhshan MH, Liptrot S, Paul J, et al. Oesophageal and gastric intestinal-type adenocarcinomas show the same male predominance due to a 17 year delayed development in females. Gut. 2009;58:16–23.

60. Cronin-Fenton DP, Murray LJ, Whiteman DC, et al. Barrett's Esophagus, Adenocarcinoma Consortium (BEACON) Investigators. Reproductive and sex hormonal factors and oesophageal and gastric junction adenocarcinoma: a pooled analysis. Eur J Cancer. 2010;46:2067–76.

61. Rubenstein JH, Taylor JB. Meta-analysis: the association of oesophageal adenocarcinoma with symptoms of gastro-oesophageal reflux. Aliment Pharmacol Ther. 2010;32:1222–7.

62. Sharma P. Barrett's esophagus. N Engl J Med. 2009;361:2548–56. DOI: 10.1056.

63. Spechler SJ. Barrett esophagus and risk of esophageal cancer: a clinical review. JAMA. 2013;310(6):627–36.

64. Wang KK, Sampliner RE. Updated guidelines 2008 for the diagnosis, surveillance and therapy of Barrett's esophagus. Am J Gastroenterol. 2008;103:788–97.

65. Gatenby P, Ramus J, Caygill C, et al. Routinely diagnosed low-grade dysplasia in Barrett's oesophagus: a population based study of natural history. Histopathology. 2009;54:814–9.
66. Reid BJ, Li X, Galipeau PC, et al. Barrett's oesophagus and oesophageal adenocarcinoma: time for a new synthesis. Nat Rev Cancer. 2010;10:87–101.
67. Schnell TG, Sontag SJ, Chejfec G, et al. Long-term non-surgical management of Barrett's esophagus with high-grade dysplasia. Gastroenterology. 2001;120:1607–19.
68. Galipeau PC, Li X, Blount P, et al. NSAIDs modulate CDKN2A, TP53, and DNA content risk for future esophageal adenocarcinoma. PLoS Med. 2007;4:e67.
69. Hoyo C, Cook MB, Kamangar F, et al. Body mass index in relation to oesophageal and oesophagogastric junction adenocarcinomas: a pooled analysis from the International BEACON Consortium. Int J Epidemiol. 2012;41:1706–18.
70. Edelstein ZR, Farrow DC, Bronner MP, et al. Central adiposity and risk of Barrett's esophagus. Gastroenterology. 2007;133:403–11.
71. Corley DA, Kubo A, Zhao W. Abdominal obesity and the risk of esophageal and gastric cardia carcinomas. Cancer Epidemiol Biomarkers Prev. 2008;17:352–8.
72. Ryan AM, Healy LA, Power DG, et al. Barrett esophagus: prevalence of central adiposity, metabolic syndrome, and a proinflammatory state. Ann Surg. 2008;247:909–15.
73. van Kruijsdijk RC, van der Wall E, Visseren FL. Obesity and cancer: the role of dysfunctional adipose tissue. Cancer Epidemiol Biomarkers Prev. 2009;18(10):2569–78.
74. Doyle SL, Donohoe CL, Finn SP, et al. IGF-1 and its receptor in esophageal cancer: association with adenocarcinoma and visceral obesity. Am J Gastroenterol. 2012;107:196–204.
75. Jacobsor BC, Somers SC, Fuchs CS, et al. Body-mass index and symptoms of gastroesophageal reflux in women. N Engl J Med. 2006;354:2340–8.
76. Conteduca V, Sansonno D, Lauletta G, et al. *H. pylori* infection and gastric cancer: state of the art (review). Int J Oncol. 2013;42:5–18.
77. Whiteman DC, Parmar P, Fahey P, et al. Australian Cancer Study. Association of *Helicobacter pylori* infection with reduced risk for esophageal cancer is independent of environmental and genetic modifiers. Gastroenterology. 2010;139:73–83.
78. Grisham MB, Jourd'heuil D, Wink DA. Review article: chronic inflammation and reactive oxygen and nitrogen metabolism–implications in DNA damage and mutagenesis. Aliment Pharmacol Ther. 2000;14 Suppl 1:3–9.
79. Sihvo EI, Salminen JT, Rantanen TK, et al. Oxidative stress has a role in malignant transformation in Barrett's oesophagus. Int J Cancer. 2002;102:551–5.
80. Calle EE, Kaaks R. Overweight, obesity and cancer: epidemiological evidence and proposed mechanisms. Nat Rev Cancer. 2004;4:579–91.
81. Trayhurn P, Bing C, Wood IS. Adipose tissue and adipokines–energy regulation from the human perspective. J Nutr. 2006;136(7 Suppl):1935S–9.
82. Turker MS, Gage BM, Rose JA, et al. A novel signature mutation for oxidative damage resembles a mutational pattern found commonly in human cancers. Cancer Res. 1999;59:1837–9.
83. Picardo SL, Maher SG, O'Sullivan JN. Barrett's to oesophageal cancer sequence: a model of inflammatory-driven upper gastrointestinal cancer. Dig Surg. 2012;29:251–60.

Endoscopic Treatment of Premalignant and Early Esophageal Malignancy

Toshitaka Hoppo and Blair A. Jobe

Introduction

Barrett's esophagus (BE) is a well-known risk factor for esophageal adenocarcinoma, and progression of metaplasia through dysplasia to adenocarcinoma is a widely accepted theory of esophageal carcinogenesis [1, 2]. High-grade dysplasia (HGD) has a high risk of progression to cancer, and esophageal resection (esophagectomy) has been recommended as a standard surgical therapy to treat HGD based on the previous studies demonstrating that the incidence of concomitant invasive cancer in the surgically resected specimens of patients with biopsy-proven HGD has been reported to be approximately 40 % [3, 4]. Esophagectomy is one of the most invasive surgeries in the upper gastrointestinal tract and is associated with high mortality and morbidity even with the recent refinement of surgical techniques and perioperative care [5, 6]. Given that lymph node involvement in patients with HGD

and T1a cancer is unlikely (<2 %), esophagectomy may be unreasonably invasive [7–9]. However, patients with HGD and T1a cancer have a chance for cure of disease, although overall prognosis of esophageal cancer is poor with 5-year survival of approximately 15 % despite multidisciplinary approaches including chemoradiation and surgical therapy [10, 11]. Therefore, it is extremely important to determine what the best approach is for this population to accomplish cure without residual or recurrent disease, while minimizing the postoperative morbidity and mortality.

With the introduction of endoscopic surveillance programs, patients with HGD and T1a cancer have been increasingly discovered. Accumulating data have demonstrated that highly selected patients with HGD and T1a cancer with low risk or no risk of lymph node involvement can be treated with esophageal-preserving approaches including endoscopic ablation (radiofrequency ablation and cryotherapy) and resection (endoscopic mucosal resection and submucosal dissection) with equivalent oncological outcomes as surgical resection [12, 13]. Esophageal-preserving approaches include any endoluminal procedure that is performed in an attempt to completely eradicate disease, while preserving the anatomical structure of esophagus. The recent advances in endoscopic technology and therapeutic techniques have made esophageal-preserving approach real. The guideline put forth by the American College of Gastroenterology (2008) states that esophagectomy is no longer

T. Hoppo, MD, PhD (✉)
Department of Surgery, Institute for the Treatment of Esophageal and Thoracic Disease, The Western Pennsylvania Hospital, 4800 Friendship Avenue, Suite 4600, Pittsburgh, PA 15224, USA
e-mail: thoppo@wpahs.org

B.A. Jobe, MD, FACS
Department of Surgery, Institute for the Treatment of Esophageal and Thoracic Disease,
The Western Pennsylvania Hospital,
Pittsburgh, PA, USA

the necessary treatment response to HGD [14]. By contrast, esophageal-preserving options have caused more confusion in the decision-making among health care providers. The optimal management of HGD and T1a cancer remains controversial. In this chapter, we focus on esophageal-preserving therapy to treat HGD and T1a cancer.

Patient Selection Based on Risk Stratification

Appropriate patient selection is crucial for esophageal-preserving therapy, and patients at high risk of lymph node involvement and/or potential progression to cancer or presence of concomitant cancer need to be accurately identified and excluded from candidates for esophageal-preserving therapy. Careful endoscopic examination of esophageal epithelium with extensive biopsies for tissue diagnosis is the first step to esophageal-preserving therapy. High-quality endoscopic images are required to detect questionable, subtle mucosal abnormalities. Several new endoscopic technologies (e.g., optical coherent tomography, autofluorescent imaging, confocal laser endomicroscopy) combined with enhancement techniques (e.g., narrowband imaging, chromoendoscopy) have been investigated; however, none of them has been routinely used in general practice. For the evaluation of accurate risk stratification, the mucosal and submucosal layers have been subdivided into thirds with each third going deeper into the esophageal wall. Currently, T1 cancers have six different layers of invasion: T1m1–m3 (m1=limited to the epithelial layer, m2=invades lamina propria, m3=invades into but not through muscularis mucosae) and T1sm1–sm3 (different thirds of the submucosa).

HGD and/or T1a Esophageal Cancer

Overall, esophageal-preserving therapy can be indicated for HGD and/or T1a adenocarcinoma with low risk or no risk of lymph node involvement or

Table 2.1 Low- and high-risk factors to consider for endoscopic resection of high-grade dysplasia (HGD) and intramucosal adenocarcinoma

Indications (low risk)	High risk
Unifocal (limited or focal), flat HGD	Multifocal HGD, HGD with nodules
Type I, IIa<2 cm, IIb, IIc<1 cm	Type I, II>3 cm, type III
Well- or moderately differentiated adenocarcinoma	Poorly differentiated adenocarcinoma
Lesions limited to the mucosa (m)	Invasion into the submucosa (sm)
No lymphovascular invasion	Presence of lymphovascular invasion

Type I, polypoid type; IIa, flat, elevated; IIb, level with the mucosa. IIc, slightly depressed; III: ulcerated type

metastatic disease. Several macro- and microscopic findings including submucosal invasion (T1b), squamous-type histology, lymphovascular invasion (L+ or V+), poor differentiation, and a nodule >3 cm in diameter have been recognized as high-risk factors for lymph node involvement [12, 13, 15, 16]. Furthermore, multifocal HGD has a significant risk of concomitant cancer ranging from 60 to 78 % [17–20]. By contrast, low-risk factors include unifocal (limited or focal) or flat HGD [17–20], type I, IIa <2 cm, IIb, IIc <1 cm, well or moderately differentiated adenocarcinoma, mucosal cancer (m), and no lymphovascular invasion (L- and V-) [12, 13]. Risk factors for HGD and T1a adenocarcinoma are summarized in Table 2.1.

Esophageal squamous cell cancer appears to be biologically more aggressive than adenocarcinoma, and the risk of lymph node involvement is higher in patients with squamous cell cancer. Patients with intraepithelial cancers (m1) and cancers invading the lamina propria (m2) have almost no risk of lymph node involvement [21–23], whereas the risk of lymph node involvement in cancers invading the muscularis mucosa (m3) and the submucosa (sm) ranges from 0 to 10 % [23] and from 50 to 55 % [22], respectively. For patients with esophageal squamous cell cancer, esophageal-preserving therapy can be indicated only for superficial (m1 and m2) cancers with well-to-moderate differentiation and no lymphovascular invasion. Patients with m3 cancers could

Table 2.2 Indications for endoscopic resection of esophageal squamous cell carcinoma (SCC)

Indications (low risk)	High risk
No consensus on the maximal size	
Well- or moderately differentiated SCC	Poorly differentiated SCC
Limited to the lamina propria (m1–2)	Invasion into the deeper layer than the muscularis mucosa (m3, sm)
No lymphovascular invasion	Presence of lymphovascular invasion

be candidates for esophageal-preserving therapy if there are no further risk factors for lymph node involvement. Risk factors for esophageal squamous cell cancer are summarized in Table 2.2.

T1b Esophageal Cancer

Once tumors invade the submucosal layer, the probability of lymph node involvement is exponentially increased due to the abundant submucosal lymphatic networks [24, 25]. Therefore, esophagectomy has been recommended as a standard of care for patients with T1b esophageal cancer. A recent review using the pooled data of 7,645 patients with T1b submucosal esophageal cancer has demonstrated that the overall rate of lymph node involvement in T1b cancers was 37 %; however, there was a substantial difference between T1sm1 and T1sm2/3 adenocarcinoma (6 % vs. 23 %/58 %, respectively), suggesting that highly selected patients with T1sm1 adenocarcinoma could be candidates for esophageal-preserving therapy [26]. This is further supported by the most recent study involving 66 patients with low-risk T1sm1 cancer (macroscopically polypoid or flat lesion, well-to-moderate differentiation and no lymphovascular invasion) demonstrating that complete remission was achieved in 97 % of patients with small nodules ≤2 cm, and long-term remission without any metachronous disease was achieved in 90 %. There were no tumor-related deaths and the estimated 5-year survival was 84 %, although one patient developed lymph node metastasis [27]. The risk of developing lymph node metas-

tasis after esophageal-preserving therapy for T1sm1 appears to be lower than the mortality rate of esophagectomy, suggesting that patients with low-risk T1sm1 adenocarcinoma could be a candidate for esophageal-preserving therapy, particularly when poor functional status and comorbid conditions make esophagectomy too risky. T1sm2 and sm3 adenocarcinoma and all T1b squamous cell carcinomas are associated with a high rate of lymph node involvement, and esophagectomy should be considered [28, 29]. It is noted that these data may not be transferable to patients at all centers delivering therapy because these data were achieved within high-volume, experienced centers.

Clinical Staging

Accurate clinical staging is essential for esophageal-preserving therapy and it is extremely important to exclude patients with potential lymph node involvement and/or metastatic disease. Therefore, all patients require positron-emission tomography/computed tomography (PET/CT), endoscopic ultrasound (EUS), and diagnostic endoscopic mucosal resection (EMR) for staging purposes, when esophageal-preserving therapy is considered. Since approximately 25 % of all patients with esophageal cancer have metastatic disease identified by PET/CT and this yield is far superior to the combination of EUS and CT scan [30, 31], PET/CT has been utilized to assess metastatic disease.

EUS has been utilized to assess tumor depth (T-stage) and lymph node involvement (N-stage). A recent meta-analysis has demonstrated that the pooled sensitivity and specificity of EUS to diagnose T1 stage cancer was 81.6 and 99.4 %, respectively [32], suggesting that EUS cannot accurately differentiate T1a from T1b esophageal cancers. To improve the diagnostic yield of T1 stage tumors, a high-frequency EUS miniprobe (20 or 30 MHz) has been introduced and investigated. A recent retrospective study demonstrated that the overall accuracy, sensitivity, and specificity to differentiate T1b from T1a cancers with high-frequency miniprobes were 73.5, 62, and 76.5 %, respectively, suggesting that even the high-frequency miniprobe still has a limited accuracy for the diagnosis of T1a cancer [33]. Other meta-analysis has demonstrated that pooled sensitivity and specificity of EUS for regional lymph node involvement were 76.4 and 72.4 %, respectively, suggesting EUS is also not satisfactory for the assessment of N-staging [34]. It is important to understand the limitation of EUS in the staging process.

Since EUS is not reliable for T- and N-staging, a diagnostic EMR for the staging purpose is essential to exclude any possibility of submucosal (T1b) or deeper invasion (>T2) and predict potential lymph node involvement based on complete histological assessment. EMR provides complete specimens including both mucosa and submucosa for histological assessment of lateral and deep margins, thereby determining the accurate T-stage (i.e., differentiating T1a from T1b). A positive lateral margin can be addressed with additional endoscopic intervention, while a positive deep margin should be considered for esophagectomy.

Endoscopic Ablation

The purpose of endoscopic ablation therapy is to eradicate disease by ablating (burning or freezing) the affected epithelium of the esophagus. Currently, radiofrequency ablation (RFA) and cryotherapy have been primarily performed as endoscopic ablation therapy. The common drawback of ablation therapy is that there is no specimen available for histological assessment.

Radiofrequency Ablation (RFA)

RFA using the Barrx™ Ablation System (Covidien, Sunnyvale, CA) has been most commonly used as ablation therapy, since the multicenter, randomized, sham-controlled trial involving 127 patients with Barrett's esophagus demonstrated that 81 % of patients with HGD had complete eradication of dysplasia with RFA compared to 19 % in the control group (no RFA) (p <0.001) and patients who underwent RFA had significantly less disease progression and fewer cancers developed during the follow-up of 12 months [35]. Either an ablation balloon catheter (Barrx™ 360 RFA Balloon Catheter) for circumferential ablation or an endoscopic mounted device (Barrx™ 90, 60, Ultra Long RFA Focal Catheter) for focal ablation can be selected based on the length, extension, and location of disease (Fig. 2.1). This system delivers a high-power, ultrashort burst of ablative energy to the abnormal esophageal epithelium, and the delivered energy provides uniform treatment to a depth of approximately 500 μm. Therefore, the depth of treatment is limited to the mucosal layer, thereby significantly reducing the risk of stricture formation. The rate of stricture formation was reported to be 6 % [35]. A further follow-up study demonstrated that patients' quality of life significantly improved after the RFA treatment, although most patients were worried about esophageal cancer and esophagectomy before the RFA treatment [36]. Due to the limited depth of treatment, RFA is not indicated for invasive cancer.

Cryotherapy

Cryotherapy involves the topical application by spraying aerosolized liquid nitrogen or carbon dioxide onto the abnormal esophageal epithelium, providing intracellular disruption and ischemia while preserving the extracellular matrix and thereby minimizing fibrosis. A prospective study involving 98 patients with HGD has demonstrated that 97 % had complete eradication of HGD with no esophageal perforation [28]. Current cryotherapy devices require a venting system such as a nasogastric tube to help excessive nitrogen gas escape out of the esophagus and stomach, thus preventing perforation of the gastrointestinal tract. Furthermore, cryotherapy is associated with several issues including its nonuniform application using a handheld catheter, the fogging of scope lens, and the prolonged duration of the therapy. Currently, a novel

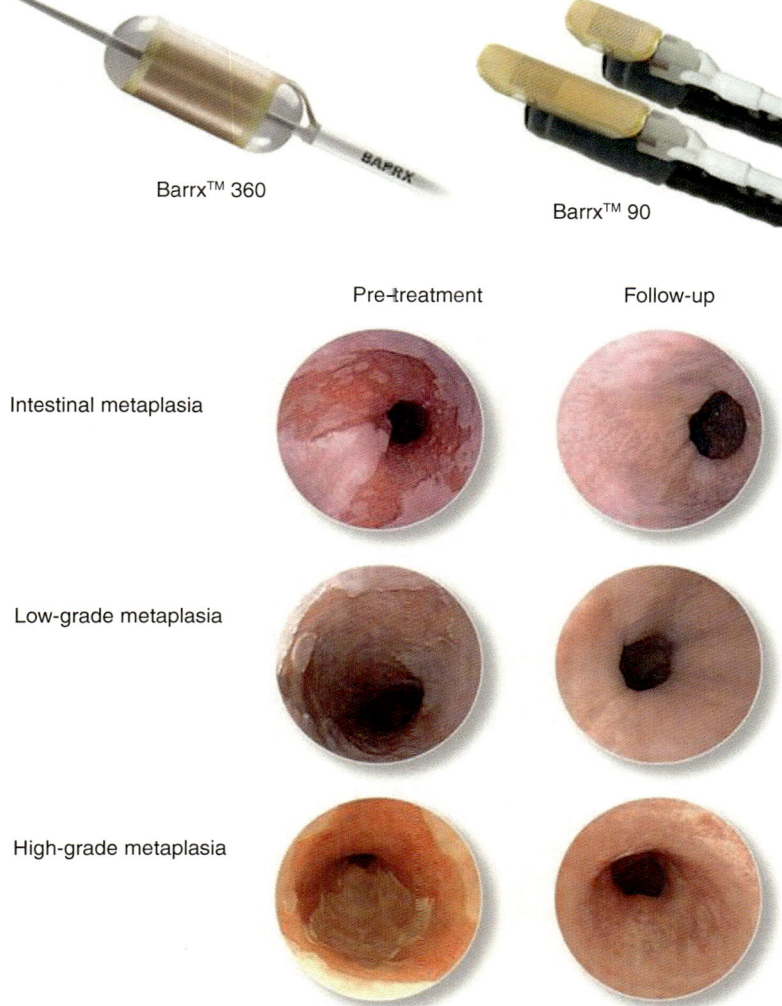

Fig. 2.1 Radiofrequency ablation therapy. The upper panels show the Barrx™ (*left*) and Barrx™ systems (*right*). The lower panel shows endoscopic findings of pre- and post-treatment for intestinal metaplasia (*top*), low-grade dysplasia (*middle*), and high-grade dysplasia (*bottom*) (Permission for use granted by Cook Medical Incorporated, Bloomington, Indiana)

Barrx™ 360

Barrx™ 90

Pre-treatment   Follow-up

Intestinal metaplasia

Low-grade metaplasia

High-grade metaplasia

through-the-scope cryoballoon device, which does not require a venting system and potentially delivers a uniform and reproducible ablation, has been under investigation, and further study to evaluate the safety and efficacy of this device is awaited.

Endoscopic Resection

The goal of endoscopic resection is to completely remove the entire segment of abnormal esophageal epithelium, thereby curing HGD and T1a cancers. Unlike endoscopic ablation therapy, endoscopic resection can provide specimens for the complete histological assessment including depth of cancer invasion, degree of cellular differentiation, and involvement of lymphatics or vessels. Currently, endoscopic mucosal resection (EMR) is used for the lesions less than 2 cm, and endoscopic submucosal dissection (ESD) is recommended for en bloc removal of lesions larger than 2 cm. The major complication associated with endoscopic resection is stricture formation, especially when more than 75 % of the esophageal circumference is involved in a single setting [29]. Small clinical series have reported that the stricture rate after circumferential EMR is up to 80 % [37, 38].

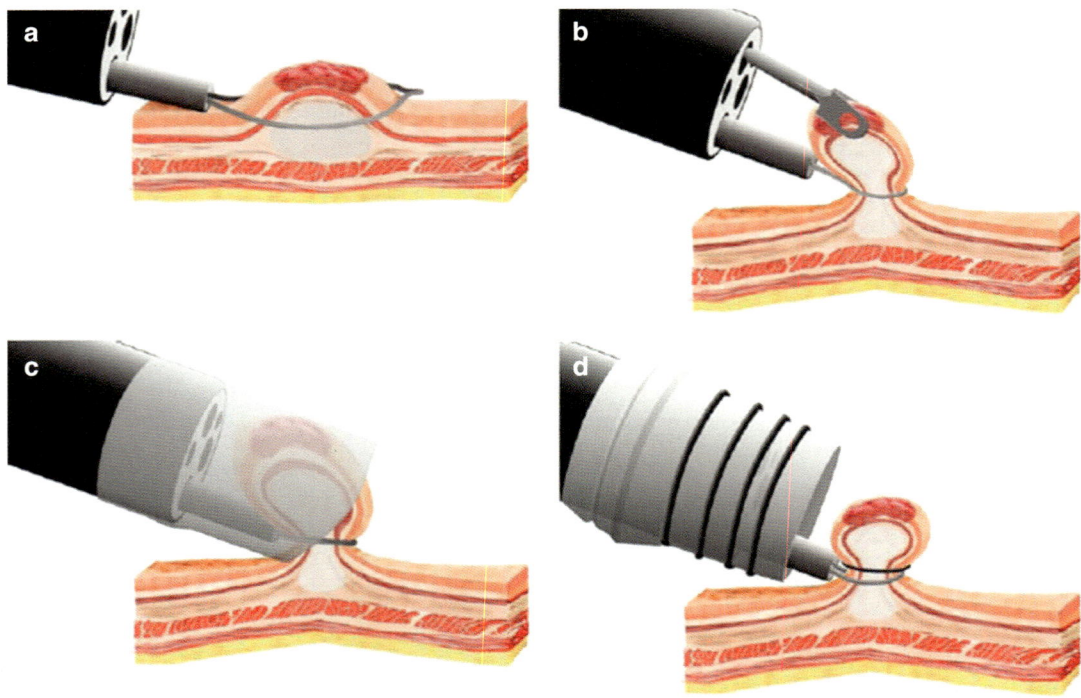

Fig. 2.2 Four types of endoscopic mucosal resection (EMR) techniques. (**a**) Snare polypectomy. (**b**) Strip biopsy technique. (**c**) The cap resection technique. (**d**) The ligate-and-cut technique (From Soetikno et al. [39] with permission)

Endoscopic Mucosal Resection (EMR)

EMR has been commonly used as both a diagnostic and therapeutic tool. There are primarily two techniques: cap resection technique and ligate-and-cut technique (Fig. 2.2) [39]. A randomized trial comparing these two techniques has demonstrated no difference in safety and efficacy between the techniques [40]. Both techniques are initiated by injecting normal saline into the submucosal space to lift the lesions away from the muscularis propria. The injection needle should be inserted into a submucosal space at the sharp angle to avoid transmural penetration of the needle. Injected saline acts as a "safety cushion" between the mucosa and muscularis propria to reduce the risk of unexpected complications such as perforation during the procedure. Additional injection of saline is sometimes required because the injected saline disappears within a few minutes. Difficulty lifting up the lesion by submucosal injection suggests invasion into the muscularis propria. For the cap resection technique, a

clear plastic cap (either straight or oblique shaped) is attached to the tip of endoscope. The oblique-shaped caps are usually used for esophageal lesions, while the straight caps are most commonly used for the lesions in the stomach and colon. The mucosal-submucosal complex is then sucked into a cap mounted on an endoscope, creating a pseudopolyp. The pseudopolyp is then resected by being captured at its base with a cautery snare which is positioned inside the cap [41]. For the ligate-and-cut technique, the only difference to the cap technique is to deploy a band to create a pseudopolyp [26, 27]. Currently, there is a novel multiband mucosectomy device available, which uses a specially designed multiple-band ligator and allows endoscopists to perform ligation and subsequent immediate resection without removal of the endoscope by passing a cautery snare through the ligator handle. The retrieved specimen is pinned to a piece of cork and placed into preservative solution prior to processing for histological assessment. EMR is indicated for lesions less than 2 cm in diameter.

Table 2.3 Risk factors potentially associated with recurrence after endoscopic resection of early esophageal cancer

Risk factors for recurrence after endoscopic resection of early esophageal cancer
1. Piecemeal resection
2. Long-segment BE
3. No ablation therapy of BE after CR
4. Time until CR achieved > 10 months
5. Multifocal neoplasia

BE Barrett's esophagus, CR complete remission

Although en-bloc resection is ideal in any situation, piecemeal resection of large lesions (>2 cm) is acceptable; however, several studies have shown that piecemeal EMR is associated with incomplete resection and compromised histological assessment, likely causing the development of metachronous lesions [42, 43].

An early retrospective study from a single institution demonstrated that 98 % of patients with HGD and T1a adenocarcinoma ($n = 115$) achieved complete response to EMR; however, 30 % of patients developed metachronous cancers during a mean follow-up of 34 months [42]. In a further study from the same institution, several factors including piecemeal resection, long-segment BE, no ablation therapy of BE after a complete response, multifocal neoplasia, and time until complete response >10 months were found to be associated with frequent tumor recurrence after endoscopic resection (Table 2.3) [43]. Based on these results, combination therapy involving focal EMR to resect nodules followed by RFA to treat any residual flat Barrett's epithelium has been investigated to minimize the development of recurrent disease. A recent multicenter, prospective study to evaluate the efficacy of this combination therapy has demonstrated that 95 % of patients with HGD or T1a adenocarcinoma ($n = 24$) had a complete response to the combination therapy and no recurrence occurred during a median follow-up of 22 months [44]. These studies emphasize the importance of intensive surveillance, the risk of metachronous lesions after endoscopic resection, the need for post-intervention intensive surveillance, and the necessity of discussing the possibility of

recurrent cancers with patients prior to the initiation of endoscopic interventions.

Endoscopic Submucosal Dissection (ESD)

ESD has been established as an advanced endoscopic resection technique to accomplish en bloc resection of lesions larger than 2 cm in diameter. ESD is expected to provide more accurate histological assessment for the lateral and deep margins of lesions and thus prevent or minimize the development of metachronous lesions. ESD employs the same concept of EMR but requires some modifications for en bloc resection of a large lesion. Each step is summarized in Fig. 2.3. ESD is initiated by a mucosal marking around the lesion by using electrocautery, thus easily identifying the location of the entire lesion after the submucosal injection (Fig. 2.4a). Subsequently, a solution is injected into the submucosal space to lift the lesion away from the muscularis propria. The injection solutions for ESD include normal saline, glycerol, and sodium hyaluronate. Sodium hyaluronate stays longer in the submucosal space than normal saline or glycerol and may be ideal for ESD. Diluted sodium hyaluronate (approximately 0.5 % solution) is usually mixed with epinephrine (0.01 mg/ml) and indigo carmine (0.04 mg/ml). The mucosal cutting is then performed to create the entry to the submucosal space by using a specialized endoscopic electocautery called "needle knife" (Fig. 2.4b, c). Several types of needle knives having different shaped tips are available, depending on the preference of endoscopists (Fig. 2.5). Once the submucosal space is entered, tension and counter-tension are maintained by a cap mounted on the tip of endoscope, which is placed in the plane between the mucosal-submucosal complex and the muscularis propria. The needle knife is then introduced through the endoscopic working channel, and the attachments and bridging vessels between the two layers are dissected. At the completion of this procedure, the lesion can be resected en bloc regardless of its size and the remaining thin layer of sm3 can be seen over the

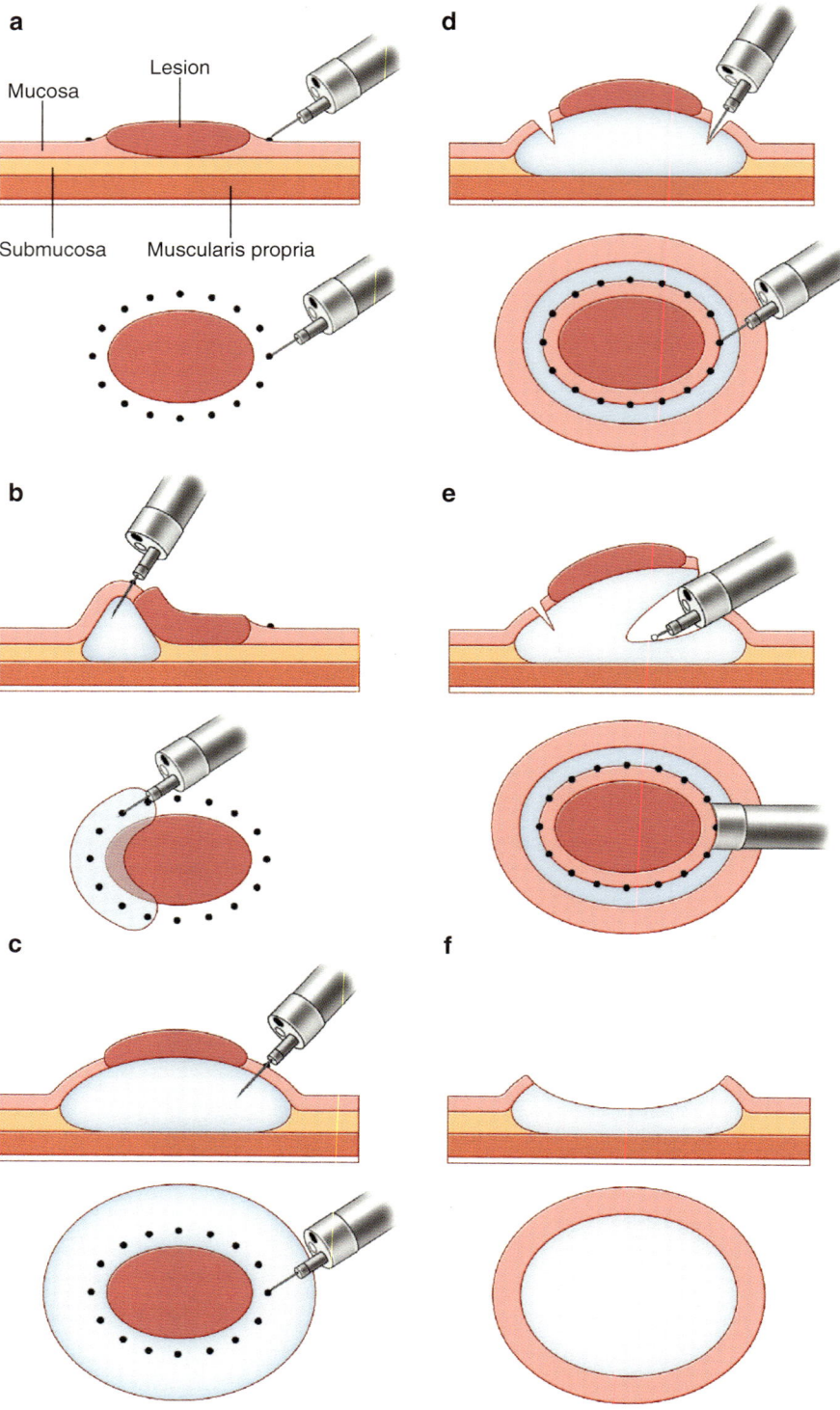

Fig. 2.3 Schematic representation of endoscopic submucosal dissection. (**a**) Mucosal markings for the incision line. (**b**) Submucosal injections of a solution. (**c**) Complete elevation of the lesion by injecting a solution into the submucosal space. (**d**) Mucosal incision around the mucosal markings. (**e**) Submucosal dissection with a needle knife through the cap attached on the tip of endoscope. (**f**) En bloc resection of the tumor. *M* mucosa, *SM* submucosa, *MP* muscularis propria

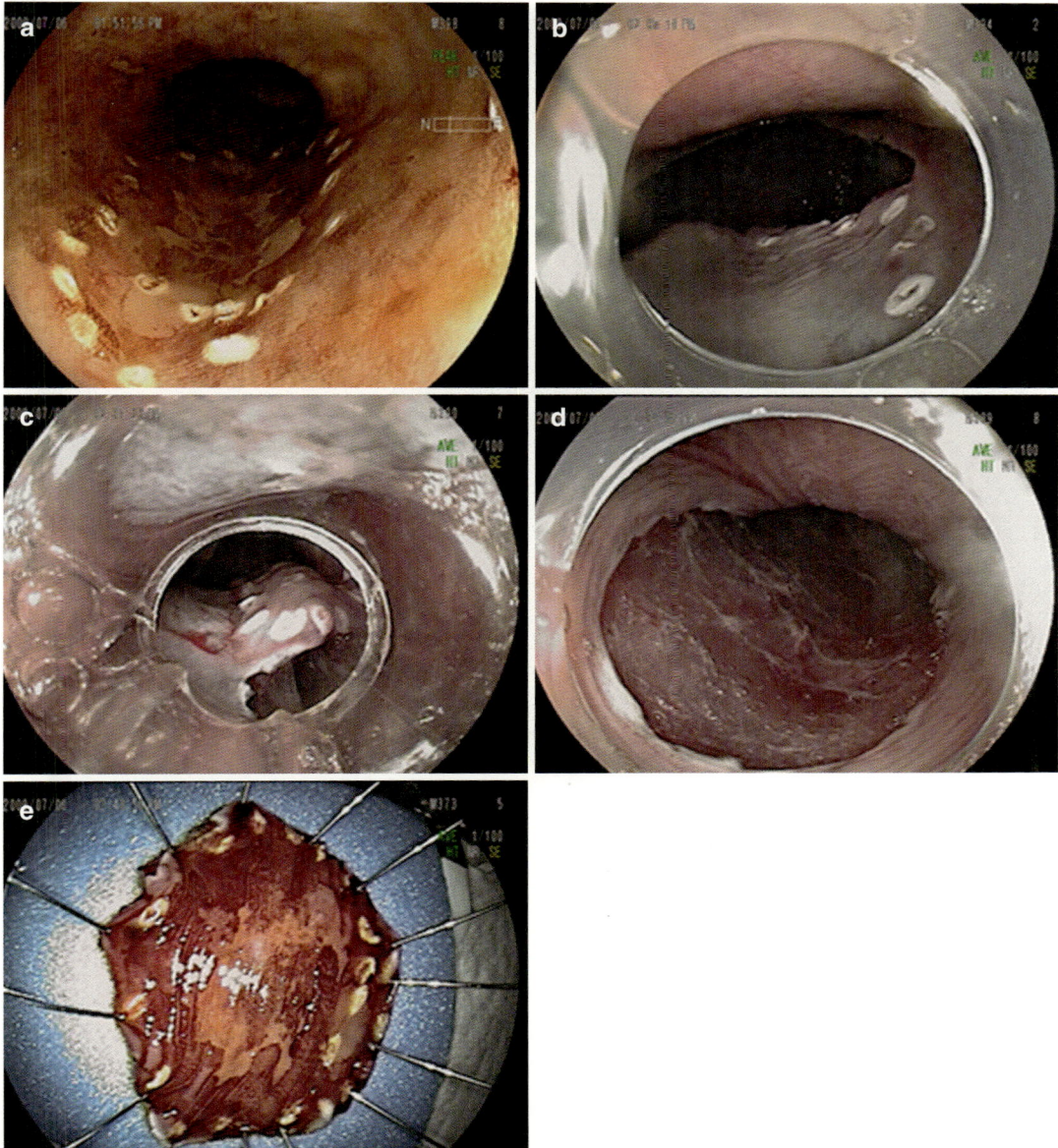

Fig. 2.4 Endoscopic submucosal dissection of early esophageal squamous cell carcinoma. (**a**) Chromoendoscopy shows the presence of an irregular unstained area in the middle esophagus. The markings are performed using an electrocautery. (**b**) After the submucosal injection of sodium hyaluronate, submucosal dissection can be performed. (**c**) Submucosal dissection is performed using the needle knife. (**d**) The tumor is resected en bloc. A thin layer of sm3 was observed over the muscle layer. (**e**) The resected specimen was spread out and pinned on a flat cork

resected area (Fig. 2.4d). It is important to maintain this thin layer of sm3, especially when repair of a perforation is required. ESD is a "one-person" procedure and does not allow for assistant hands. It is therefore important to maintain adequate counter-traction on the mucosa to be resected throughout the procedure. For this purpose, it may be better to start with a partial mucosal incision rather than a circumferential mucosal incision, maintaining the continuity of the lesion to the esophageal epithelium as "counter-traction," and mucosal incision and

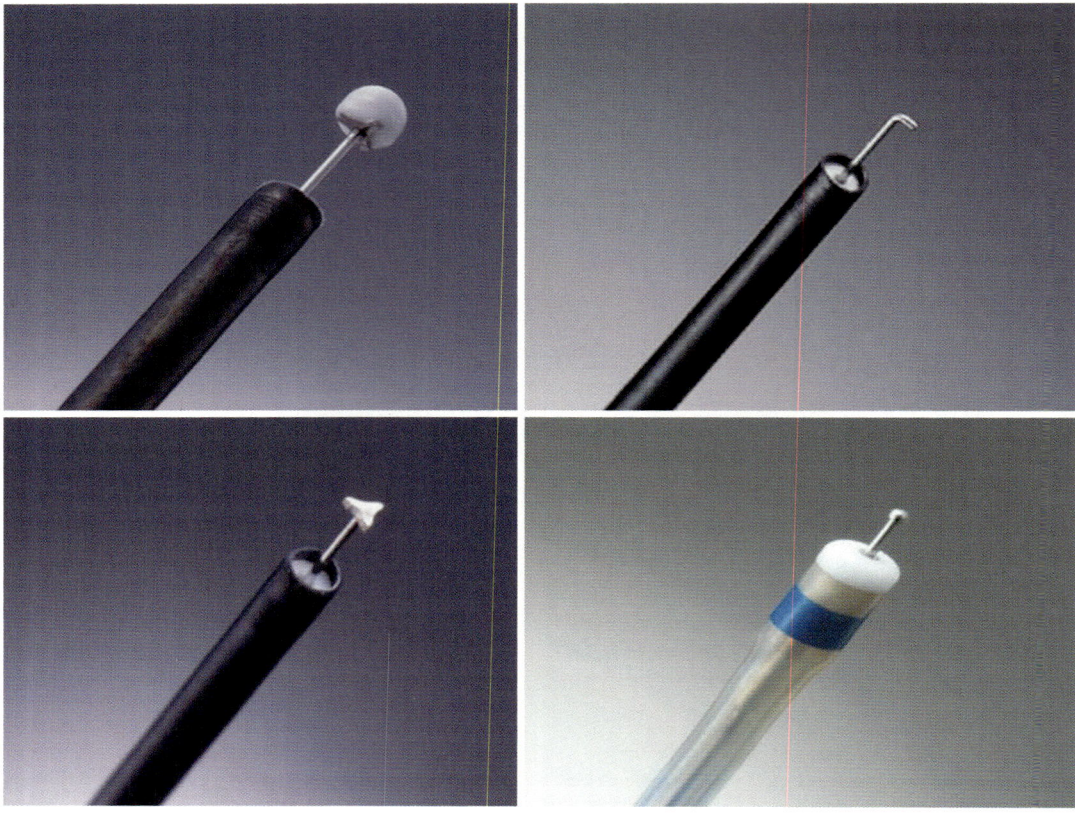

Fig. 2.5 Different types of needle knife for endoscopic submucosal dissection. *Upper left*: insulation-tipped diathermic electrosurgical knife (IT knife). *Upper right*: hook knife. *Lower left*: triangle-tip knife (TT knife). *Lower right*: dual knife

submucosal dissection should be repeated step by step. The advantage of gravity should be considered; submucosal dissection should be started from the upper portion of the lesion so that the dissected mucosa is pulled down by gravity, spontaneously exposing the submucosal layer. It is also worth considering repositioning patients to obtain the advantage of gravity.

ESD is expected to be superior to EMR because of the availability of en bloc resection specimens, although no randomized controlled study comparing ESD with EMR is available. Since ESD has not been routinely performed to treat patients with HGD and T1a cancers, the available data to show the efficacy of ESD in this setting are limited. In a study to evaluate the long-term outcomes of 84 patients with superficial esophageal squamous cell cancer who underwent

ESD, a Japanese group reported that en bloc resection and complete resection were achieved in 100 and 88 % of patients, respectively, and the 5-year cause-specific survival of patients with T1a cancers was 100 % [45]. Major complications including perforation occurred in 4 % of patients, and 18 % developed benign esophageal stricture requiring dilation [45]. This suggests that ESD could be a reasonable option for cure of HGD and T1a cancers. The perforation rate during ESD is reported to be higher than that during EMR (4–10 % vs. 0.3–0.5 %, respectively) [46–50]. Perforation is easily identified during the procedure, and a small perforation can be addressed by deploying endoclips [41, 42]. A large perforation requires an emergent surgery to avoid peritonitis and/or mediastinitis. Furthermore, stricture formation is the other major complication of ESD. Strictures are more likely to occur after ESD for esophageal lesions (up to 26 %) [29, 43, 44]. It should be noted that ESD for BE and esophageal adenocarcinoma may be technically more difficult than ESD for gastric cancer or esophageal squamous cell cancer because of its location in the distal esophagus close to the gastroesophageal junction and the submucosal scarring due to reflux-induced inflammation. Because of the high rates of perforation and stricture and steep learning-curve, ESD has not been widely accepted especially for esophageal lesions in the United States.

Management After Esophageal-Preserving Therapy

It should be emphasized that intensive endoscopic surveillance and strict acid suppression with high-dose proton pump inhibitors (PPI) and nocturnal H2 blockers after intervention are critical for successful esophageal-preserving therapy. Strict acid suppression establishes an acid-free environment in the treated area, thus facilitating the healing process to the normal "neosquamous" lining. There has been no consensus on surveillance protocols following esophageal-preserving therapy; however, the guidelines issued by the American Society for Gastrointestinal Endoscopy (ASGE) states that surveillance endoscopy for patients with HGD should undergo every 3 months for at least 1 year with multiple large capacity biopsy specimens obtained at 1 cm intervals. After 1 year, if there is no detection of recurrence, the interval of surveillance may be lengthened if there are no dysplastic changes on two subsequent endoscopies performed at 3-month intervals [51]. Since BE is caused by long-term acid exposure to the distal esophagus, a surgical repair of underlying gastroesophageal reflux disease (GERD) should be considered in order to eliminate all acid exposure to the esophageal epithelium, thus liberating patients from acid suppression therapy. Although the ASGE guideline states that antireflux surgery should not be advised with the rationale that the procedure will prevent esophageal cancer [51], it may be reasonable to continue intensive surveillance every 3 months up to 1 year following esophageal-preserving therapy, and then consider antireflux surgery if there is no evidence of recurrence. Long-term endoscopic surveillance per the ASGE guidelines is still required even after antireflux surgery is performed. BE refractory to endoscopic intervention may be caused by persistent, significant acid exposure to the treated area, and early antireflux surgery may be considered.

Upper endoscopy has been performed under conscious sedation, causing significant direct (e.g., personnel, facility) and indirect (e.g., off work, third-party transportation) costs. In addition, most complications are associated with conscious sedation. With the recent advances in optic technology, small-caliber endoscopes have been developed and introduced to perform transnasal endoscopy. Transnasal endoscopy can be performed in the office setting without intravenous sedation, and our previous study has demonstrated the equivalent efficacy and accuracy and better patients' tolerance compared to conventional endoscopy [52]. There is a small-caliber endoscope available, which has a disposable sheath with an incorporated coaxial biopsy channel placed over it. Therefore, there is no need for post-procedure endoscope processing as required for sedated endoscopy, and the cost can be significantly reduced. This technology may allow us perform a low-cost, safe, and intensive surveillance of patients who undergo esophageal-preserving therapy.

Long-Term Outcome of Esophageal-Preserving Therapy

The long-term outcome data of esophageal-preserving therapy to treat HGD and T1a cancers are still limited. In a single large prospective study involving 349 patients with HGD and T1a adenocarcinoma who underwent esophageal-preserving therapies such as ablation and endoscopic resection, 96.6 % achieved complete response and only 3.7 % required surgery during a mean follow-up of 5 years without tumor-related deaths. In addition, patients who underwent RFA for persistent or recurrent BE had a lower incidence of metachronous neoplasia compared to those who did not undergo RFA (16.5 % vs. 28.3 %) [43]. This suggests that additional ablation therapy for remaining BE may minimize the development of metachronous neoplasia. The rates of bleeding and stenosis were 12 and 4.3 %, respectively.

Several studies have demonstrated a low complication rate and a good disease-specific 5-year survival rate for the endoscopic resection of esophageal squamous cell carcinoma [53–55]. The most recent retrospective cohort study involving 51 patients with either squamous dysplasia or T1a squamous cell cancer who underwent repeated EMR until complete local remission was achieved, 91 % of patients had complete remission, and the disease-specific 5-year survival rate was 95 %. Minor bleeding occurred in 17 % of patients and 3 patients (6 %) developed mild stenosis requiring dilation, although there was no perforation. During the follow-up period, local disease recurrence was observed in 26 % of patients [53].

Future Prospective

With the advances in endoscopic technologies and techniques, aggressive endoscopic resection is technically feasible. However, the main concern is a post-procedure stricture formation. To prevent or minimize stricture formation after aggressive endoscopic resection, novel approaches such as biologic scaffold materials composed of xenogeneic extracellular matrix (ECM) and cell-sheet technology have been investigated in the context of regenerative medicine. ECM has been shown to remodel the default tissue via neo-epithelialization rather than scar formation [54, 55] and to successfully minimize a stricture formation after aggressive, circumferential endoscopic resection both in preclinical [56] and clinical settings [57]. Cell-sheet technology is a tissue engineering approach to attempt reconstructing tissue without scaffold [58]. Epithelial cells obtained from patients' oral mucosal tissue are cultured on temperature-responsive culture plates. By

reducing the temperature below 32 °C, the cultured cells spontaneously detach from the culture plate without any proteolytic enzyme as a "cell sheet". Transplantable, autologous epithelial cell sheets have been applied onto the treated area after aggressive ESD and shown to successfully minimize stricture formation in the clinical setting [59]. Regenerative medicine approaches may make more aggressive endoscopic resection possible, although further studies are required.

Conclusion

Highly selected patients with HGD and T1a cancers can be treated endoscopically. Based on the risk stratification and accurate clinical staging, patients with potential lymph node involvement and/or metastatic disease need to be excluded. At present, patients with HGD and T1a adenocarcinoma or early squamous cell carcinoma (m1 and m2) with low risk or no risk of lymph node involvement can be a candidate for esophageal-preserving therapy. Highly selected patients with T1sm1 adenocarcinoma could be a candidate for esophageal-preserving therapy, particularly when poor functional status and comorbid conditions make esophagectomy too risky. Intensive surveillance and strict acid suppression therapy are required after esophageal-preserving therapy. Since BE is caused by GERD, antireflux surgery should be considered once the treated area is determined to be stable.

References

1. Jankowski JA, Wright NA, Meltzer SJ, et al. Molecular evolution of the metaplasia-dysplasia-adenocarcinoma sequence in the esophagus. Am J Pathol. 1999;154(4): 965–73.
2. Werner M, Mueller J, Walch A, Hofler H. The molecular pathology of Barrett's esophagus. Histol Histopathol. 1999;14(2):553–9.
3. Collard JM. High-grade dysplasia in Barrett's esophagus. The case for esophagectomy. Chest Surg Clin N Am. 2002;12(1):77–92.
4. Falk GW, Rice TW, Goldblum JR, Richter JE. Jumbo biopsy forceps protocol still misses unsuspected cancer in Barrett's esophagus with high-grade dysplasia. Gastrointest Endosc. 1999;49(2):170–6.

5. Birkmeyer JD, Siewers AE, Finlayson EV, et al. Hospital volume and surgical mortality in the United States. N Engl J Med. 2002;346(15):1128–37.

6. Halm EA, Lee C, Chassin MR. Is volume related to outcome in health care? A systematic review and methodologic critique of the literature. Ann Intern Med. 2002;137(6):511–20.

7. Oh DS, Hagen JA, Chandrasoma PT, et al. Clinical biology and surgical therapy of intramucosal adenocarcinoma of the esophagus. J Am Coll Surg. 2006; 203(2):152–61.

8. Rice TW, Blackstone EH, Adelstein DJ, et al. Role of clinically determined depth of tumor invasion in the treatment of esophageal carcinoma. J Thorac Cardiovasc Surg. 2003;125(5):1091–102.

9. Rice TW, Zuccaro Jr G, Adelstein DJ, Rybicki LA, Blackstone EH, Goldblum JR. Esophageal carcinoma: depth of tumor invasion is predictive of regional lymph node status. Ann Thorac Surg. 1998;65(3):787–92.

10. Pohl H, Sirovich B, Welch HG. Esophageal adenocarcinoma incidence: are we reaching the peak? Cancer Epidemiol Biomarkers Prev. 2010;19(6):1468–70.

11. Siegel R, Naishadham D, Jemal A. Cancer statistics, 2012. CA Cancer J Clin. 2012;62(1):10–29.

12. Ell C, May A, Pech O, et al. Curative endoscopic resection of early esophageal adenocarcinomas (Barrett's cancer). Gastrointest Endosc. 2007;65(1):3–10.

13. Pech O, May A, Gossner L, et al. Curative endoscopic therapy in patients with early esophageal squamouscell carcinoma or high-grade intraepithelial neoplasia. Endoscopy. 2007;39(1):30–5.

14. Wang KK, Sampliner RE. Updated guidelines 2008 for the diagnosis, surveillance and therapy of Barrett's esophagus. Am J Gastroenterol. 2008;103(3):788–97.

15. Bolton WD, Hofstetter WL, Francis AM, et al. Impact of tumor length on long-term survival of pT1 esophageal adenocarcinoma. J Thorac Cardiovasc Surg. 2009; 138(4):831–6.

16. Stein HJ, Feith M, Bruecher BL, Naehrig J, Sarbia M, Siewert JR. Early esophageal cancer: pattern of lymphatic spread and prognostic factors for long-term survival after surgical resection. Ann Surg. 2005;242(4):566–73; discussion 573–5.

17. Buttar NS, Wang KK, Sebo TJ, et al. Extent of high-grade dysplasia in Barrett's esophagus correlates with risk of adenocarcinoma. Gastroenterology. 2001;120(7): 1630–9.

18. Levine DS, Haggitt RC, Blount PL, Rabinovitch PS, Rusch VW, Reid BJ. An endoscopic biopsy protocol can differentiate high-grade dysplasia from early adenocarcinoma in Barrett's esophagus. Gastroenterology. 1993;105(1):40–50.

19. Schnell TG, Sontag SJ, Chejfec G, et al. Long-term nonsurgical management of Barrett's esophagus with high-grade dysplasia. Gastroenterology. 2001;120(7): 1607–19.

20. Weston AP, Sharma P, Topalovski M, Richards R, Cherian R, Dixon A. Long-term follow-up of Barrett's high-grade dysplasia. Am J Gastroenterol. 2000;95(8): 1888–93.

21. Araki K, Ohno S, Egashira A, Saeki H, Kawaguchi H, Sugimachi K. Pathologic features of superficial esophageal squamous cell carcinoma with lymph node and distal metastasis. Cancer. 2002;94(2):570–5.

22. Eguchi T, Nakanishi Y, Shimoda T, et al. Histopathological criteria for additional treatment after endoscopic mucosal resection for esophageal cancer: analysis of 464 surgically resected cases. Mod Pathol. 2006;19(3):475–80.

23. Tajima Y, Nakanishi Y, Ochiai A, et al. Histopathologic findings predicting lymph node metastasis and prognosis of patients with superficial esophageal carcinoma: analysis of 240 surgically resected tumors. Cancer. 2000;88(6):1285–93.

24. Rice TW. Pro: esophagectomy is the treatment of choice for high-grade dysplasia in Barrett's esophagus. Am J Gastroenterol. 2006;101(10):2177–9.

25. Sepesi B, Watson TJ, Zhou D, et al. Are endoscopic therapies appropriate for superficial submucosal esophageal adenocarcinoma? An analysis of esophagectomy specimens. J Am Coll Surg. 2010;210(4): 418–27.

26. Gockel I, Sgourakis G, Lyros O, et al. Risk of lymph node metastasis in submucosal esophageal cancer: a review of surgically resected patients. Expert Rev Gastroenterol Hepatol. 2011;5(3):371–84.

27. Manner H, Pech O, Heldmann Y, et al. Efficacy, safety, and long-term results of endoscopic treatment for early-stage adenocarcinoma of the esophagus with low-risk sm1 invasion. Clin Gastroenterol Hepatol. 2013;11(6):630–5.

28. Shaheen NJ, Greenwald BD, Peery AF, et al. Safety and efficacy of endoscopic spray cryotherapy for Barrett's esophagus with high-grade dysplasia. Gastrointest Endosc. 2010;71(4):680–5.

29. Katada C, Muto M, Manabe T, Boku N, Ohtsu A, Yoshida S. Esophageal stenosis after endoscopic mucosal resection of superficial esophageal lesions. Gastrointest Endosc. 2003;57(2):165–9.

30. Gananadha S, Hazebroek EJ, Leibman S, et al. The utility of FDG-PET in the preoperative staging of esophageal cancer. Dis Esophagus. 2008;21(5):389–94.

31. Meyers BF, Downey RJ, Decker PA, et al. The utility of positron emission tomography in staging of potentially operable carcinoma of the thoracic esophagus: results of the American College of Surgeons Oncology Group Z0060 trial. J Thorac Cardiovasc Surg. 2007; 133(3):738–45.

32. Puli SR, Reddy JB, Bechtold ML, Antillon D, Ibdah JA, Antillon MR. Staging accuracy of esophageal cancer by endoscopic ultrasound: a meta-analysis and systematic review. World J Gastroenterol. 2008;14(10): 1479–90.

33. Chemaly M, Scalone O, Durivage G, et al. Miniprobe EUS in the pretherapeutic assessment of early esophageal neoplasia. Endoscopy. 2008;40(1):2–6.

34. Sgourakis G, Gockel I, Lyros O, Hansen T, Mildenberger P, Lang H. Detection of lymph node metastases in esophageal cancer. Expert Rev Anticancer Ther. 2011;11(4):601–12.

35. Shaheen NJ, Sharma P, Overholt BF, et al. Radiofrequency ablation in Barrett's esophagus with dysplasia. N Engl J Med. 2009;360(22):2277–88.

36. Shaheen NJ, Peery AF, Hawes RH, et al. Quality of life following radiofrequency ablation of dysplastic Barrett's esophagus. Endoscopy. 2010;42(10):790–9.

37. Seewald S, Ang TL, Omar S, et al. Endoscopic mucosal resection of early esophageal squamous cell cancer using the Duette mucosectomy kit. Endoscopy. 2006;38(10):1029–31.

38. Soehendra N, Seewald S, Groth S, et al. Use of modified multiband ligator facilitates circumferential EMR in Barrett's esophagus (with video). Gastrointest Endosc. 2006;63(6):847–52.

39. Soetikno RM, Gotoda T, Nakanishi Y, Soehendra N. Endoscopic mucosal resection. Gastrointest Endosc. 2003;57(4):567–79.

40. May A, Gossner L, Behrens A, et al. A prospective randomized trial of two different endoscopic resection techniques for early stage cancer of the esophagus. Gastrointest Endosc. 2003;58(2):167–75.

41. Inoue H, Endo M, Takeshita K, Yoshino K, Muraoka Y, Yoneshima H. A new simplified technique of endoscopic esophageal mucosal resection using a cap-fitted panendoscope (EMRC). Surg Endosc. 1992;6(5):264–5.

42. May A, Gossner L, Pech O, et al. Local endoscopic therapy for intraepithelial high-grade neoplasia and early adenocarcinoma in Barrett's oesophagus: acute-phase and intermediate results of a new treatment approach. Eur J Gastroenterol Hepatol. 2002;14(10):1085–91.

43. Pech O, Behrens A, May A, et al. Long-term results and risk factor analysis for recurrence after curative endoscopic therapy in 349 patients with high-grade intraepithelial neoplasia and mucosal adenocarcinoma in Barrett's oesophagus. Gut. 2008;57(9):1200–6.

44. Pouw RE, Wirths K, Eisendrath P, et al. Efficacy of radiofrequency ablation combined with endoscopic resection for barrett's esophagus with early neoplasia. Clin Gastroenterol Hepatol. 2010;8(1):23–9.

45. Ono S, Fujishiro M, Niimi K, et al. Long-term outcomes of endoscopic submucosal dissection for superficial esophageal squamous cell neoplasms. Gastrointest Endosc. 2009;70(5):860–6.

46. Fujishiro M, Yahagi N, Kakushima N, et al. Endoscopic submucosal dissection of esophageal squamous cell neoplasms. Clin Gastroenterol Hepatol. 2006;4(6):688–94.

47. Gotoda T. A large endoscopic resection by endoscopic submucosal dissection procedure for early gastric cancer. Clin Gastroenterol Hepatol. 2005;3(7 Suppl 1): S71–3.

48. Kato M. Endoscopic submucosal dissection (ESD) is being accepted as a new procedure of endoscopic treatment of early gastric cancer. Intern Med. 2005; 44(2):85–6.

49. Ono H. Early gastric cancer: diagnosis, pathology, treatment techniques and treatment outcomes. Eur J Gastroenterol Hepatol. 2006;18(8):863–6.

50. Yokoi C, Gotoda T, Hamanaka H, Oda I. Endoscopic submucosal dissection allows curative resection of locally recurrent early gastric cancer after prior endoscopic mucosal resection. Gastrointest Endosc. 2006; 64(2):212–8.

51. Hirota WK, Zuckerman MJ, Adler DG, et al. ASGE guideline: the role of endoscopy in the surveillance of premalignant conditions of the upper GI tract. Gastrointest Endosc. 2006;63(4):570–80.

52. Jobe BA, Hunter JG, Chang EY, et al. Office-based unsedated small-caliber endoscopy is equivalent to conventional sedated endoscopy in screening and surveillance for Barrett's esophagus: a randomized and blinded comparison. Am J Gastroenterol. 2006;101(12): 2693–703.

53. Ciocirlan M, Lapalus MG, Hervieu V, et al. Endoscopic mucosal resection for squamous premalignant and early malignant lesions of the esophagus. Endoscopy. 2007;39(1):24–9.

54. Inoue H, Fukami N, Yoshida T, Kudo SE. Endoscopic mucosal resection for esophageal and gastric cancers. J Gastroenterol Hepatol. 2002;17(4):382–8.

55. Takeshita K, Tani M, Inoue H, et al. Endoscopic treatment of early oesophageal or gastric cancer. Gut. 1997;40(1):123–7.

56. Nieponice A, McGrath K, Qureshi I, et al. An extracellular matrix scaffold for esophageal stricture prevention after circumferential EMR. Gastrointest Endosc. 2009;69(2):289–96.

57. Badylak SF, Hoppo T, Nieponice A, Gilbert TW, Davison JM, Jobe BA. Esophageal preservation in five male patients after endoscopic inner-layer circumferential resection in the setting of superficial cancer: a regenerative medicine approach with a biologic scaffold. Tissue Eng Part A. 2011;17(11–12): 1643–50.

58. Yamato M, Utsumi M, Kushida A, Konno C, Kikuchi A, Okano T. Thermo-responsive culture dishes allow the intact harvest of multilayered keratinocyte sheets without dispase by reducing temperature. Tissue Eng. 2001;7(4):473–80.

59. Takagi R, Yamato M, Kanai N, et al. Cell sheet technology for regeneration of esophageal mucosa. World J Gastroenterol. 2012;18(37):5145–50.

The Volume-Outcome Relationship, Standardized Clinical Pathways, and Minimally Invasive Surgery for Esophagectomy

Sheraz R. Markar and Donald E. Low

Volume-Outcome Relationship Associated with the Surgical Treatment of Esophageal Cancer

Esophagectomy remains an important component of treatment for locoregional esophageal cancer. Despite recent advancements in surgical technique and perioperative care, esophagectomy remains one of the most demanding surgical procedures associated with a highly variable rate of morbidity and mortality (3–14 %) and a poor overall survival (5 year survival of 20–30 %) [1–3]. Recent studies examining the volume-outcome relationship for esophageal resection suggest that high-volume institutions with a larger caseload and appropriate infrastructure are better prepared to deliver consistently high-quality outcomes [4–6].

Some studies have suggested that hospital volume does not influence perioperative mortality following esophagectomy [6, 7]. However, in 2012, a pooled analysis of nine relevant publications comprising 27,843 patients who underwent esophagectomy from 2000 to 2011 demonstrated

that esophagectomy performed at low-volume centers was associated with an increase in the incidence of inhospital (8.48 % vs. 2.82 %) and 30-day mortality (2.09 % vs. 0.73 %) [8]. There was insufficient evidence to provide a meaningful analysis of the effect of hospital volume on length of hospital stay and postoperative complications. Furthermore, hospital volume has not currently been demonstrated to have any significant influence on long-term survival following esophagectomy [9]. Therefore, the present published data would suggest that high hospital esophagectomy volume is associated with a reduction in mortality; however, there is insufficient data to comment on other important variables including long-term survival, complications, and quality of life following surgery.

It remains unclear whether hospital or surgeon volume is the most important factor determining clinical outcome following esophagectomy. Some studies have suggested that surgeon volume does not influence clinical outcome following esophagectomy [10, 11]; however, others suggest high surgeon volume is associated with a reduced incidence of postoperative complications and reduced length of hospital stay [12]. It is important to acknowledge the variability in esophagectomy surgical approaches (e.g., transhiatal, Ivor-Lewis, 3-stage, minimally invasive, etc.), and this heterogeneity may not be accurately characterized in clinical coding and thus fails to allow for subset esophageal procedural analysis to elucidate subtle variations in outcome.

S.R. Markar, MRCS(Eng), MA, MSc (✉)
Department of Thoracic Surgery,
Virginia Mason Medical Center,
1100 Ninth Avenue, Seattle, WA 98111, USA
e-mail: sheraz_markar@hotmail.com

D.E. Low, FACS, FRCS(c)
Department of General, Thoracic, and Vascular Surgery,
Virginia Mason Medical Center,
Seattle, WA, USA

S.N. Hochwald, M. Kukar (eds.), *Minimally Invasive Foregut Surgery for Malignancy: Principles and Practice*,
DOI 10.1007/978-3-319-09342-0_3, © Springer International Publishing Switzerland 2015

It is therefore possible that the improvements seen in postoperative mortality following esophagectomy in recent years may either be the result of individual surgeon performance, evolution in surgical technique, or improvements in perioperative care associated with high-volume esophageal surgical units, e.g., improved intensive care units and monitoring, physiotherapy, and multidisciplinary team input.

More recently, some groups have highlighted the volume outcome analysis as a means to provide a system guiding evidence-based hospital referral. The Leapfrog Group is a consortium of public and private healthcare stakeholders in the USA aiming to leverage purchasing power to improve and ensure healthcare quality and inform consumers regarding hospital performance [13]. However, recent follow-up studies have demonstrated that although a greater proportion of esophageal resections were performed in hospitals meeting a given evidence-based hospital referral volume metric in the 7 years in which Leapfrog has been collecting data, this shift had a negligible impact on postoperative outcome [14, 15]. In countries with a socialized healthcare system, e.g., the UK, Netherlands, and Sweden, the demonstrable improvements in clinical outcome associated with high institutional procedural volume have driven the push towards centralization of esophageal cancer services to high-volume institutions, which has translated into a reduction in observed perioperative mortality [16, 17]. Management of patients with esophageal cancer at high-volume institutions lends itself towards a true multidisciplinary approach to the treatment of these patients. Presentation and assessment of these patients at a multidisciplinary tumor board, with appropriate allocation of neoadjuvant or adjuvant therapies along with attention to additional issues including appropriate staging, nutrition, and improvement in enrollment in national clinical trials, are important components of the multimodality nature of management of these esophageal cancer patients.

In major oncological procedures such as esophagectomy, greater procedural volume whether surgeon or institutional has been shown to be associated with a reduction in perioperative mortality.

Countries that have used the volume-outcome relationship as a means to centralize esophageal cancer services to high-volume centers have seen this centralization of surgical services translate into a reduction in perioperative mortality in more recent years. The treatment of esophageal malignancy remains a highly challenging issue associated with significant pre-, intra-, and postoperative challenges, and high-volume centers provide the appropriate multidisciplinary infrastructure to reduce the potential impact of these challenges upon clinical outcome.

Impact of the Application of Standardized Clinical Pathways on Outcomes Associated with Esophageal Resection

Standardized clinical care pathways allow the introduction of a targeted goal-directed approach to postoperative recovery following major surgery. They provide a template for all medical personnel interacting with these patients and can outline an individualized goal-directed treatment approach and recovery for each patient. A multidisciplinary approach to the formulation, implementation, and evolution of standardized care pathways is important to facilitate success.

Clinical pathways are usually multifaceted and aimed at optimizing every aspect of a patient's treatment including preoperative assessment, procedural selection, intraoperative management, and postoperative care. These pathways once well established can provide a framework for quality improvement, improving postoperative outcomes and reducing costs [18–20]. Formal clinical care pathways have been successfully introduced in oncological colorectal surgery to provide a targeted goal-directed patient recovery, which has translated into a reduction in morbidity and in length of hospital stay [21–23].

In the past esophageal surgeons have been hesitant to apply multidisciplinary clinical pathways to enhance recovery following esophagectomy, due to the complex nature of the surgery and the associated rate of morbidity. However, in

Table 3.1   The effect of enhanced recovery on clinical outcome following esophagectomy

Author	ECP patients	LOS (PC) (days)	LOS (ECP) (days)	Mortality (PC) (%)	Mortality (ECP) (%)	Morbidity (PC) (%)	Morbidity (ECP) (%)
Zehr et al. (1991–1997) [24]	96	13.6±6.9	9.5±2.8	3.6	0	–	–
Cerfolio et al. (1999–2003)[20]	90	–	7 (median)	–	4.4	–	26.6
Low et al. (1991–2006) [25]	340	–	11.5 (6–49)	–	0.3	–	45
Jiang et al. (2006–2007) [26]	114	–	7 (5–28)	–	2.6	–	16.7
Tomaszek et al.[a] (2004–2008) [27]	110	9 (4–107)	7 (5–54)	4.6[b]	4.6[b]	42.8[b]	42.8[b]
Munitiz et al. (1998–2008) [19]	74	13 (8–106)	9 (5–98)	5	1	38	31
Preston et al. (2011–2012) [28]	12	17 (12–30)	7 (6–37)	0	0	75	33.3
Li et al. (2009–2011) [29]	59	10 (9–17)	8 (7–17)	0	2	62	59
Tang et al. (2008–2010) [30]	36	15 (IQR: 12–24)	11 (IQR: 8–15.5)	3.7	5.6	25.9	16.7
Blom et al. (2008–2010) [31]	103	15 (12–26)	14 (11–20)	1	4	68	71

PC previous care, *ECP* esophagectomy clinical pathway

[a]Compared a conventional preexisting pathway group to an alternative pathway group

[b]Results for both grouped analyzed together

more recent years, there has been expanding evidence to suggest that the principles of enhanced recovery can be applied to esophagectomy, resulting in a reduction in morbidity, length of hospital stay, and overall costs [19, 20, 24–31] (Table 3.1).

Esophagectomy clinical pathways optimally are initiated at the time of patient's initial referral, where an initial telephone interview with the patient typically done by the cancer nurse specialist will help to initiate the process of assessment of the patient's general physiological fitness and nutritional status. Furthermore, this interview provides an opportunity to inform patients and family regarding the relevant steps in their clinical staging investigations and allocation to multimodality therapy and introduce the concept of goal-directed recovery following surgery. The oncology nurse coordinator has an important role in making initial contact with the patient and in coordinating the staging investigations along with appointments with surgery, oncology, and substitutory dietary services, as well as arranged

physiological testing. The role of the oncology nurse coordinator has evolved and been assigned greater importance over the past 20 years, as they provide a point of contact for the patient during their initial consultation, staging investigations, treatment, and recovery. The importance of the initial interview by the nurse coordinator is routinely highlighted in patient satisfaction surveys following treatment.

All patients presenting with potentially resectable esophageal cancer should be discussed at a multidisciplinary tumor board, and this includes an assessment of patient demographics including comorbidities, tumor characteristics, and nutritional assessment to allow appropriate allocation of multimodality treatment.

Neoadjuvant chemoradiotherapy followed by surgery has been shown to improve survival in patients with esophageal cancer when compared to surgery alone [32–34]. However, patients must be carefully selected and, in some cases, optimized to be able to tolerate the entire course of treatment involved in trimodality therapy.

Table 3.2 Evolution in patient demographics; age and medical comorbidities at Virginia Mason Medical Center, Seattle, WA, USA (1991–2012)

Variable	1991–1996 (Group 1)	1997–2002 (Group 2)	2003–2007 (Group 3)	2008–2012 (Group 4)	P value
Case no.	92	159	161	183	
Patient age	64 (16–90)	64 (15–89)	66 (32–89)	66 (37–90)	0.17
M:F ratio (%)	74 (80.4)	134 (84.3)	127 (78.9)	141 (77)	0.63
BMI	26 (18–38)	25 (17–41)	26 (18–45)	27 (17–42)	0.03
Charlson (– age)	2 (0–4)	2 (0–6)	2 (0–5)	2 (0–7)	0.005
Charlson (+age)	4 (0–7)	4 (0–9)	5 (1–8)	5 (0–10)	0.02
ASA	3 (1–4)	3 (2–4)	3 (2–4)	3 (1–5)	0.07
Arrhythmia (%)	9 (9.8)	11 (6.9)	14 (8.7)	21 (11.5)	0.83
IHD (%)	12 (13.0)	34 (21.4)	19 (11.8)	31 (16.9)	0.51
Diabetes (%)	2 (2.2)	2 (1.3)	3 (1.9)	29 (15.8)	0.0004
Hypertension (%)	11 (12.0)	29 (18.2)	39 (24.2)	90 (49.2)	<0.0001
Liver disease (%)	0 (0)	2 (1.3)	3 (1.9)	9 (4.9)	0.03
Renal insufficiency (%)	1 (1.1)	1 (0.6)	6 (3.7)	6 (3.3)	0.43
COPD (%)	7 (7.6)	11 (6.9)	4 (2.5)	19 (10.4)	0.60
DVT/PE (%)	0 (0)	0 (0)	0 (0)	11 (6)	0.02
PVD (%)	1 (1.1)	3 (1.9)	4 (2.5)	8 (4.4)	0.28

Nutritional assessment prior to commencing multimodality treatment of esophageal cancer is important to ensure patient compliance and completion of therapy. In patients with major issues with dysphagia, odynophagia ,or loss of appetite resulting in significant loss of weight, the patient should be considered for placement of removable endoscopic esophageal stent for obstructive symptoms or pretreatment jejunostomy to facilitate nutritional support during neoadjuvant treatment. In the current era approximately 20 % of patients at our institution receive a pretreatment jejunostomy to address potential nutritional issues and improve tolerance and completion of neoadjuvant treatment. Other groups have reported the successful utilization of percutaneous radiologically sited gastrostomy tubes as an alternative to jejunostomy to address these pretreatment nutritional issues [35]. However, we prefer jejunostomies as we believe they are safer, less likely to compromise the gastric conduit, and can be placed in conjunction with another procedure such as diagnostic laparoscopy or port-a-cath placement. Routine pretreatment nutritional assessment is one illustration of the importance of these clinical pathways, especially when they are initiated at the time of referral and then form the

framework to optimize every aspect of the patient's treatment and recovery.

Pretreatment patient education allows appropriate management of patient expectations and empowers patients and their families to work with their primary caregivers to achieve treatment and recovery landmarks within a goal-directed pathway. Management of patient expectations is an important component of any clinical pathway, as preoperative education must foster patient understanding and commitment to the pathway goals. This issue becomes more important as health systems move towards centralization of complex cancer services, which will inevitably result in patients traveling for especially complex surgical procedures. Within our own institutional esophagectomy series, 48 % of patients travel from more than 150 miles and 26 % from more than 400 miles. We also aim to communicate decisions made at multidisciplinary tumor board to the patient and primary care practitioner within 24 h of the tumor board meeting.

In recent years there have been significant changes in the demographics of patients considered for surgical resection for esophageal cancer at high-volume institutions, with an increase in average age, body mass index, and the incidence of medical comorbidities (Table 3.2). Previous

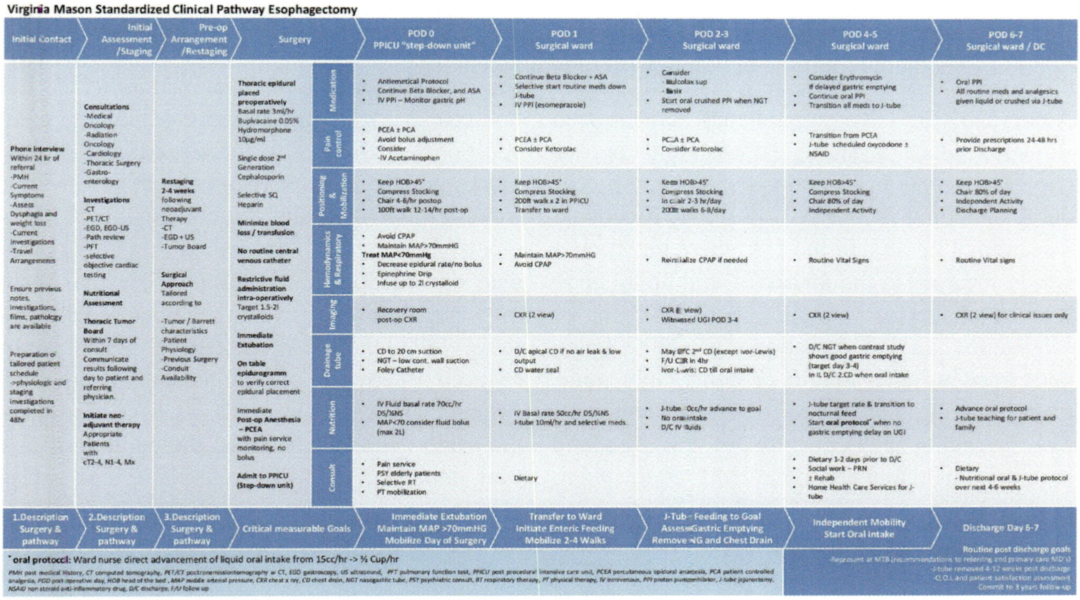

Virginia Mason Standardized Clinical Pathway Esophagectomy

	Initial Contact	Initial Assessment /Staging	Pre-op Arrangement /Restaging	Surgery	POD 0 PPICU "step-down unit"	POD 1 Surgical ward	POD 2-3 Surgical ward	POD 4-5 Surgical ward	POD 6-7 Surgical ward / DC
(overview)	Phone Interview: Within 24 hr of referral; -PMH; -Current Symptoms; -Assess Dysphagia and weight loss; -Current investigations; -Travel Arrangements. Ensure previous notes, investigations, films, pathology are available. Preparation of tailored patient schedule ->physiologic and staging investigations completed in 48hr	Consultations: -Medical Oncology; -Radiation Oncology; -Cardiology; -Thoracic Surgery; -Gastroenterology. Investigations: -CT; -PET/CT; -EGD, EGD-US; -Path review; -PFT; -selective objective cardiac testing. Nutritional Assessment. Thoracic Tumor Board: Within 7 days of consult. Communicate results following day to patient and referring physician. Initiate neo-adjuvant therapy Appropriate Patients with cT2-4, N1-3, Mx	Restaging 2-4 weeks following neoadjuvant Therapy: -CT; -EGD + US; -Tumor Board. Surgical Approach Tailored according to: -Tumor / Barrett characteristics; -Patient Physiology; -Previous Surgery; -Conduit Availability						
Medication				Thoracic epidural placed preoperatively; Basal rate 3ml/hr; Bupivacaine 0.05%; Hydromorphone 10µg/ml. Single dose 2nd Generation Cephalosporin. Selective SQ Heparin	Antiemetic Protocol; Continue Beta Blocker, and ASA; IV PPI – Monitor gastric pH	Continue Beta Blocker + ASA; Selective start routine meds down J-tube; IV PPI (esomeprazole)	Consider - bulcolax sup - lasix; Start oral crushed PPI when NGT removed	Consider Erythromycin if delayed gastric emptying; Continue oral PPI; Transition all meds to J-tube	Oral PPI; All routine meds and analgesics given liquid or crushed via J-tube
Pain control				Minimize blood loss / transfusion	PCEA ± PCA; Avoid bolus adjustment; Consider -IV Acetaminophen	PCEA ± PCA; Consider Ketorolac	PCA ± PCA; Consider Ketorolac	Transition from PCEA; J-tube scheduled oxycodone ± NSAID	Provide prescriptions 24-48 hrs prior Discharge
Positioning & Mobilization				Single dose 2nd Generation Cephalosporin; Selective SQ Heparin	Keep HOB>45°; Compress Stocking; Chair 4-6/hr postop; 100ft walk 12-14/hr post-op	Keep HOB>45°; Compress Stocking; 200ft walk x 2 in PPICU; Transfer to ward	Keep HOB>45°; Compress Stocking; In chair 2-3 hr/day; 200ft walks 6-8/day	Keep HOB>45°; Compress Stocking; Chair 80% of day; Independent Activity	Keep HOB>45°; Chair 80% of day; Independent Activity; Discharge Planning
Hemodynamic & Respiratory				No routine central venous catheter; Restrictive fluid administration intra-operatively Target 1.5-2l crystalloids. Avoid CPAP; Maintain MAP>70mmHG; Treat MAP<70mmHG; Decrease epidural rate/no bolus; Epinephrine Drip; Infuse up to 2l crystalloid	Maintain MAP>70mmHG; Avoid CPAP		Reinitialize CPAP if needed	Routine Vital Signs	Routine Vital signs
Imaging				Immediate Extubation	Recovery room post-op CXR	CXR (2 view)	CXR (2 view); Witnessed UGI POD 3-4	CXR (2 view)	CXR (2 view) for clinical issues only
Drainage tube				On table epidurogram to verify correct epidural placement	CD to 20 cm suction; NGT – low cont. wall suction; Foley Catheter	D/C apical CD if no air leak & low output; CD water seal	May @°C 2nd CD (except ivor-Lewis); F/U CXR in 4hr; ivor-Lewis: CD till oral intake	D/C NGT when contrast study shows good gastric emptying (target day 3-4); In IL D/C 2.CD when oral intake	
Nutrition				Immediate Post-op Anesthesia; -PCEA with pain service monitoring, no bolus	IV Fluid basal rate 70cc/hr D5/NS; MAP<70 consider fluid bolus (max 2L)	IV Basal rate 50cc/hr D5/NS; J-tube 10ml/hr and selective meds.	J-tube 0cc/hr advance to goal; No oral intake; D/C IV fluids	J-tube target rate & transition to nocturnal feed; Start oral protocol* when no gastric emptying delay on UGI	Advance oral protocol; J-tube teaching for patient and family
Consult				Admit to PPICU (Step-down unit); Pain service; PST elderly patients; Selective RT; PT mobilization	Dietary			Dietary 1-2 days prior to D/C; Social work – PRN; ± Rehab; Home Health Care Services for J-tube	Dietary - Nutritional oral & J-tube protocol over next 4-6 weeks
(goals)	1.Description Surgery & pathway	2.Description Surgery & pathway	3.Description Surgery & pathway	Critical measurable Goals	Immediate Extubation; Maintain MAP >70mmHG; Mobilize Day of Surgery	Transfer to Ward; Initiate Enteric Feeding; Mobilize 2-4 Walks	J-Tub- Feeding to Goal; Assess Gastric Emptying; Remove NG and Chest Drain	Independent Mobility; Start Oral Intake	Discharge Day 6-7; Routine post discharge goals

* oral protocol: Ward nurse direct advancement of liquid oral intake from 15cc/hr -> ⅓ Cup/hr

PMH past medical history, CT computed tomography, PET/CT positron emission tomography w CT, EGD gastroscopy, US ultrasound, PFT pulmonary function test, PPICU post procedural intensive care unit, PCEA percutaneous epidural anastesia, PCA patient controlled analgesia, POD post-operative day, HOB head of the bed, MAP middle arterial pressure, CXR chest x ray, CD chest drain, NGT nasogastric tube, PST psychiatric consult, RT respiratory therapy, PT physical therapy, IV intravenous, PPI proton pumpinhibitor, J-tube jejunostomy, NSAID non steroid anti-inflammatory drug, D/C discharge, F/U follow up

-Reassessment at MTB recommendations to referring and primary care MD'd
-J-tube removed 4-12 weeks post discharge
-Q.O.L and patient satisfaction assessment
-Commit to 5 years follow-up

Fig. 3.1 Esophagectomy clinical pathway (From Markar et al. [38] with permission)

reports of enhanced recovery protocols have specifically highlighted the challenges that elderly patients undergoing esophagectomy represent. Cerfolio et al. [20] demonstrated that 75 % of patients over 70 years of age failed their 'fast track' protocol. Moskovitz et al. [36] in a series of 31 patients undergoing esophagectomy over the age of 80 years demonstrated significant poorer outcomes with a longer length of hospital stay (26 (21.1–30.8) vs. 17.9 (16–19.8)) and a greater incidence of perioperative mortality (19.4 % vs. 7.3 %) compared to those under 80 years. However, we have previously published from our own institutional series that selected patients over the age of 80 years can undergo surgical treatment for esophageal cancer within a standardized clinical pathway and have a similar clinical outcome to younger patients, with no incidences of inhospital or 30-day mortality in a series of 32 patients over 80 years [37].

A multidisciplinary commitment to the continued revision of these standardized clinical pathways is important to ensure continued evolution and improvement in clinical outcomes. A standardized esophagectomy clinical pathway was first introduced in 1991 at the Virginia Mason Medical Center, Seattle, WA, USA, and has undergone five revisions to date. These revisions have specifically involved all members of the healthcare team including from surgery, anesthesiology, intensive care unit staff, ward nursing, dietetics, and cancer nurse coordinators.

Specific goals within the pathway that evolved during the past 20-year period (see Fig. 3.1) include:

- Improving patient education regarding pathway targets
- Adapting surgical approach according to individual presenting patient characteristics
- Developing approaches to minimizing blood loss and perioperative fluid administration
- Optimizing perioperative pain regimens to maintain targeted postoperative hemodynamics but facilitating postoperative mobilization goals to ultimately mobilize patients on the day of surgery
- Assessment and monitoring of nutrition prior to neoadjuvant therapy and esophagectomy
- Earlier application of enteric feeding and nasogastric tube removal
- Modifying targeted discharge goals from 12–14 days in the early 1990s to 6–7 days in the current era.

Minimally Invasive vs. Open Esophagectomy

A minimally invasive surgical approach has been shown to reduce physiological stress and improve clinical outcome in several major surgical procedures including colorectal, liver, and pancreatic resections [39–41]. In the UK, there has been a steady increase in the uptake of minimally invasive esophagectomy (MIE), with 24.7 % of esophageal cancer resections in 2009 being performed using a hybrid or completely minimally invasive approach [42]. A robust comparative review or meta-analysis of the literature regarding the relative merits of MIE compared to a standard open approach would be challenging due to several inherent limitations of the publications on this subject. The definition of MIE is highly variable and includes laparoscopic abdominal phase with open thoracotomy, open abdominal phase and thoracoscopic approach to thoracic dissection, and totally minimally invasive esophagectomy. Together with the continued variation in open approaches to esophagectomy, this makes direct objective comparison more challenging than in other surgical procedures and the widespread applicability of such comparisons somewhat questionable.

Pooled analyses of the available evidence have identified potential benefits to MIE over open approaches including reduced overall morbidity including respiratory morbidity and length of hospital stay; however, a minimally invasive approach does not appear to influence perioperative mortality [43–45]. It is important to note that these systematic reviews and pooled analyzes are largely based on poor-quality evidence with significant heterogeneity in reported results (Table 3.3) and very limited data regarding long-term survival following MIE. Furthermore, there is significant heterogeneity in the definition of complications following esophagectomy, which is an important limitation when attempting to draw objective conclusions based upon the limited existing evidence [68].

Minimally invasive esophagectomy has also been associated with an increase in the incidence of gastric conduit failure, which may be related to methodologies for laparoscopic fashioning of the gastric conduit [69, 70]. The variability in surgical approaches and the variability in the documentation of postoperative outcomes create additional challenges to the comparison of outcomes with MIE, implementation of MIE within training programs, and the conducting of high-quality randomized controlled trials [71]. To date one randomized controlled trial has been published comparing MIE with open esophagectomy [49] and demonstrated a significantly reduced incidence of pulmonary infection in patients who underwent MIE (9 % vs. 29 %). In the same cohort of patients, the authors of this trial demonstrated the acute-phase and stress responses were better preserved in the MIE group, which may underline the fewer clinical manifestations of respiratory infections seen in the MIE group [72]. Furthermore Luketich et al. published a large series of over 1,000 minimally invasive esophagectomies with a 30-day mortality rate of 1.7 %, median length of hospital stay of 8 (6–14) days, and anastomotic leak rate of 5 % [73]. These outstanding results from this single-institution study compare favorably to any published open series. This does provide evidence to suggest that a minimally invasive approach to esophagectomy can be introduced in high-volume centers without deterioration in outcomes that was seen with the introduction of a minimally invasive approach to other complex surgical procedures including hepatectomy and pancreatectomy. The current data suggests that in accomplished high-volume centers minimally invasive esophagectomy can be performed safely and it may have some advantages with respect to pulmonary morbidity, and can produce equal oncological outcomes as reflected by lymph node yields. However, it is important to note that the average MIE results from the published literature do suggest a high level of variability in clinical outcomes associated with MIE (Table 3.3), and further large national or multi-institutional randomized controlled trials are required to document the risks, benefits, and long-term survival following MIE in comparison to open esophagectomy, before a consensus on this important issue is reached.

Table 3.3 Comparison of minimally invasive vs. open esophagectomy

Author	Patient no. (MIF/HMIE)	Patient no. (open)	Inhospital mortality (MIE/HMIE) (%)	Inhospital mortality (open) (%)	Anastomotic leak (MIE/HMIE) (%)	Anastomotic leak (open) (%)	Lymph node yield (MIE/HMIE)[a]	Lymph node yield (open)[a]
Bailey et al. [46]	39	31	5.0	6.0	NA	NA	16±1.2	17±1.4
Ben-David et al. [47]	100	32	1.0	5.0	4.0	12.5	14 (8–31)	NA
Berger et al. [48]	65	53	7.7	7.5	14.0	11.0	20	9
Biere[x] et al. [49]	53	56	3.0	2.0	12.0	7.0	20 (3–44)	21 (7–47)
Blazeby et al. [50]	124	68	1.6	3.0	NA	NA	20.5–34.7	29
Briez et al. [51]	140	140	1.4	7.1	5.7	4.3	22 (8–53)	22 (6–56)
Gao et al. [52]	96	78	NA	3.8	7.3	7.7	17.8	18.0
Hamouda et al. [53]	51	24	0	0	7.8	8.0	12 (Early Gp) 23 (Late Gp)	24
Javidfar et al. [54]	92	165	3.2	4.2	5.0	4.0	17 (IQR: 12.5–24.5)	11 (IQR: 7–16)
Kunisaki et al. [55]	92	79	NA	NA	8.7	NA	34.3	29
Lee et al. [56]	74	64	NA	NA	13.5	28.0	14.6 (HMIE) 14.0 (MIE)	18.4
Nafteux et al. [57]	65	101	3.1	2.0	7.7	9.9	12 (HGD/1a) 14 (1b)	17 (HGD/1a) 18 (1b)
Noble et al. [58]	53	53	2.0	2.0	9	4	18 (7–52)	19 (7–50)
Parameswaran et al. [59]	67	19	4.5	5.3	13.4 (GCF)	10.5 (GCF)	NA	NA
Safranek et al. [60]	75	46	4.0	2.2	14.7	2.2	14	15
Scheepers et al. [61]	50	60	NA	NA	NA	NA	14 (8–24)	10 (8–22)
Schroder et al. [62]	238	181	2.9	6.1	7.6	9.4	27	32.3
Schoppmann et al. [63]	31	31	0	0	3.2	25.8	17.9±7.8	20.5±12.6
Sihag et al. [64]	38	76	NA	NA	0	2.6	19 (15–28)	21 (16–27)
Smithers et al. [65]	332	114	2.1	2.6	5.4	8.7	17 (2–59) (HMIE) 17 (9–33) (MIE)	16 (1–44)
Yamasaki et al. [66]	109	107	0	1.9	5.5	3.7	19.3	20.8
Zingg et al. [67]	56	98	3.6	6.1	20.0	12.8	5.7	6.7

Biere[x] only randomized controlled trial included

HMIE hybrid minimally invasive esophagectomy, MIE total minimally invasive esophagectomy, NA not available, HGD high-grade dysplasia, GCF gastric conduit failure

[a]Lymph node yield given as mean/median ±range (where available)

References

1. Kohn GP, Galanako JA, Meyes MO, Feins RH, Farrell TM. National trends in esophageal surgery – are outcomes as good as we believe? J Gastrointest Surg. 2009;13(11):1900–10.
2. National Oesophago-Gastric cancer audit 2013; an audit of the care received by people with Oesophago-Gastric Cancer in England and Wales. https://catalogue.ic.nhs.uk/publications/clinical/oesophago-gastric/nati-clin-audi-supp-prog-oeso-gast-canc-2013/clin-audi-supp-prog-oeso-gast-2013-rep.pdf.
3. Ra J, Paulson EC, Kucharczuk J, et al. Postoperative mortality after esophagectomy for cancer: development of a preoperative risk prediction model. Ann Surg Oncol. 2008;15:1577–84.
4. Anderson O, Ni Z, Moller H, Coupland VH, Davies EA, Allum WH, et al. Hospital volume and survival in oesophagectomy and gastrectomy for cancer. Eur J Cancer. 2011;47:2408–14.
5. Finks JF, Osbourne NH, Birkmeyer JD. Trends in hospital volume and operative mortality for high-risk surgery. N Engl J Med. 2011;364(22):2128–37.
6. Kozower BD, Stukenborg GJ. Hospital esophageal cancer resection volume does not predict patient mortality risk. Ann Thorac Surg. 2012;93(5):1690–6.
7. LaPar DJ, Kron IL, Jones DR, Stukenborg GJ, Kozower BD. Hospital procedure volume should not be used as a measure of surgical quality. Ann Surg. 2012;256(4):606–15.
8. Markar SR, Karthikesalingam A, Thrumurthy S, Low DE. Volume-outcome relationship in surgery for esophageal malignancy: systematic review and meta-analysis 2000–2011. J Gastrointest Surg. 2012;16:1055–63.
9. Derogar M, Sadr-Azodi O, Johar A, Lagergren P, Lagergren J. Hospital and surgeon volume in relation to survival after esophageal cancer surgery in a population-based study. J Clin Oncol. 2013;31(5):551–7.
10. Wouters MW, Gooiker GA, van Sandick JW, Tollenaar RA. The volume-outcome relation in the surgical treatment of esophageal cancer: a systematic review and meta-analysis. Cancer. 2012;118(7):1754–63.
11. Rutegard M, Lagergren J, Rouvelas I, Lagergren P. Surgeon volume is a poor proxy for skill in esophageal cancer surgery. Ann Surg. 2009;249(2):256–61.
12. Yasunaga H, Matsuyama Y, Ohe K, Japan Surgical Society. Effects of hospital and surgeon case-volumes on postoperative complications and length of stay after esophagectomy in Japan. Surg Today. 2009;39(7):566–71.
13. The Leapfrog Group. Fact sheet. Available at www.leapfroggroup.org.
14. Massarweh NN, Flum DR, Symons RG, Varghese TK, Pellegrini CA. A critical evaluation of the impact of Leapfrog's evidence-based hospital referral. J Am Coll Surg. 2011;212(2):150–9.
15. Varghese Jr TK, Wood DE, Farjah F, Oelschlager BK, Symons RG, MacLeod KE, Flum DR, Pellegrini CA. Variation in esophagectomy outcomes in hospitals meeting Leapfrog volume outcome standards. Ann Thorac Surg. 2011;91(4):1003–9.
16. Coupland VH, Lagergren J, Luchtenborg M, Jack RG, Allum W, Holmberg L, Hanna GB, Pearce N, Moller H. Hospital volume, proportion resected and mortality from oesophageal and gastric cancer: a population-based study in England, 2004–2008. Gut. 2013;62(7):961–6.
17. Dikken JL, van Sandick JW, Allum WH, et al. Differences in outcomes of oesophageal and gastric cancer surgery across Europe. Br J Surg. 2013;100:83–94.
18. Lovely JK, Maxson PM, Jacob AK, Cima RR, Horlocker TT, Hebl JR, Harmesen WS, Huebner M, Larson DW. Case-matched series of enhanced versus standard recovery pathway in minimally invasive colorectal surgery. Br J Surg. 2012;99:120–6.
19. Munitiz V, Martinez-de-Haro LF, Ortiz A, Ruiz-de-Angulo D, Pastor P, Parrilla P. Effectiveness of a written clinical pathway for enhanced recovery after transthoracic (Ivor Lewis) oesophagectomy. Br J Surg. 2010;97:714–8.
20. Cerfolio RJ, Bryant AS, Bass CS, Alexander JR, Bartolucci AA. Fast tracking after Ivor Lewis esophagogastrectomy. Chest. 2004;126:1187–94.
21. Gustafsson UO, Scott MJ, Schwenk W, Demartines N, Roulin D, Francis N, McNaught CE, Macfie J, Liberman AS, Soop M, et al. Guidelines for perioperative care in elective colonic surgery: Enhanced Recovery After Surgery (ERAS((R))) Society recommendations. World J Surg. 2013;37(2):259–84.
22. Aarts MA, Okrainec A, Glicksman A, Pearsall E, Victor JC, McLeod RS. Adoption of enhanced recovery after surgery (ERAS) strategies for colorectal surgery at academic teaching hospitals and impact on total length of hospital stay. Surg Endosc. 2012;26(2):442–50.
23. Rotter T, Kinsman L, James E, Machotta A, Gothe H, Willis J, Snow P, Kugler J. Clinical pathways: effects on professional practice, patient outcomes, length of stay and hospital costs. Cochrane Database Syst Rev. 2010;(3):CD006632.
24. Zehr KJ, Dawson PB, Yang SC, Heitmiller RF. Standardized clinical care pathways for major thoracic cases reduce hospital costs. Ann Thorac Surg. 1998;66(3):914–9.
25. Low DE, Kunz S, Schembre D, Otero H, Malpass T, His A, Song G, Hinke R, Kozarek RA. Esophagectomy – it's not just about mortality anymore: standardize perioperative clinical pathways improve outcomes in patients with esophageal cancer. J Gastrointest Surg. 2007;11:1395–402.
26. Jiang K, Cheng L, Wang JJ, Li JS, Nie J. Fast track clinical pathway implications in esophagogastrectomy. World J Gastroenterol. 2009;15:496–501.
27. Tomaszek SC, Cassivi SD, Allen MS, Shen KR, Nichols 3rd FC, Deschamps C, Wigle DA. An alternative postoperative pathway reduces length of hospitalisation following oesophagectomy. Eur J Cardiothorac Surg. 2010;37:807–13.
28. Preston SR, Markar SR, Baker CR, Soon Y, Singh S, Low DE. Impact of a multidisciplinary standardized

clinical pathway on perioperative outcomes in patients with oesophageal cancer. Br J Surg. 2013;100:105–12.

29. Li C, Ferri LE, Mulder DS, Ncuti A, Neville A, Lee L, Kaneva P, Watson D, Vassiliou M, Carli F, Feldman LS. An enhanced recovery pathway decreases duration of stay after esophagectomy. Surgery. 2012;152:606–14.

30. Tang J, Humes DJ, Gemmil E, Welch NT, Parsons SL, Catton JA. Reduction in length of stay for patients undergoing oesophageal and gastric resections with implementation of enhanced recovery packages. Ann R Coll Surg Engl. 2013;95:323–8.

31. Blom RL, van Heijl M, Bemelman WA, Hollmann MW, Klinkenbijl JH, Busch OR, van Berge Henegouwen MI. Initial experiences of an enhanced recovery protocol in esophageal surgery. World J Surg. 2013;37:2372–8.

32. van Hagen P, Hulshof MC, van Lanschot JJ, et al. Preoperative chemoradiotherapy for esophageal or junctional cancer. N Engl J Med. 2012;366:2074–84.

33. Sjoquist KM, Burmeister BH, Smithers BM, Zalcberg JR, Simes RJ, Barbour A, et al. Survival after neoadjuvant chemotherapy or chemoradiotherapy for resectable oesophageal carcinoma: an updated meta-analysis. Lancet Oncol. 2011;12:681–92.

34. Courrech Staal EFW, Aleman BMP, Boot H, van Velthuysen MLF, van Tinteren H, van Sandick JW. Systematic review of the benefits and risks of neoadjuvant chemoradiation for oesophageal cancer. Br J Surg. 2010;97:1482–96.

35. Tessier W, Piessen G, Briez N, et al. Percutaneous radiological gastrostomy in esophageal cancer patients: a feasible and safe access for nutritional support during multimodal therapy. Surg Endosc. 2013;27:633–41.

36. Moskovitz AH, Rizk NP, Venkatraman E, et al. Mortality increases for octogenarians undergoing esophagogastrectomy for esophageal cancer. Ann Thorac Surg. 2006;82:2031–6.

37. Markar SR, Low DE. Physiology not chronology, dictates outcomes after esophagectomy for esophageal cancer: outcomes in patients 80 years and older. Ann Surg Oncol. 2013;20:1020–6.

38. Markar SR, Schmidt H, Kunz S, Bodnar A, Hubka M, Low DE. Evolution of standardized clinical pathways: refining multidisciplinary care and process to improve outcomes of the surgical treatment of esophageal cancer. J Gastrointest Surg. 2014;18(7):1238–46.

39. Grailey K, Markar SR, Karthikesalingam A, Aboud R, Ziprin P, Faiz O. Laparoscopic versus open colorectal resection in the elderly population. Surg Endosc. 2013;27:19–30.

40. Venkat R, Edil BH, Schulick RD, Lidor AO, Makary MA, Wolfgang CL. Laparoscopic distal pancreatectomy is associated with significantly less overall morbidity compared to the open technique: a systematic review and meta-analysis. Ann Surg. 2012;255:1048–59.

41. Fancellu A, Rosman AS, Sanna V, Nigri GR, Zorcolo L, Pisano M, Melis M. Meta-analysis of trials comparing minimally-invasive and open liver resections for hepatocellular carcinomas. J Surg Res. 2011;171:e33–45.

42. Mamidanna R, Bottle A, Aylin P, et al. Short-term outcomes following open versus minimally invasive esophagectomy for cancer in England: a population-based national study. Ann Surg. 2012;255:197–203.

43. Butler N, Collins S, Memon B, et al. Minimally invasive oesophagectomy: current status and future direction. Surg Endosc. 2011;25:2071–83.

44. Sgourakis G, Gockel I, Radtke A, et al. Minimally invasive versus open esophagectomy: meta-analysis of outcomes. Dig Dis Sci. 2010;55:3031–40.

45. Nagpal K, Ahmed K, Vats A, et al. Is minimally invasive surgery beneficial in the management of esophageal cancer? A meta-analysis. Surg Endosc. 2010;24:1621–9.

46. Bailey L, Khan I, Willows E, et al. Open and laparoscopically assisted oesophagectomy: a prospective comparative study. Eur J Cardiothorac Surg. 2013;43:268–73.

47. Ben-David K, Sarosi GA, Cendan JC, et al. Decreasing morbidity and mortality in 100 consecutive minimally invasive esophagectomies. Surg Endosc. 2012;26:162–7.

48. Berger AC, Bloomenthal A, Weksler B, et al. Oncologic efficacy is not compromised, and may be improved with minimally invasive esophagectomy. J Am Coll Surg. 2011;212:560–6.

49. Biere SS, van Berge Henegouwen MI, Maas KW, et al. Minimally invasive versus open oesophagectomy for patients with oesophageal cancer: a multicentre, open-label, randomised controlled trial. Lancet. 2012;379:1887–92.

50. Blazeby JM, Blencowe NS, Titcomb DR, et al. Demonstration of the IDEAL recommendations for evaluating and reporting surgical innovation in minimally invasive oesophagectomy. Br J Surg. 2011;98:544–51.

51. Briez N, Piessen G, Torres F, et al. Effects of hybrid minimally invasive oesophagectomy on major postoperative pulmonary complications. Br J Surg. 2012;99:1547–53.

52. Gao Y, Wang Y, Chen L, et al. Comparison of open three-field and minimally-invasive esophagectomy for esophageal cancer. Interact Cardiovasc Thorac Surg. 2011;12:366–9.

53. Hamouda AH, Forshaw MJ, Tsigritis K, et al. Perioperative outcomes after transition from conventional to minimally invasive Ivor-Lewis esophagectomy in a specialized center. Surg Endosc. 2010;24:865–9.

54. Javidfar J, Bacchetta M, Yang JA, et al. The use of a tailored surgical technique for minimally invasive esophagectomy. J Thorac Cardiovasc Surg. 2012;143:1125–9.

55. Kunisaki C, Kosaka T, Ono HA, et al. Significance of thoracoscopy-assisted surgery with a minithoracotomy and hand-assisted laparoscopic surgery for esophageal cancer: the experience of a single surgeon. J Gastrointest Surg. 2011;15:1939–51.

56. Lee JM, Cheng JW, Lin MT, et al. Is there any benefit to incorporating a laparoscopic procedure into minimally invasive esophagectomy? The impact on perioperative results in patients with esophageal cancer. World J Surg. 2011;35:790–7.

57. Nafteux P, Moons J, Coosemans W, et al. Minimally invasive oesophagectomy: a valuable alternative to

open oesophagectomy for the treatment of early oesophageal and gastro-oesophageal junction carcinoma. Eur J Cardiothorac Surg. 2011;40:1455–63.

58. Noble F, Kelly JJ, Bailey IS, et al. A prospective comparison of totally minimally invasive versus open Ivor Lewis esophagectomy. Dis Esophagus. 2013;26: 263–71.

59. Parameswaran R, Titcomb DR, Blencowe NS, et al. Assessment and comparison of recovery after open and minimally invasive esophagectomy for cancer: an exploratory study in two centers. Ann Surg Oncol. 2013;20:1970–7.

60. Safranek PM, Cubitt J, Booth MI, et al. Review of open and minimal access approaches to oesophagectomy for cancer. Br J Surg. 2010;97:1845–53.

61. Scheepers JJ, van der Peet DL, Veenhof AA, et al. Influence of circumferential resection margin on prognosis in distal esophageal and gastroesophageal cancer approached through the transhiatal route. Dis Esophagus. 2009;22:42–8.

62. Schroder W, Holscher AH, Bludau M, et al. Ivor-Lewis esophagectomy with and without laparoscopic conditioning of the gastric conduit. World J Surg. 2010;34:738–43.

63. Schoppmann SF, Prager G, Langer F, et al. Fifty-five minimally invasive Esophagectomies: a single centre experience. Anticancer Res. 2009;29:2719–25.

64. Sihag S, Wright CD, Wain JC, et al. Comparison of perioperative outcomes following open versus minimally invasive Ivor Lewis oesophagectomy at a single, high-volume centre. Eur J Cardiothorac Surg. 2012; 42:430–7.

65. Smithers BM, Gotley DC, Martin I, et al. Comparison of the outcomes between open and minimally invasive esophagectomy. Ann Surg. 2007;245:232–40.

66. Yamasaki M, Miyata H, Fujiwara Y, et al. Minimally invasive esophagectomy for esophageal cancer: comparative analysis of open and hand-assisted laparoscopic abdominal lymphadenectomy with gastric conduit reconstruction. J Surg Oncol. 2011;104:623–8.

67. Zingg U, McQuinn A, DiValentino D, et al. Minimally invasive versus open esophagectomy for patients with esophageal cancer. Ann Thorac Surg. 2009;87:911–9.

68. Blencowe NS, Strong S, McNair AG, Brookes ST, Crosby T, Griffin SM, Blazeby JM. Reporting of short-term clinical outcomes after esophagectomy: a systematic review. Ann Surg. 2012;255:658–66.

69. Wajed SA, Veeramootoo D, Shore AC. Surgical optimization of the gastric conduit for minimally invasive oesophagectomy. Surg Endosc. 2012;26:271–6.

70. Nguyen NT, Nguyen XT, Reavis KM, et al. Minimally invasive esophagectomy with and without gastric ischemic conditioning. Surg Endosc. 2012;26:1637–41.

71. Hanna GB, Arya S, Markar S. Variation in the standard of minimally invasive esophagectomy for cancer – systematic review. Semin Thorac Cardiovasc Surg. 2012;24:176–87.

72. Maas KW, Biere SS, van Hoogstraten IM, et al. Immunological changes after minimally invasive or conventional esophageal resection for cancer: a randomized trial. World J Surg. 2014;38(1):131–7.

73. Luketich JD, Pennathur A, Awais O, et al. Outcomes after minimally invasive esophagectomy: review of over 1000 patients. Ann Surg. 2012;256:95–103.

Goals of Surgical Therapy for Esophageal Cancer

A. Koen Talsma, J. Shapiro, Bas P.L. Wijnhoven, and J. Jan B. Van Lanschot

Introduction

Operative resection of esophageal cancer is probably one of the most challenging procedures in surgery. Partly this is because it encompasses two or even three body compartments: chest and abdomen with or without neck. Moreover, its position immediately adjacent to vital structures (trachea, bronchi, aorta, and heart) warrants a careful dissection. With the recent introduction of minimally invasive esophagectomy, the operation has become technically even more demanding. This chapter describes the surgeon's main goals when performing a potentially curative esophagectomy for esophageal cancer, regardless of the surgical approach that is chosen. The various indicators that have been identified to promote oncological control in open surgery will be discussed as well as the tools that help to prevent complications.

In fact, these same goals have to be set for minimally invasive esophagectomy.

A.K. Talsma, MD, MSc (✉) • J. Shapiro, MD
B.P.L. Wijnhoven, MD, PhD
J.J.B. Van Lanschot, MD, PhD
Department of Surgery, Erasmus Medical Center,
15 Gravendykwal 230, Suite H-812,
Rotterdam, 2040, 3000 CA, The Netherlands
e-mail: koentalsma@hotmail.com

Pretreatment Work-Up and Staging

Multidisciplinary Approach

In patients with esophageal cancer, a great variety of treatment options are available. For proper medical decision making, accurate pretreatment staging is of crucial importance. Early (mucosal) lesions, for example, can be cured with endoscopic mucosal resection, thus avoiding conventional surgery. At the other end of the clinical spectrum, accurate pretreatment staging is also essential to avoid futile attempts at radical treatment for patients that are in fact incurable due to distant metastases and to guide effective palliation that can be achieved with endoscopic stenting or intraluminal brachytherapy. Discussion of all patients with esophageal malignancies in a multidisciplinary tumor board is recommended because it is associated with improved outcomes after surgery [1, 2]. In a considerable number of patients, the diagnostic work-up or treatment plan is altered after careful evaluation in a multidisciplinary tumor board [3]. Adenocarcinomas arising at the esophagogastric junction can pose a specific problem for guiding the choice between neoadjuvant chemo- versus chemoradiotherapy and between subtotal esophagectomy versus extended gastrectomy. At present, Siewert type I and II tumors are treated as esophageal cancers while type III tumors are generally treated as gastric cancers.

Patient Selection: Does the General Condition of the Patient Allow for Extensive Surgery?

The pretreatment assessment should not only focus on tumor staging but also on optimization of the patient's general condition. The success of a specific treatment modality does not only depend on the tumor stage but also on the fitness of the patient. Surgery for esophageal and junctional cancer has a high risk of postoperative (especially pulmonary) complications. Several risk scoring systems have been developed as predictors of poor postoperative outcome. These scoring systems can be used for the individual patient to guide treatment choice. Moreover, these scoring systems can be used to correct for case-mix differences when comparing performance between hospitals. The prognostic value of the available models however is generally limited. Worldwide, the most widely used and most simple classification is that of the American Society of Anesthesiologists [4] but has been criticized for being subjective. The POSSUM [5] and Charlson score [6] are more comprehensive but are also more cumbersome to calculate [7]. Several series have shown that POSSUM and esophageal(O)-POSSUM [8] overestimate post-operative mortality in gastroesophageal cancer patients [9–11]. The Portsmouth(P)-POSSUM showed less overestimation and may be the most useful predictor of likely postoperative mortality in these types of patients [12]. Older age (e.g., >80 years) per se is not a contraindication for upper GI surgery, but older patients have increased postoperative mortality and decreased long-term survival after esophageal resection for cancer [13, 14]. Substantial weight loss before surgery was also a negative prognostic factor in several studies [15, 16].

Tumor Selection: Can the Tumor Be Radically Resected and Potentially Cured?

Over the past decades, long-term survival results have substantially improved. Besides centralization of surgical procedures, early cancer detection, and use of neoadjuvant therapy, improved patient and tumor selection based on novel staging modalities accounts for this improvement [17, 18].

Guidelines for pretreatment staging of patients with esophageal and junctional cancer recommend a number of investigations, including endoscopy with biopsy; endoscopic ultrasonography (EUS); computed tomography (CT) of neck, chest, and abdomen; and external ultrasonography (US) of the neck with fine-needle aspiration (FNA) of suspected lymph nodes. In addition, positron emission tomography (PET) can also be a useful staging modality, albeit not yet mandatory in, e.g., Dutch, UK, and US guidelines. In case of an advanced tumor above the carina, bronchoscopy is advised to confirm or exclude invasion of the tracheobronchial tree. Clinical and histopathological staging is generally based on the tumor/node/metastasis (TNM) classification developed by the Union Internationale Contre le Cancer (UICC) and the American Joint Committee on Cancer (AJCC) [19]. The most important change in the latest (7th) edition is that the concept of non-regional lymph nodes has been abandoned and that staging of tumors in the esophagus, at the esophagogastric junction, and in the stomach has been harmonized. The number of positive lymph nodes is now more important than their location.

EUS

EUS is superior to any current diagnostic modality for imaging of the primary tumor and its immediate surroundings (T- and N-stage) due to its ability to identify the component layers of the esophageal wall [20, 21]. The main problem with EUS is failure to pass in 1 out of 5 patients [22]. FNA of suspected nodes is only indicated when the results will change the treatment plan (e.g., radiation field). EUS can identify metastatic lymph nodes at the celiac trunk but is not accurate in detecting distant metastases, with the exception of hematogenous metastases in the left liver lobe and left adrenal gland. FNA of the celiac nodes is technically feasible in 95 % of patients [23].

CT and External US

Spiral CT and external US are used for the detection of distant hematogenous and lymphatic metastases (M-stage). Probably, PET scanning can replace US of the neck, although it is generally recommended to confirm suspected lymph nodes by US-FNA to exclude false positivity of the PET scan (e.g., due to sarcoidosis) [24]. The ability to accurately predict locoregional resectability is especially important before embarking upon a thoracoscopic or laparoscopic surgical approach to minimize the risk of accidental damage. For this purpose, CT continues to play an important role. Invasion into adjacent organs is unlikely when a periesophageal fat plane can be recognized, but when absent, it cannot be taken as absolute evidence of invasion. This accounts for the overestimation of tumor invasion into trachea, aorta, and pericardium.

PET

PET is a noninvasive imaging technique which is increasingly used in the staging of various tumor types, including esophageal cancer [25, 26]. The increased glucose metabolism of malignant cells is the driving force for the uptake of fluorine-18-fluorodeoxyglucose (FDG), which is the most common radiotracer used for oncological PET studies. In addition to qualitative staging (esp. detection of distant metastases), PET is able to quantify FDG uptake in malignant tissue by calculating the standardized uptake value (SUV) of the primary tumor. After extensive "conventional" diagnostic work-up, additional PET scanning yields a diagnosis of distant dissemination in an additional 10 % of patients, especially in case of T3 tumors [27]. The simultaneous, combined PET and CT scan is able to localize and classify hotspots more accurately than PEt alone.

Intraoperative Staging by Laparoscopy and Sentinel Node Biopsy

Although inconsistently applied, a systematic review has recommended the use of staging laparoscopy in junctional cancer patients [28], especially for demonstrating low-volume peritoneal disease.

The value of sentinel node (SN) sampling in esophageal cancer is less clear than for, e.g., breast cancer and malignant melanoma. In a British study, 96 % of SN biopsies accurately detected lymph node metastatic disease [29]. In another study, however, so-called skip lesions were identified in 55 % of resected two-field lymphadenectomy specimens [30–32]. Currently, a multicenter trial in Japan is being performed, in which the extent of lymph node dissection during gastric surgery is tailored depending on the SN biopsy [33].

Restaging

After completion of neoadjuvant therapy, patients can be restaged to evaluate response to treatment and to detect any progression of disease before proceeding to surgery. The assessment of nodal disease following chemoradiotherapy by EUS and CT is disappointing because viable tumor cannot be readily distinguished from fibrotic tissue [32, 34]. Studies with PET especially when measuring SUV before and after chemotherapy have been encouraging [35, 36]. Unfortunately, tumor response assessment by PET after neoadjuvant chemoradiotherapy is hampered by radiation-induced inflammation.

Future Developments

Recently, more research has focused on staging techniques that address the biological behavior of tumors which is important in the response to chemoradiotherapy and likelihood of recurrence. This can be achieved by PET scanning with novel radiotracers such as (18)F FLT 3-deoxy-3-fluorothymidine or (11)C-choline [37, 38]. Other studies focus on MRI as a potential noninvasive technique for locoregional staging of esophageal cancer [39]. Encouraging results have been achieved in the rapidly improving technology of in vivo intraoperative imaging as well [40].

Definitive Chemoradiotherapy: An Alternative for Potentially Curative Resection?

In recent years two randomized controlled trials compared definitive chemoradiotherapy (dCRT) to neoadjuvant chemoradiotherapy plus surgery (nCRT + S). Both studies employed a non-inferiority design to test the chance that patients in both treatment paradigms have a significantly different survival.

The first study by Stahl et al. [41] included 172 patients between 1994 and 2002 from 11 German centers. It compared dCRT (without salvage surgery) with nCRT+S for "locally advanced" (i.e., T3–4, N0-1, M0) esophageal squamous cell carcinomas. Two-year survival was 35.4 and 39.9 % in the dCRT arm and nCRT+S arm, respectively (P=0.007). Freedom from local progression was worse in the dCRT arm (40.7 % vs. 64.3 %, respectively; HR 2.1 P=.003). A significant difference was found in treatment-related mortality: 3.5 % in the dCRT arm and 12.8 % in the nCRT+S arm (χ^2, P=.03). In summary, there was no difference in overall survival; however, local failure was more common, and treatment-related death was less common in the dCRT arm.

The second randomized controlled trial (FFCD 9102) [42] compared dCRT to nCRT+S in patients who had an objective clinical response or an improvement of dysphagia after neoadjuvant chemoradiotherapy (259/444, 58.3 %). Two-year survival rates for the dCRT arm and nCRT+S arm were 39.8 and 33.6 %, respectively (P=0.03, i.e., the chance that the actual difference is >10 %). Three-month mortality (0.8 % vs. 9.3 %, P=0.003) favored the dCRT arm, whereas locoregional relapse (43.0 % vs. 33.6 %, HR 1.63, P=0.03) favored the nCRT+S arm.

Both studies suffered from major drawbacks (e.g., inadequate power and lack of standardized chemoradiotherapy protocols), thus precluding more general conclusions from these data. This ambiguity towards dCRT is reflected in clinical practice where in most countries dCRT is reserved only for those patients who are deemed unfit for surgery.

Surgical Performance Indicators: On Which Parameters Should MIE Be Judged?

Resection Margins

The main goal in the surgical treatment for esophageal cancer is the complete removal of the primary tumor and affected lymph nodes. As esophageal cancer easily spreads longitudinally via the submucosal lymphatics, the incidence of intramucosal and submucosal metastases is reportedly high (Fig. 4.1a, b). The completeness of resection of the primary tumor and its intramural metastases can be described with respect to the proximal, distal, and circumferential resection margin and is a well-known determinant of long-term survival in several studies [43–46]. Previous studies have investigated the required length of macroscopic proximal and distal resection margins in order to minimize anastomotic recurrence. A reasonable margin is 10 cm for larger tumors and 4 cm for more localized tumors [47]. When only a short proximal resection margin can be obtained through the thoracic exposure (especially for a squamous cell carcinoma), a cervical extension with subtotal esophagectomy is advisable. An adenocarcinoma of the lower esophagus requires an extensive sleeve resection of the lesser curve and fundus to minimize positive distal resection margins.

An esophageal resection can be suboptimal due because of an involved circumferential margin. The definition of circumferential resection margin (CRM) involvement remains controversial. The College of American Pathologists (CAP) and the Royal College of Pathologists (RCP) use different definitions for CRM involvement. Microscopic tumor involvement (R1 resection) is defined by CAP as tumor found at the cut circumferential resection margin, while it is defined by RCP as any tumor within 1 mm of the circumferential resection plane. Recently, a systematic review was published of 14 studies involving 2,433 patients. Rates of CRM involvement were 15.3 and 36.5 % according to the CAP and RCP criteria, respectively. It was shown that CRM involvement is an important predictor of poor prognosis and that the CAP criteria had a greater (negative) prognostic power than the RCP criteria [48]. It can be difficult and time-consuming to identify a positive circumferential resection margin in a large T3 tumor, and it has been suggested that this should preferably be done in accordance with the CAP criteria (tumor is found at the inked lateral margin of resection) [49]. There has been a significant decrease in

Fig. 4.1 (a) The lymphatics of the esophagus are distributed in the form of a submucosal and a paraesophageal plexus that can both drain directly into the periesophageal lymph nodes. (b) Longitudinal spread of tumor to involve submucosal lymphatic plexus (From Elsevier; Raja et al. [116] with permission)

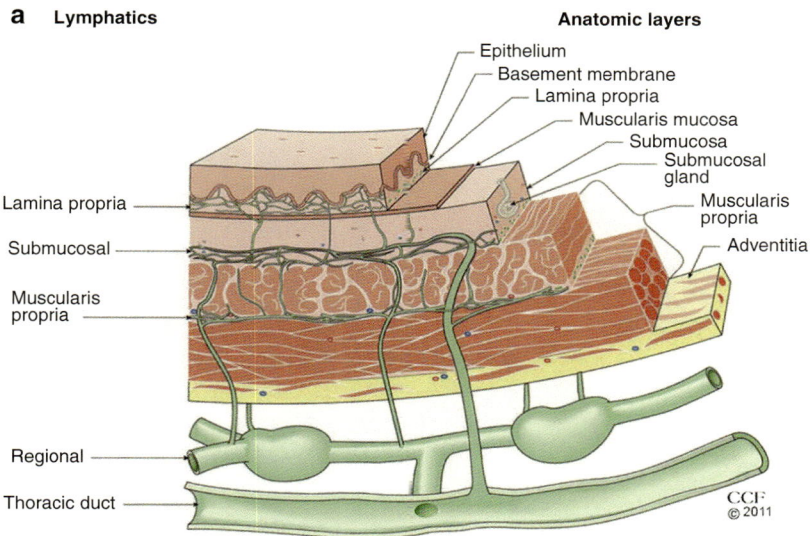

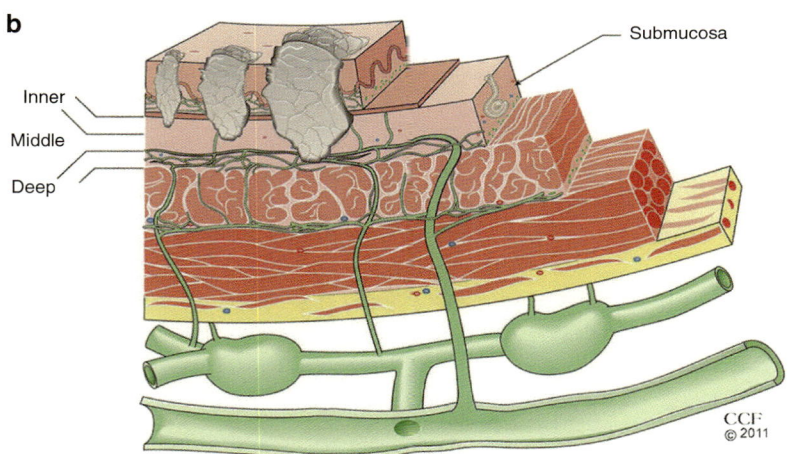

CRM involvement especially with the introduction of neoadjuvant chemoradiotherapy [17, 50]. After neoadjuvant chemotherapy CRM involvement still has prognostic importance [51].

Lymphadenectomy

As esophageal cancer readily spreads longitudinally in the submucosal lymphatics, early dissemination to lymph nodes in the chest and abdomen may be involved in cancer of all parts of the esophagus. And even skip metastases, defined as positive distant lymph nodes

in combination with negative regional lymph nodes, are encountered relatively frequently [52]. Lymphatic dissemination occurs not only in a chaotic pattern but also at an early stage. Some 30 % of the T1b tumors (with infiltration limited to the submucosa) already have positive lymph nodes involved [53]. Ideally, a complete resection of all locoregional nodes draining the esophagus should include the two or three fields (see above) in addition to the easily accessible periesophageal and perigastric lymph nodes (Fig. 4.2). In a survey among surgeons around the world, the technically challenging three-field lymphadenectomy was performed

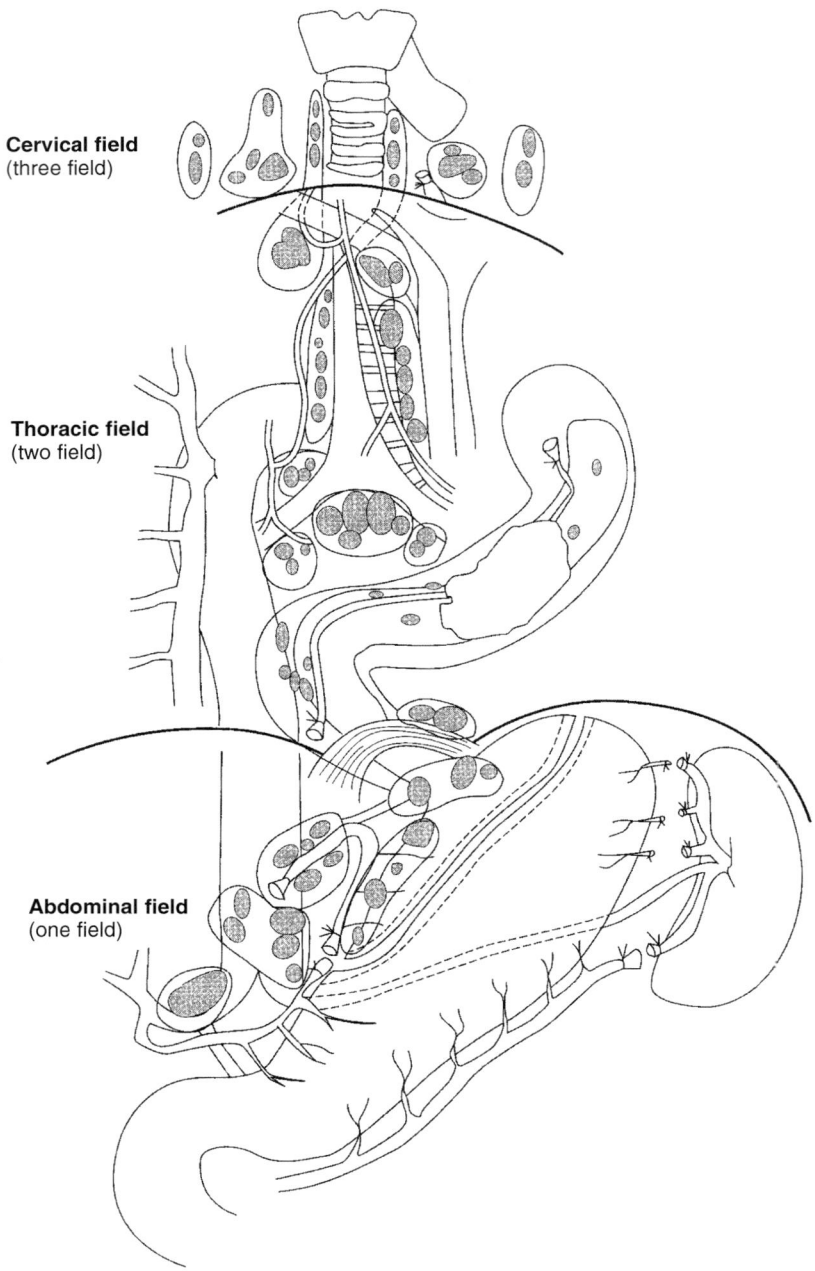

Fig. 4.2 Extent of resection and fields of lymph node dissection routinely carried out for cancer of the esophagus (From Griffin and Raimes [117] with permission)

Cervical field (three field)

Thoracic field (two field)

Abdominal field (one field)

routinely by only 12 % of the responders [54]. A SEER analysis showed that the median number of total lymph nodes resected in over 5,600 esophagectomies was only eight nodes [55]. Lymphadenectomy can be performed safely during minimally invasive surgery, and it has been shown that minimally invasive and robotic esophagectomy have similar lymph node retrieval compared to open techniques [56–58].

For staging purposes it is clear that an extended lymphadenectomy is superior to a limited dissection. It has, therefore, been suggested by the 7th edition of the TNM staging system that for staging purposes, the total number of resected and identified lymph nodes should be at least 15 nodes. The therapeutic impact of an extended lymphadenectomy is still a matter of debate in esophageal cancer surgery [59]. Some authors state that surgery has reached its limit, while others believe that the course of the disease can be influenced positively by aggressive surgery with an extended lymphadenectomy. One of the hypotheses supporting the benefits of extended lymphadenectomy is the clearance of micrometastases that can be present in up to 50 % of histology-negative nodes. This hypothesis is supported by the correlation of micrometastases in routine lymph node-negative patients with a poor outcome [60, 61].

More skeptical authors believe that the therapeutic impact of an increased lymph node harvest per se is limited and it is probably not the type of operation performed that makes a difference but rather the stage of the disease at the time of operation [56]. According to this view, lymph node metastases are markers of systemic disease and removal of the primary lesion alone will yield the same survival [62]. The spurious effect of extended lymphadenectomy might then be caused by stage migration which occurs if positive nodes in the extended field change N-stage. This results in the so-called Will Rogers phenomenon or stage purification and leads to unreliable stage-by-stage comparisons of survival. For that reason some authors prefer to use the lymph node ratio (i.e., the number of positive nodes over the number of removed nodes) rather than the absolute number of positive nodes [63, 64].

Several prospective trials have been performed comparing survival after esophagectomy with or without extended lymphadenectomy. In the largest RCT (HIVEX trial), comparing limited transhiatal esophagectomy and extended transthoracic esophagectomy with two-field lymphadenectomy, 5-year survival was not significantly different [65, 66]. The survival benefit of an extended lymphadenectomy by a transthoracic approach was limited to a subgroup of patients with low burden of nodal disease (1–8 nodes positive on pathological examination of the resection specimen). The identification of this group makes the pretreatment staging very challenging. Unfortunately, unlike in

breast cancer, the sentinel node concept has not become popular in esophageal surgery [29, 31]. Several studies have confirmed the higher morbidity after thoracotomy than after transhiatal approach: more pulmonary complications, more recurrent nerve injuries, and higher early mortality [67–69].

Meta-analysis of the available literature data did not show differences in survival between transhiatal and transthoracic operations. Other studies compared fields of dissection, for example, the single-center studies by Lerut et al. [70] and Altorki et al. [71] that suggested a potential survival benefit for three-field lymphadenectomy.

Finally, there are studies that investigated the absolute number of nodes dissected. This has led to different recommendations regarding the optimal extent of lymphadenectomy ranging from 16 to 30 nodes. In a population of 4,627 patients in the Worldwide Esophageal Cancer Collaboration (WECC), extent of lymphadenectomy was not associated with increased survival for patients with extremes of esophageal cancer (TisN0M0 and 7 or more nodes positive) and those with well-differentiated pN0 cancer [72]. For all other cancers, 5-year survival improved with increasing extent of lymphadenectomy. Based on these WECC data, a stage-dependent extent of lymphadenectomy was recommended. This is comparable to the findings of the HIVEX trial that showed a better survival after a transthoracic approach in the subgroup of patients with 1–8 nodes positive [66]. Rizk et al. identified 18 nodes resected as the minimum necessary for accurate staging and for eliminating an effect of lymphadenectomy on survival [73]. In the study by Altorki et al., effect of lymphadenectomy on survival was lost after 25 nodes for early stage and after 16 nodes in stage III and IV cancers [71]. Peyre et al. investigated an international database of 2,303 esophagectomies in which survival was maximized with 23 nodes resected [74].

Nowadays, multimodality treatment of esophageal cancer has been widely accepted. As neoadjuvant chemoradiotherapy (CRT) is known to "sterilize" nodes, it is unclear whether the recommendations for number of lymph nodes from the surgery-alone era still stand. Extended lymphadenectomy seems to be beneficial, particularly in patients who are not downstaged regarding pathological tumor depth (ypT) and those with persistent nodal metastases (ypN+) [75, 76]. The effect of lymphadenectomy is influenced by tumor response after CRT, and the survival benefit is stronger in patients without a complete pathological response (non-pCR) compared to those with pCR [77].

Morbidity: Prevention of Complications

The typical esophageal cancer patient suffers from several comorbidities including obesity (especially in adenocarcinoma) and cardiopulmonary diseases (in both squamous and adenocarcinoma) that put the patient at increased risk for postoperative complications. Serious intraoperative and postoperative complications can occur with minimally invasive as well as open techniques, also depending on the need of a thoracic phase of the operation. Overall, complication rates are reported in over 50 % of esophagectomy series, with incidence varying between 17 and 74 % [78, 79]. Postoperative complications have been directly linked to a variety of other outcome parameters including mortality, readmission rate, early cancer recurrence, survival, length of hospital stay, costs and resource utilization, and quality of life [80–83]. The most important issues in the management of perioperative complications are prevention and early detection. However, a clear understanding of the relationships between complications, their recognition, management, and how they influence subsequent mortality is hampered by the lack of standardized definitions [84, 85]. Finally, early detection and proper management of postoperative complications is of crucial importance. It has been shown repeatedly that the so-called failure to rescue largely explains the difference in mortality rates between low-volume and high-volume hospitals for complicated surgery including esophagectomy [86].

The exact role for minimally invasive techniques is still not fully clear. The increased magnification offered by thoracoscopy might decrease complications, but lack of tactile control is probably a contributory factor to the increase of intraoperative injuries. It is unlikely that minimally invasive methods will reduce mortality rates since in experienced centers death after open esophagectomy is already a rare event. Minimally invasive esophagectomy (MIE) might be proven superior for other endpoints such as blood loss, duration of ICU or hospital stay, need for analgesics, and pulmonary function. The best available evidence comes from a recently published RCT (TIME trial) showing that MIE is accompanied by less pulmonary complications [87]. This trial has been criticized because of the lack of a clear definition of "pulmonary complications" as the primary endpoint [88]. Moreover, an unexplained increase of recurrent nerve injuries was present in the open group.

Respiratory Complications
Respiratory failure is a major problem after esophagectomy. Several studies have reported that about half of the inhospital deaths after esophagectomy is due to pneumonia, which is the most frequent general complication after surgery [89]. Preventive measures include preoperative respiratory training, cessation of smoking, and continuous postoperative pain control by epidural analgesia in order to avoid restrictive respiration and insufficient coughing. Micro-aspiration as a consequence of impaired swallowing coordination because of a cervical anastomosis also plays a role in the pathophysiology of bronchopneumonias. Another reason for postoperative respiratory impairment is a large pleural effusion, which should be drained if provoking extended atelectasis. Avoiding the need for a combined thoracotomy and laparotomy may potentially reduce postoperative pain, ventilator dependence, and cardiopulmonary complications [90]. In a study comparing thoracoscopic resection with a historical cohort, the overall incidence of pulmonary complications was reduced from 33 to 20 % [91]. Probably cardiopulmonary complications do not depend on the incision size only. The benefit of smaller port sites that are needed during minimally invasive surgery may be offset by the

lengthened time of operation and single-lung ventilation. The use of a prone position also plays a role but will be discussed elsewhere.

Recurrent Laryngeal Nerve Injury

More recurrent laryngeal nerve injuries when using thoracoscopy have been reported, which might be attributed to the use of diathermia. Others claim that the use of minimally invasive techniques has lowered the incidence of hoarseness because of the magnified view [87].

Anastomotic Leakage

Lack of standardization of definitions is a problem when reporting on complications. In a recent meta-analysis, anastomotic leakage was reported in most of the publications, but it was defined in only a minority with 22 differing definitions [84]. Early disruption of the esophagogastric anastomosis is the result of a technical problem and immediate reexploration is frequently indicated for correction. Many different suturing and (semi-)mechanical techniques have been described. The semimechanical side-by-side technique claims a lower leakage rate compared to a hand-sewn anastomosis, but has not been tested in a randomized trial [92, 93]. Leakage is more frequent in the neck than in the chest, but the associated mortality might be lower, especially after a transhiatal approach [94]. If a transmural necrosis of the gastric conduit is suspected, this can be diagnosed by endoscopy and when present is also an indication for surgery with formation of a cervical esophagostomy, resection of the gastric tube, and placement of a feeding jejunostomy. After rehabilitation of the patient, a colonic interposition can be performed at a secondary stage. Late disruptions become manifest generally between postoperative day 5 and 10 and are most frequently due to ischemia. They can be managed nonoperatively in most cases with aggressive drainage using radiologically guided drains or endoluminal vacuum therapy [95]. Self-expandable stents can be inserted in these situations but can have the disadvantage of migration or further necrosis due to tissue compression ultimately leading to, e.g., neoesophago-tracheal fistula formation.

Chylothorax

The incidence of accidental thoracic duct leakage can be diminished by intraoperative identification and ligation of the duct. Reported incidence of chylothorax varies between 3 and 10 % and is seen more often in patients who undergo transthoracic esophagectomy and in patients who have more positive nodes. Patients with chyle leakage have more pulmonary complications. Conservative therapy (initial parenteral feeding and subsequent enteral diet with medium-chain triglycerides (MCT)) is often successful, but operative therapy should be seriously considered in patients with a persistently high daily output of more than 2 L after 2 days of optimal conservative therapy [96].

Cardiac Arrhythmias

Cardiac arrhythmias are not uncommon in the postoperative phase. Atrial fibrillation (AF) is seen in 15–20 % of patients and requires further investigation because it can be an early manifestation of, e.g., mediastinitis due to intrathoracic anastomotic leakage. AF can also be associated with hypervolemia, preexistent pulmonary or cardiac disease, and dilation of the gastric conduit.

Mortality and Quality Control

Definitions

There is an increasing interest in comparing institutional performance. For surgical procedures postoperative mortality rate is generally used, because it is a relatively objective measure and reflects the summation of the most severe postoperative complications. Currently it is unclear which definition of postoperative mortality best reflects surgical quality of care. The 30-day operative mortality (30DM) and the inhospital mortality (IHM) after esophageal resection are well documented and vary from 4 % for specialized centers to > 10 % for nationwide registries [97]. Few studies report on mortality beyond 30 days. Damhuis et al. however showed in the Dutch Cancer Registry that 43 % of inhospital deaths after surgery for esophageal cancer occurred 30 days or more after the operation [98]. Therefore, 90-day mortality (90DM) might be preferred as a performance indicator. Using a longer time period after the operation for defining postoperative mortality may thus provide a better definition of quality of surgery [99]. Extending the mortality period beyond 30 days and beyond inhospital stay has the advantage that patients who die because of surgery-related complications outside the hospital are included as well.

Not only short-term outcomes but also long-term survival should be part of the benchmark as both aspects are relevant for comparing surgical performance. Both surgery-related deaths and cancer recurrence-related deaths are reflections of surgical quality of care. Less radical surgical resections will generally result in lower postoperative morbidity and mortality but will generally give less favorable oncological outcomes.

Case Mix Correction

Even after agreement on a uniform definition of postoperative mortality, direct comparison of crude mortality rates between hospitals can be misleading as they do not take into account the case-mix difference, i.e., the differences in physiological condition and tumor stages of patients. Sophisticated models have been developed for prediction of 30DM and IHM [8, 14, 67, 100–104] after esophageal surgery, but models for 90DM have been mostly based on large multi-institutional databases with only few parameters available [105].

Outcome-Volume Relationship and Registration

Over the past decades, better long-term survival results have been presented, evolving from 18 % 5-year survival in the era from 1980 to 1990 to 48 % in the most recently published RCT (Table 4.1) [17, 65, 99, 106, 107]. It is suggested that many factors are responsible for this positive effect, including large hospital volume, early tumor detection, improved patient selection based on novel staging modalities, increased use of neoadjuvant therapy, better surgical and anesthesiological techniques, and improved standardized

Table 4.1 Several studies over previous decades showing improved long-term survival after esophageal resection

Study	Randomization	Survival
Muller et al., 1990 [106]	N/A	5-year survival 10 %
Walsh et al., 1996 [107]	Multimodality therapy versus surgery	3-year survival 32 %
Hulscher et al. 2002, Omloo et al. 2007 [65, 66]	Transthoracic versus transhiatal approach	5-year survival 36 %
Van Hagen, 2013 [17]	Multimodality therapy versus surgery	5-year survival 47 %

perioperative clinical pathways [18, 108]. In many countries around the world, it has been decided that high-risk surgical procedures such as esophagectomy should be restricted to facilities with a yearly minimum volume [109, 110]. It has been demonstrated that the incidence of postoperative complications is similar across hospitals but that the associated mortality rates are lowest in high-volume centers, which generally show a lower "failure to rescue" [86, 111]. Centralization is currently implemented widely. Also auditing has been implemented as a way of improvement of care. Of course this results in an additional registration burden for the surgeon, but comparing individual or institutional results with the benchmark has proven valuable in other types of cancer surgery, such as for rectal cancer [112, 113]. For esophageal cancer, variables of interest are, for example, hospital mortality, radicality (R-status), extent of lymph node dissection, length of hospital stay, application of neoadjuvant therapy, availability of PET-CT, and the presence of a well-structured MDT. The quality indicators can be divided in structural, process, and outcome measures, respectively (Table 4.2) [114]. Heterogeneity and lack of standardized definitions of the outcome of interest are a problem here as well. In a review of esophagectomy outcomes from 164 NSQIP (National Surgical Quality Improvement Project) hospitals, it was demonstrated that even following case mix adjustment, results between centers

Table 4.2 Performance indicators that have been identified in esophageal cancer surgery

Quality-of-care indicators
Structural measures
Hospital volume
Surgeon volume
Centralization
Process measures
Discussion in multidisciplinary board
Age
Preoperative quality of life
Staging (FDG-PET vs. FDG-PET)
Lymphadenectomy
Neoadjuvant chemoradiation
Surgical approach
Outcome measures
Postoperative complications
Radicality of resection
Number of resected lymph nodes

From Courrech Staal et al. [114] with permission

varied by 161 % for 30-day mortality and 84 % for serious morbidity [67].

Finally, comparing the quality of infrequent operations such as esophagectomies is difficult, besides issues of definition and case-mix correction, because of another complex element in comparing surgical performance, i.e., the problem of sample size [115].

Conclusion/Take Home Messages

- Discussion of all patients with esophageal malignancies in a multidisciplinary tumor board is recommended and is associated with improved outcomes after surgery.
- ASA, (O)-POSSUM, and Charlson are the preoperative risk scoring systems that are often used in esophageal surgery.
- The most important change in the most recent 7th edition of the TNM staging system is that the concept of non-regional lymph nodes has been abandoned and that staging of esophageal cancer has been harmonized with gastric cancer.
- After extensive "conventional" diagnostic work-up, additional PET scanning yields a

diagnosis of distant dissemination in an additional 10 % of patients, especially in case of T3 tumors.
- The goals that have been achieved in open esophageal surgery should also act as targets for minimally invasive esophagectomy, being a lymph node retrieval of at least 15 nodes, R0 resection (>1 mm margin), and operative mortality <5 %.
- Neoadjuvant chemoradiotherapy decreases the incidence of a tumor-positive circumferential margin.
- Meta-analysis of the available literature data did not show differences in survival between transhiatal and transthoracic operations. The survival benefit of an extended lymphadenectomy by a transthoracic approach seems to be limited to a subgroup of patients with low burden of nodal disease.
- Overall, complication rates are reported in over 50 % of esophagectomy series, with incidences varying between 17 and 74 %. Postoperative complications have been directly linked to a variety of other outcome parameters including mortality, readmission rate, early cancer recurrence, survival, length of hospital stay, resource utilization, and quality of life.
- It has been suggested that MIE is accompanied by less pulmonary complications.
- The 30-day operative mortality (30DM) and the inhospital mortality (IHM) after esophageal resection vary from 4 % for specialized centers to >10 % for nationwide registries.
- Many factors are responsible for the better long-term survival rates that have been achieved over the previous decades, including large hospital volume, early tumor detection, improved patient selection based on novel staging modalities, increased use of neoadjuvant therapy, better surgical and anesthesiological techniques, and improved standardized perioperative clinical pathways.
- The lack of standardized definitions of complications and mortality has hampered outcome assessment after open and minimally invasive esophagectomy.

References

1. Stephens MR, et al. Multidisciplinary team management is associated with improved outcomes after surgery for esophageal cancer. Dis Esophagus. 2006; 19(3):164–71.

2. Davies AR, et al. The multidisciplinary team meeting improves staging accuracy and treatment selection for gastro-esophageal cancer. Dis Esophagus. 2006;19(6):496–503.

3. van Hagen P, et al. Impact of a multidisciplinary tumour board meeting for upper-GI malignancies on clinical decision making: a prospective cohort study. Int J Clin Oncol. 2013;18(2):214–9.

4. Keats AS. The ASA classification of physical status–a recapitulation. Anesthesiology. 1978;49(4): 233–6.

5. Prytherch DR, et al. POSSUM and Portsmouth POSSUM for predicting mortality. Physiological and Operative Severity Score for the enUmeration of Mortality and morbidity. Br J Surg. 1998;85(9): 1217–20.

6. Hall WH, et al. An electronic application for rapidly calculating Charlson comorbidity score. BMC Cancer. 2004;4:94.

7. Chandra A, Mangam S, Marzouk D. A review of risk scoring systems utilised in patients undergoing gastrointestinal surgery. J Gastrointest Surg. 2009;13(8): 1529–38.

8. Tekkis PP, et al. Risk-adjusted prediction of operative mortality in oesophagogastric surgery with O-POSSUM. Br J Surg. 2004;91(3):288–95.

9. Lagarde SM, et al. Evaluation of O-POSSUM in predicting in-hospital mortality after resection for oesophageal cancer. Br J Surg. 2007;94(12):1521–6.

10. Lai F, et al. Evaluation of various POSSUM models for predicting mortality in patients undergoing elective oesophagectomy for carcinoma. Br J Surg. 2007; 94(9):1172–8.

11. Bosch DJ, et al. Comparison of different risk-adjustment models in assessing short-term surgical outcome after transthoracic esophagectomy in patients with esophageal cancer. Am J Surg. 2011;202(3):303–9.

12. Dutta S, Horgan PG, McMillan DC. POSSUM and its related models as predictors of postoperative mortality and morbidity in patients undergoing surgery for gastro-oesophageal cancer: a systematic review. World J Surg. 2010;34(9):2076–82.

13. Cijs TM, et al. Outcome of esophagectomy for cancer in elderly patients. Ann Thorac Surg. 2010;90(3): 900–7.

14. Koppert LB, et al. Impact of age and co-morbidity on surgical resection rate and survival in patients with oesophageal and gastric cancer. Br J Surg. 2012;99(12):1693–700.

15. Polee MB, et al. Prognostic factors for survival in patients with advanced oesophageal cancer treated with cisplatin-based combination chemotherapy. Br J Cancer. 2003;89(11):2045–50.

16. Masoomi H, et al. Predictive factors of acute respiratory failure in esophagectomy for esophageal malignancy. Am Surg. 2012;78(10):1024–8.

17. van Hagen P, et al. Preoperative chemoradiotherapy for esophageal or junctional cancer. N Engl J Med. 2012;366(22):2074–84.

18. Stein HJ, Siewert JR. Improved prognosis of resected esophageal cancer. World J Surg. 2004;28(6):520–5.

19. Sobin LH, Compton CC. TNM seventh edition: what's new, what's changed: communication from the International Union Against Cancer and the American Joint Committee on Cancer. Cancer. 2010;116(22): 5336–9.

20. Kelly S, et al. A systematic review of the staging performance of endoscopic ultrasound in gastro-oesophageal carcinoma. Gut. 2001;49(4):534–9.

21. van Vliet EP, et al. Staging investigations for oesophageal cancer: a meta-analysis. Br J Cancer. 2008; 98(3):547–57.

22. Vickers J, Alderson D. Influence of luminal obstruction on oesophageal cancer staging using endoscopic ultrasonography. Br J Surg. 1998;85(7):999–1001.

23. Reed CE, et al. Esophageal cancer staging: improved accuracy by endoscopic ultrasound of celiac lymph nodes. Ann Thorac Surg. 1999;67(2):319–21; discussion 322.

24. Omloo JM, et al. Additional value of external ultrasonography of the neck after CT and PET scanning in the preoperative assessment of patients with esophageal cancer. Dig Surg. 2009;26(1): 43–9.

25. van Westreenen HL, et al. Systematic review of the staging performance of 18F-fluorodeoxyglucose positron emission tomography in esophageal cancer. J Clin Oncol. 2004;22(18):3805–12.

26. Blom RL, et al. PET/CT-based metabolic tumour volume for response prediction of neoadjuvant chemoradiotherapy in oesophageal carcinoma. Eur J Nucl Med Mol Imaging. 2013;40(10):1500–6.

27. van Westreenen HL, et al. Limited additional value of positron emission tomography in staging oesophageal cancer. Br J Surg. 2007;94(12):1515–20.

28. Gouma DJ, et al. Laparoscopic ultrasonography for staging of gastrointestinal malignancy. Scand J Gastroenterol Suppl. 1996;218:43–9.

29. Lamb PJ, et al. Sentinel node biopsy to evaluate the metastatic dissemination of oesophageal adenocarcinoma. Br J Surg. 2005;92(1):60–7.

30. Schroder W, et al. Localization of isolated lymph node metastases in esophageal cancer–does it influence the sentinel node concept? Hepatogastroenterology. 2007; 54(76):1116–20.

31. Grotenhuis BA, et al. The sentinel node concept in adenocarcinomas of the distal esophagus and gastroesophageal junction. J Thorac Cardiovasc Surg. 2009;138(3):608–12.

32. Kalha I, et al. The accuracy of endoscopic ultrasound for restaging esophageal carcinoma after chemoradiation therapy. Cancer. 2004;101(5):940–7.

33. Kitagawa Y, et al. Sentinel node mapping for gastric cancer: a prospective multicenter trial in Japan. J Clin Oncol. 2013;31(29):3704–10.

34. Ribeiro A, et al. Endoscopic ultrasound restaging after neoadjuvant chemotherapy in esophageal cancer. Am J Gastroenterol. 2006;101(6):1216–21.

35. Westerterp M, et al. Esophageal cancer: CT, endoscopic US, and FDG PET for assessment of response to neoadjuvant therapy–systematic review. Radiology. 2005;236(3):841–51.

36. Swisher SG, et al. 2-Fluoro-2-deoxy-D-glucose positron emission tomography imaging is predictive of pathologic response and survival after preoperative chemoradiation in patients with esophageal carcinoma. Cancer. 2004;101(8):1776–85.

37. Smyth EC, Shah MA. Role of (1)(8)F 2-fluoro-2-deoxyglucose positron emission tomography in upper gastrointestinal malignancies. World J Gastroenterol. 2011;17(46):5059–74.

38. Han D, et al. Comparison of the diagnostic value of 3-deoxy-3-18F-fluorothymidine and 18F-fluorodeoxyglucose positron emission tomography/computed tomography in the assessment of regional lymph node in thoracic esophageal squamous cell carcinoma: a pilot study. Dis Esophagus. 2012;25(5):415–26.

39. Riddell AM, et al. The appearances of oesophageal carcinoma demonstrated on high-resolution, T2-weighted MRI, with histopathological correlation. Eur Radiol. 2007;17(2):391–9.

40. Kijanka M, et al. Rapid optical imaging of human breast tumour xenografts using anti-HER2 VHHs site-directly conjugated to IRDye 800CW for image-guided surgery. Eur J Nucl Med Mol Imaging. 2013;40(11):1718–29.

41. Stahl M, et al. Chemoradiation with and without surgery in patients with locally advanced squamous cell carcinoma of the esophagus. J Clin Oncol. 2005;23(10):2310–7.

42. Bedenne L, et al. Chemoradiation followed by surgery compared with chemoradiation alone in squamous cancer of the esophagus: FFCD 9102. J Clin Oncol. 2007;25(10):1160–8.

43. Dexter SP, et al. Circumferential resection margin involvement: an independent predictor of survival following surgery for oesophageal cancer. Gut. 2001;48(5):667–70.

44. Scheepers JJ, et al. Influence of circumferential resection margin on prognosis in distal esophageal and gastroesophageal cancer approached through the transhiatal route. Dis Esophagus. 2009;22(1):42–8.

45. Rao VS, et al. Comparison of circumferential resection margin clearance criteria with survival after surgery for cancer of esophagus. J Surg Oncol. 2012;105(8):745–9.

46. O'Neill JR, et al. Defining a positive circumferential resection margin in oesophageal cancer and its implications for adjuvant treatment. Br J Surg. 2013;100(8):1055–63.

47. Skinner DB. En bloc resection for neoplasms of the esophagus and cardia. J Thorac Cardiovasc Surg. 1983;85(1):59–71.

48. Chan DS, et al. Systematic review and meta-analysis of the influence of circumferential resection margin involvement on survival in patients with operable oesophageal cancer. Br J Surg. 2013;100(4):456–64.

49. Verhage RJ, et al. How to define a positive circumferential resection margin in T3 adenocarcinoma of the esophagus. Am J Surg Pathol. 2011;35(6):919–26.

50. Sujendran V, et al. Effect of neoadjuvant chemotherapy on circumferential margin positivity and its impact on prognosis in patients with resectable oesophageal cancer. Br J Surg. 2008;95(2):191–4.

51. Khan OA, Cruttenden-Wood D, Toh SK. Is an involved circumferential resection margin following oesphagectomy for cancer an important prognostic indicator? Interact Cardiovasc Thorac Surg. 2010;11(5):645–8.

52. Prenzel KL, et al. Prognostic relevance of skip metastases in esophageal cancer. Ann Thorac Surg. 2010;90(5):1662–7.

53. Westerterp M, et al. Outcome of surgical treatment for early adenocarcinoma of the esophagus or gastroesophageal junction. Virchows Arch. 2005;446(5):497–504.

54. Boone J, et al. International survey on esophageal cancer: part I surgical techniques. Dis Esophagus. 2009;22(3):195–202.

55. Schwarz RE, Smith DD. Clinical impact of lymphadenectomy extent in resectable esophageal cancer. J Gastrointest Surg. 2007;11(11):1384–93; discussion 1393–4.

56. Herbella FA, Patti MG. Minimally invasive esophagectomy. World J Gastroenterol. 2010;16(30):3811–5.

57. Weksler B, et al. Robot-assisted minimally invasive esophagectomy is equivalent to thoracoscopic minimally invasive esophagectomy. Dis Esophagus. 2012;25(5):403–9.

58. Pennathur A, Luketich JD. Minimally invasive esophagectomy: short-term outcomes appear comparable to open esophagectomy. Ann Surg. 2012;255(2):206–7.

59. Hulscher JB, et al. Transthoracic versus transhiatal resection for carcinoma of the esophagus: a meta-analysis. Ann Thorac Surg. 2001;72(1):306–13.

60. Lagarde SM, et al. Prognostic factors in adenocarcinoma of the esophagus or gastroesophageal junction. J Clin Oncol. 2006;24(26):4347–55.

61. Izbicki JR, et al. Prognostic value of immunohistochemically identifiable tumor cells in lymph nodes of patients with completely resected esophageal cancer. N Engl J Med. 1997;337(17):1188–94.

62. Orringer ME, Marshall B, Iannettoni MD. Transhiatal esophagectomy for treatment of benign and malignant esophageal disease. World J Surg. 2001;25(2):196–203.

63. Siewert JR, et al. Histologic tumor type is an independent prognostic parameter in esophageal cancer: lessons from more than 1,000 consecutive resections

at a single center in the Western world. Ann Surg. 2001;234(3):360–7; discussion 368–9.

64. van Sandick JW, et al. Indicators of prognosis after transhiatal esophageal resection without thoracotomy for cancer. J Am Coll Surg. 2002;194(1):28–36.

65. Hulscher JB, et al. Extended transthoracic resection compared with limited transhiatal resection for adenocarcinoma of the esophagus. N Engl J Med. 2002;347(21):1662–9.

66. Omloo JM, et al. Extended transthoracic resection compared with limited transhiatal resection for adenocarcinoma of the mid/distal esophagus: five-year survival of a randomized clinical trial. Ann Surg. 2007;246(6):992–1000; discussion 1000–1.

67. Merkow RP, et al. Short-term outcomes after esophagectomy at 164 American College of Surgeons National Surgical Quality Improvement Program hospitals: effect of operative approach and hospital-level variation. Arch Surg. 2012;147(11):1009–16.

68. Boshier PR, Anderson O, Hanna GB. Transthoracic versus transhiatal esophagectomy for the treatment of esophagogastric cancer: a meta-analysis. Ann Surg. 2011;254(6):894–906.

69. Fujita H, et al. Mortality and morbidity rates, postoperative course, quality of life, and prognosis after extended radical lymphadenectomy for esophageal cancer. Comparison of three-field lymphadenectomy with two-field lymphadenectomy. Ann Surg. 1995; 222(5):654–62.

70. Lerut T, et al. Three-field lymphadenectomy for carcinoma of the esophagus and gastroesophageal junction in 174 R0 resections: impact on staging, disease-free survival, and outcome: a plea for adaptation of TNM classification in upper-half esophageal carcinoma. Ann Surg. 2004;240(6):962–72; discussion 972–4.

71. Altorki NK, et al. Total number of resected lymph nodes predicts survival in esophageal cancer. Ann Surg. 2008;248(2):221–6.

72. Rizk NP, et al. Optimum lymphadenectomy for esophageal cancer. Ann Surg. 2010;251(1):46–50.

73. Rizk N, et al. The prognostic importance of the number of involved lymph nodes in esophageal cancer: implications for revisions of the American Joint Committee on Cancer staging system. J Thorac Cardiovasc Surg. 2006;132(6):1374–81.

74. Peyre CG, et al. The number of lymph nodes removed predicts survival in esophageal cancer: an international study on the impact of extent of surgical resection. Ann Surg. 2008;248(4):549–56.

75. Stiles BM, et al. Worldwide Oesophageal Cancer Collaboration guidelines for lymphadenectomy predict survival following neoadjuvant therapy. Eur J Cardiothorac Surg. 2012;42(4):659–64.

76. Torgersen Z, et al. Prognostic implications of lymphadenectomy in esophageal cancer after neo-adjuvant therapy: a single center experience. J Gastrointest Surg. 2011;15(10):1769–76.

77. Chao YK, et al. Lymph node dissection after chemoradiation in esophageal cancer: a subgroup analysis of patients with and without pathological response. Ann Surg Oncol. 2012;19(11):3500–5.

78. Dunst CM, Swanstrom LL. Minimally invasive esophagectomy. J Gastrointest Surg. 2010;14 Suppl 1:S108–14.

79. Courrech Staal EF, et al. Systematic review of the benefits and risks of neoadjuvant chemoradiation for oesophageal cancer. Br J Surg. 2010;97(10):1482–96.

80. Kassin MT, et al. Risk factors for 30-day hospital readmission among general surgery patients. J Am Coll Surg. 2012;215(3):322–30.

81. Hii MW, et al. Impact of postoperative morbidity on long-term survival after oesophagectomy. Br J Surg. 2013;100(1):95–104.

82. Derogar M, et al. Influence of major postoperative complications on health-related quality of life among long-term survivors of esophageal cancer surgery. J Clin Oncol. 2012;30(14):1615–9.

83. Lagarde SM, et al. Postoperative complications after esophagectomy for adenocarcinoma of the esophagus are related to timing of death due to recurrence. Ann Surg. 2008;247(1):71–6.

84. Blencowe NS, et al. Reporting of short-term clinical outcomes after esophagectomy: a systematic review. Ann Surg. 2012;255(4):658–66.

85. Koch CG, et al. What are the real rates of postoperative complications: elucidating inconsistencies between administrative and clinical data sources. J Am Coll Surg. 2012;214(5):798–805.

86. Ghaferi AA, Birkmeyer JD, Dimick JB. Variation in hospital mortality associated with inpatient surgery. N Engl J Med. 2009;361(14):1368–75.

87. Biere SS, et al. Minimally invasive versus open oesophagectomy for patients with oesophageal cancer: a multicentre, open-label, randomised controlled trial. Lancet. 2012;379(9829):1887–92.

88. Law S. Is minimally invasive preferable to open oesophagectomy? Lancet. 2012;379(9829):1856–8.

89. Tandon S, et al. Peri-operative risk factors for acute lung injury after elective oesophagectomy. Br J Anaesth. 2001;86(5):633–8.

90. Law S, et al. Predictive factors for postoperative pulmonary complications and mortality after esophagectomy for cancer. Ann Surg. 2004;240(5):791–800.

91. Akaishi T, et al. Thoracoscopic en bloc total esophagectomy with radical mediastinal lymphadenectomy. J Thorac Cardiovasc Surg. 1996;112(6):1533–40; discussion 1540–1.

92. Orringer MB, Marshall B, Iannettoni MD. Eliminating the cervical esophagogastric anastomotic leak with a side-to-side stapled anastomosis. J Thorac Cardiovasc Surg. 2000;119(2):277–88.

93. Collard JM, et al. Terminalized semimechanical side-to-side suture technique for cervical esophagogastrostomy. Ann Thorac Surg. 1998;65(3):814–7.

94. van Heijl M, et al. Intrathoracic manifestations of cervical anastomotic leaks after transhiatal and transthoracic oesophagectomy. Br J Surg. 2010;97(5): 726–31.

95. Weidenhagen R, et al. Anastomotic leakage after esophageal resection: new treatment options by endoluminal vacuum therapy. Ann Thorac Surg. 2010; 90(5):1674–81.
96. Lagarde SM, et al. Incidence and management of chyle leakage after esophagectomy. Ann Thorac Surg. 2005;80(2):449–54.
97. Dikken JL, et al. Effect of hospital volume on postoperative mortality and survival after oesophageal and gastric cancer surgery in the Netherlands between 1989 and 2009. Eur J Cancer. 2012;48(7):1004–13.
98. Damhuis RA, et al. Comparison of 30-day, 90-day and in-hospital postoperative mortality for eight different cancer types. Br J Surg. 2012;99(8):1149–54.
99. Jamieson GG, et al. Postoperative mortality following oesophagectomy and problems in reporting its rate. Br J Surg. 2004;91(8):943–7.
100. Wright CD, et al. Predictors of major morbidity and mortality after esophagectomy for esophageal cancer: a Society of Thoracic Surgeons General Thoracic Surgery Database risk adjustment model. J Thorac Cardiovasc Surg. 2009;137(3):587–95; discussion 596.
101. Morita M, et al. In-hospital mortality after a surgical resection for esophageal cancer: analyses of the associated factors and historical changes. Ann Surg Oncol. 2011;18(6):1757–65.
102. Lagarde SM, et al. Prognostic nomogram for patients undergoing oesophagectomy for adenocarcinoma of the oesophagus or gastro-oesophageal junction. Br J Surg. 2007;94(11):1361–8.
103. Lagarde SM, et al. Preoperative prediction of the occurrence and severity of complications after esophagectomy for cancer with use of a nomogram. Ann Thorac Surg. 2008;85(6):1938–45.
104. Grotenhuis BA, et al. Validation of a nomogram predicting complications after esophagectomy for cancer. Ann Thorac Surg. 2010;90(3):920–5.
105. Dikken JL, et al. Influence of hospital type on outcomes after oesophageal and gastric cancer surgery. Br J Surg. 2012;99(7):954–63.
106. Muller JM, et al. Surgical therapy of oesophageal carcinoma. Br J Surg. 1990;77(8):845–57.
107. Walsh TN, et al. A comparison of multimodal therapy and surgery for esophageal adenocarcinoma. N Engl J Med. 1996;335(7):462–7.
108. Low DE, et al. Esophagectomy–it's not just about mortality anymore: standardized perioperative clinical pathways improve outcomes in patients with esophageal cancer. J Gastrointest Surg. 2007;11(11):1395–402; discussion 1402.
109. Dikken JL, et al. Differences in outcomes of oesophageal and gastric cancer surgery across Europe. Br J Surg. 2013;100(1):83–94.
110. Markar SR, et al. Volume-outcome relationship in surgery for esophageal malignancy: systematic review and meta-analysis 2000–2011. J Gastrointest Surg. 2012;16(5):1055–63.
111. Patti MG, et al. A hospital's annual rate of esophagectomy influences the operative mortality rate. J Gastrointest Surg. 1998;2(2):186–92.
112. van Gijn W, et al. Nationwide outcome registrations to improve quality of care in rectal surgery. An initiative of the European Society of Surgical Oncology. J Surg Oncol. 2009;99(8):491–6.
113. Birgisson H, et al. Improved survival in cancer of the colon and rectum in Sweden. Eur J Surg Oncol. 2005;31(8):845–53.
114. Courrech Staal EF, et al. Quality-of-care indicators for oesophageal cancer surgery: a review. Eur J Surg Oncol. 2010;36(11):1035–43.
115. Dimick JB, Welch HG, Birkmeyer JD. Surgical mortality as an indicator of hospital quality: the problem with small sample size. JAMA. 2004;292(7):847–51.
116. Raja S, et al. Esophageal submucosa: the watershed for esophageal cancer. J Thorac Cardiovasc Surg. 2011;142(6):1403–11.
117. Griffin S, Raimes SA. A companion to specialist surgical practice: oesophagogastric surgery. 4th ed. Elsevier; 2009. p 97.

Wesley A. Papenfuss and Todd L. Demmy

Introduction

Surgery of the esophagus continues to be challenging with significant morbidity and mortality. Despite advances in anesthetic and surgical techniques, morbidity can be as high as 50 % and mortality as high as 10 %. Directing complex gastrointestinal procedures to specialized centers has improved outcomes significantly [1, 2].

Esophageal cancer patients are likely to have significant comorbid disease including cardiac, respiratory, and hepatic disease, diabetes, and malnutrition. Properly assessing and optimizing these comorbidities is essential to preoperative planning.

This chapter will focus on the medical evaluation of the esophageal surgery patient including nutritional optimization in the neoadjuvant setting.

Surgical Evaluation

The oncologic evaluation of the esophageal cancer patient is well described elsewhere [3]. Briefly, evaluations of anatomy and resectability are the

most important aspects. All patients should have appropriate staging tests including CT of chest, abdomen, and pelvis with integrated PET imaging to exclude metastatic disease. A mid/upper esophagus tumor generally requires bronchoscopy to rule out tracheal invasion that precludes resection.

Initial or repeat upper endoscopy may be needed to confirm or refine the pathologic diagnosis, define the proximal extent of Barrett's esophagus, evaluate neoadjuvant treatment response, document residual esophageal/gastric disease, and evaluate the proposed reconstructive conduit. Colonoscopy may be appropriate when considering alternative conduits for reconstruction.

Imaging indicating overt metastatic disease or invasion of "unresectable" organs such as the pulmonary vein, aorta, and trachea generally establishes unresectability. Preoperative visceral angiography may be useful for those at risk for mesenteric artery stenosis such as patients with known coronary artery disease [4]. Overall, the benefits of angiography are controversial.

Medical Evaluation

Comorbid conditions are common among patients undergoing esophagectomy for cancer; for instance, they are at risk for cardiopulmonary disorders, hepatic disease, and variable degrees of malnutrition. The following section discusses the assessment and management of patients with coexisting diseases (see Table 5.1)

W.A. Papenfuss, MD
Department of Surgical Oncology,
Roswell Park Cancer Institute,
Elm & Carlton Streets, Buffalo, NY 14263, USA

T.L. Demmy, MD (⊠)
Department of Thoracic Surgery,
Roswell Park Cancer Institute,
Elm & Carlton Streets, Buffalo, NY, USA
e-mail: todd.demmy@roswellpark.org

Table 5.1 Preoperative medical evaluation prior to esophageal cancer surgery

	Cardiac disease	Pulmonary disease	Liver disease	VTE	Nutrition	Frailty
Risk factors	CAD Prior MI Angina Diabetes Hypertension	COPD/asthma Exercise intolerance Prior lung surgery	ETOH Hepatitis Stigmata Varices seen on imaging	Hx of VTE Immobility Malignancy Chemotherapy	>10 % Weight loss Albumin<3.5 BMI<18	Age>65 Impaired gait Recent chemotherapy/surgery Chronic disease
Evaluation	EKG Echo Exercise stress testing	Pulmonary function testing	Childs score	As clinically indicated	Dietitian consult	Frailty testing
Intervention	Coronary angiography/intervention Risk factor modification B-blockers Statins	Smoking cessation Respiratory training Oral hygiene		Appropriate anticoagulation Inferior vena cava filter placement prior to surgery	Pre-op supplement TPN Stent Feeding tube	Physical/occupational therapy Dietitian consult Polypharmacy evaluation Psychiatric/neurologic evaluation
Relative contraindication	Uncorrected myocardial ischemia VO_2 max<11 ml/kg/min	FEV1<70 % FVC<80 %	Childs A or worse Portal hypertension		Inability to maintain weight	

Cardiac

Arrhythmia is common after esophagectomy, occurring in 20–30 % of patients [5]. The most common arrhythmia is atrial fibrillation occurring in 10–20 % of cases [6, 7] It is associated with an increased hospital length of stay and increased risk of postoperative death. A retrospective review of esophagectomy found an association between male gender, age greater than 65 years, history of COPD, history of cardiac disease, and neoadjuvant therapy with an increased risk of postoperative atrial fibrillation [7, 8]. Therefore, patients at increased risk of arrhythmia should be evaluated and appropriate optimization considered preoperatively. Patients on beta blockade should have this continued, electrolytes repleted, and statin therapy considered.

There continues to be debate over postoperative arrhythmia prevention [9]. A prospective randomized trial of amiodarone initiated at the time of general anesthesia induction found a significant decrease in post-esophagectomy atrial fibrillation (15 % versus 40 %), with no increased adverse effects [9]. However, amiodarone use can cause pneumonitis in 10–15 % of patients leading to death in 10 % of those affected. For this reason, amiodarone use should be reserved for patients at high risk for postoperative atrial fibrillation (e.g., age > 70 or cardiac disease) and low risk for pulmonary injury.

Myocardial infarction is uncommon after esophagectomy (1–2 %). However, patients should be assessed for their risk for postoperative MI according to the ACC AHA guidelines [10]. Esophageal surgery is considered intermediate risk with a 1–5 % chance of perioperative MI. Preoperative assessment may include EKG, echocardiography, exercise stress testing, and coronary angiography as appropriate. For patients with limited fitness at centers with cardiopulmonary exercise testing, a VO$_2$ max less than 11 ml/kg/min predicts complications following esophagectomy [11].

The use of perioperative beta-blockers and statins deserves mention. While the addition of beta-blockers as prophylaxis against postoperative events is controversial, patients who are already on these drugs should have them continued in the perioperative setting [12]. Statin use may reduce the risk of myocardial infarction as well as the risk of postoperative atrial flutter in patients undergoing noncardiac surgery [13]. Their use should be considered in patients deemed to be at elevated risk of postoperative cardiovascular events.

Pulmonary

Pulmonary complications are the most frequent complication following esophagectomy occurring in 20–40 % of patients. Despite the advances in minimally invasive surgery, all patients should be prepared for possible thoracotomy. Pulmonary testing should be considered in patients who have a history of smoking, pulmonary disease, or signs and symptoms suggestive of an underlying pulmonary disorder. Patients with compromised pulmonary function as evidenced by FVC < 80 % and FEV1 < 70 % predicted have been shown to have an increased risk of pulmonary complications [14]. Patients who are identified to have an increased risk of pulmonary complications may benefit from preoperative rehab or training [15, 16].

Preoperative interventions can prevent postoperative pneumonia. Smoking cessation at least 1 month prior to surgery has been associated with decreased incidence of pneumonia following thoracic surgery. Smoking cessation, respiratory training (incentive spirometry, respiratory muscle stretching, deep diaphragm breathing, and effective cough), and attention to oral hygiene/plaque removal decrease pulmonary complications following esophagectomy [17]. Minimally invasive esophagectomy causes fewer pulmonary complications. In an open-label, randomized trial, minimally invasive esophagectomy greatly decreased inpatient pulmonary complications (29 versus 9 % open) [18].

Hepatic Disease

Patients with liver disease are at an increased risk of mortality following surgery. Alcohol use contributing to squamous cell esophageal cancer risk factors may also induce cirrhosis and liver dysfunction. While varices may be seen on preoperative imaging, liver dysfunction may be occult until the perioperative setting. Mortality approaches 100 % in patients with Childs C criteria. Even Childs A patients have mortality as high as 10 % following esophagectomy [19]. In a review of 18 known cirrhotics undergoing esophagectomy, Tachibana et al. found an overall 16.7 % mortality (versus 5.7 % in noncirrhotics). One-year and 3-year survivals were also significantly less [20]. The presence of cirrhosis should be considered in all patients who have a history of liver disease, overt physical signs on examination, irregularities on liver function tests or imaging, or known risk factors. Liver biopsy may be necessary to confirm the diagnosis.

Age

Using a specific age exclusion for esophagectomy is controversial [21]. Age-related comorbidities foster complications which are tolerated poorly because of concomitant reductions in organ reserve. There are recent reports in the literature regarding the safety of esophagectomy performed in elderly patients. Pultrum et al. report their experience performing extended esophageal resection via thoracolaparotomy at a high volume center. While there was no difference in overall survival, perioperative morbidity was predictably higher in patients greater than or equal to 70 years, particularly in regard to pulmonary, cardiac, and infectious complications [22]. This report has been criticized as potentially difficult to reproduce because few centers could achieve the authors' case volumes [21]. A recent pooled analysis of 25 studies revealed that elderly patients were less likely to receive neoadjuvant therapy and more likely to experience inhospital mortality and pulmonary and cardiac complications [23].

More important than age is overall patient frailty. Multiple factors have been described and shown to be associated with postoperative outcomes (Table 5.2) [24]. A prospective study found the degree of frailty to be associated with the rate

Table 5.2 Frailty in the surgical patient

Functional factors	Medical factors
Difficulty with activities of daily living	Diabetes
Weight loss	Pulmonary disease (COPD, pneumonia)
Body mass index	Cardiac disease (CHF, MI, hypertension)
Grip strength	Peripheral vascular disease
Gait speed	Cerebral vascular disease (TIA, CVA)
History of falls	Delirium
	History of depression

of postoperative complications [25]. In a recent study of esophagectomy patients in the NSQIP database, both morbidity and mortality increased with the presence of 1 of 11 NSQIP-measured preoperative variables as determined by a modified frailty index. As the number of items present in the frailty index increased from zero to five, the rate of a serious complication requiring ICU admission increased from 18 to 61 %. Mortality rate increased from 1.8 to 23.1 % [26].

In summary, age alone should not preclude esophagectomy but should be considered in the context of the patients overall functional status, frailty index, and associated comorbid conditions.

Obesity

Obesity is an epidemic problem causing an increased incidence of distal esophageal cancer. Therefore, surgeons can expect to encounter more obese patients with esophageal cancer. Obese patients have higher rates of diabetes and underlying cardiac and pulmonary diseases. Preoperative evaluation of the obese patient may require echocardiography, cardiopulmonary exercise testing, pulmonary function testing (with special attention to functional residual capacity), evaluation for obstructive sleep apnea, risk modification for venous thromboembolism (VTE), and optimizing glycemic control for patients with a HgA1c > 8 % [27–29].

The incremental contribution of obesity to perioperative morbidity and mortality is controversial. Obesity itself has not been related to increased morbidity and mortality in patients undergoing surgery for intra-abdominal cancer [30]. However, anastomotic and wound complications increase in obese patients with diabetes [31–33]. In addition, several studies report no detrimental effect on survival in the obese esophageal cancer patient [33–35]. Minimally invasive esophagectomy in the obese patient is also feasible with similar morbidity and mortality but longer operative times [36]. Like age, obesity, per se, should not preclude open or minimally invasive esophagectomy; however, care must be taken when managing coexistent comorbidities.

Venous Thromboembolism

Thromboembolic events occur in 14–32 % of patients undergoing neoadjuvant therapy for esophageal cancer [37, 38]. Such patients require extended anticoagulation therapy for treatment and prevention of end-organ damage, which may delay time to surgery. Decisions regarding the timing of surgery, the role of perioperative anticoagulation, and IVC filter placement need to be made on a case-by-case basis. Current guidelines suggest the use of inferior vena cava filters in patients with residual DVT and a contraindication to anticoagulation, recurrent DVT or PE despite anticoagulation, and patients undergoing major surgery within 2 months of a thromboembolic event [39]. Removal of the filter should be considered once the patient is deemed appropriate to resume anticoagulation and is easiest performed within 10–14 days of placement [39]. Inferior vena cava filter placement in patients with recent DVT/PE before planned esophagectomy may decrease the risk of fatal perioperative pulmonary embolism.

Prior Surgical History

Minimally invasive esophagectomy requires operating in both the abdominal and thoracic cavities and is made more complex by previous surgical procedures in these regions. Previous thoracotomies, upper abdominal (e.g., anti-reflux or ulcer) surgeries, and prior head and neck procedures deserve mention.

Orringer et al. reported their experience performing transhiatal esophagectomy for benign disease in patients having had prior operation for GERD or hiatal hernia. Thoracotomy was necessary in 16.6 % and a colonic conduit was required in 10.6 % of patients [40]. MIE has also been reported in patients after thoracotomy for end-stage achalasia [41].

Esophageal cancer after bariatric surgery is uncommon. However, with the increased use of bariatric surgery, we can expect reports to increase. A recent series describes an experience of five minimally invasive esophagectomies following gastric bypass. Four had undergone laparoscopic Roux-en-y gastric bypass and one patient had open bypass. One patient required colonic interposition for reconstruction after esophagectomy. There was no mortality in their series. The previously bypassed stomach is utilized as the new gastric conduit, while the Roux limb is utilized for jejunostomy tube placement [42].

Prior head and neck surgery can complicate esophagectomy depending on the planned surgical approach. A cervical anastomosis may prove challenging given prior dissection or radiation within the operative field. For this reason, a thoracic dissection and anastomosis should be considered in these patients.

Nutritional Assessment and Optimization

Patients with esophageal cancer frequently present with dysphagia and variable degrees of weight loss prior to diagnosis. For this reason, nutritional assessment before any treatment is imperative.

Assorted methods can assess the nutritional status of cancer patients. Clinical parameters include weight loss, dietary change as a marker for dysphagia, and gastrointestinal symptoms including nausea, vomiting, diarrhea, and anorexia. Physical exam findings suggestive of malnutrition include loss of subcutaneous fat,

Table 5.3 Factors associated with malnutrition

Weight loss > 10 %
BMI < 20 kg/m^2
Albumin < 3.5 g/dL
Prealbumin < 10 mg/dL
Degree of dysphagia
Gastrointestinal symptoms
Muscle wasting
Loss of subcutaneous fat
Ascites
Edema

Table 5.4 Advantages and disadvantages of different methods of enteral support

	Advantages	Disadvantages
Gastrostomy	Ease of placement Bolus feeds	Potential injury to conduit
Jejunostomy	Evaluate for metastatic disease	Unable to bolus (requires pump)
	Able to use post-resection	Usually surgically placed
Esophageal stent	Immediate relief of dysphagia	Retrosternal pain
	Improved quality of life	Requires removal before resection
		Migration/ perforation

muscle wasting, edema, and ascites as signs of protein calorie malnutrition (see Table 5.3). Laboratory evaluations include assessments of rapid turnover proteins including albumin (half-life 20 days), prealbumin (half-life 2–3 days), and transferrin (half-life 8–10 days) [43].

Weight loss greater than 10 % over 3–6 months and greater than 5 % over 1 month suggests significant malnutrition [44]. Preoperative nutritional supplementation, provided as TPN, was found to be beneficial only in the most malnourished [45]. Immuno-enhanced enteral supplementation has been studied with the hope of decreasing morbidity and mortality following major surgery for gastrointestinal cancer. A randomized controlled trial that utilized preoperative immunotherapy (supplementation of omega 3 fatty acids) failed to demonstrate a significant difference in length of stay or morbidity in esophagectomy patients [46]. However, a meta-analysis of studies using immunonutrition in the perioperative setting for patients undergoing elective gastrointestinal cancer operations showed shorter length of stay and fewer postoperative infectious complications [47]. At this time, the use of immunonutrition in the perioperative setting remains controversial. Severely malnourished patients may benefit but should be treated for approximately 2 weeks preoperatively [48, 49].

Often, esophageal cancer patients need additional nutritional support. Enteral is preferred over parenteral nutrition to avoid infectious complications. This is especially important when multimodality therapy is considered. The ability to maintain nutritional status fosters completion of multimodality regimens [50, 51]. This can be

accomplished in a number of ways: esophageal stenting, gastrostomy, or jejunostomy. Each of these methods has its own advantages and disadvantages (see Table 5.4).

Gastrostomy can be achieved endoscopically and by interventional radiology techniques or surgical placement. The use of gastrostomy before esophagectomy is somewhat controversial due to the risks of injuring the future gastric conduit or its blood supply. In general, percutaneous endoscopic gastrostomy tubes have low complication rates, and esophagectomies following placements have not been associated with increased conduit-related complications [52]. Transoral placement poses its own difficulties due to an obstructing tumor. Additionally, a recent study identified g-tube site metastasis in 9.4 % of patients undergoing endoscopic placement in esophageal cancer [53].

Percutaneous radiologic gastrostomy (PRG) is a radiologic technique whereby the stomach is accessed under radiologic guidance. PRG has the theoretical advantage of avoiding the primary malignancy during placement of the feeding tube. PRG was placed successfully in 96.3 % of patients, and there were no conduit-related complications attributable to the procedure in all resected patients [54]. Open or laparoscopic gastrostomy tube placement allows for direct visualization of tube placement and avoids injury to other organs or the future conduit vasculature.

Jejunostomy placement has been described by percutaneous [55] and endoscopic means but is usually accomplished surgically. The advantage of a laparoscopic approach is that it allows for an assessment of undetected peritoneal surface metastasis while avoiding manipulation of the future gastric conduit. If metastatic disease is encountered at the time of laparoscopy, then a permanent gastrostomy tube can be placed at that time. Laparoscopic placement has been shown to be feasible and safe without significant postoperative sequelae [56]. Choice of jejunal tube location requires careful consideration as not to hinder future surgical therapy.

Esophageal stent placement for preoperative nutritional optimization of the esophageal cancer patient is another option. Several recent trials have demonstrated their use in the near obstructed patient destined for neoadjuvant chemoradiotherapy [57–59]. In addition to providing nutrition, stenting palliated obstructive symptoms leading to an improved quality of life [60]. The choice of stent is very important. Self-expanding metal stents are difficult to remove and are generally used in patients ineligible for definitive esophageal resection. Self-expanding silicone stents are preferred for patients treated with operative/curative intent. They provide immediate relief of obstruction and are easier to remove before or at the time of planned surgical resection. Stent migration is uncommon but managed easily endoscopically. Gastrointestinal perforation is rare.

Deciding between modalities requires considering specific case factors. When compared to jejunostomy, stent placement was associated with improved dysphagia scores, improved weight gain, fewer interruptions in neoadjuvant therapy, improvement in albumin levels, and less percentage of body weight lost [43, 60]. Gastrostomy tubes may be more convenient for the patient but have the unlikely possibility of damaging the gastric conduit precluding its use.

Our preferred approach to the patient requiring nutritional support for planned neoadjuvant therapy is laparoscopic jejunostomy placement. This allows for evaluation of the future gastric conduit, direct anatomic assessment of GE junction tumors, and the ability to rule out metastatic peritoneal disease. Thoughtful placement of the jejunostomy will not complicate the future operative approach. In the event of metastatic disease, a gastrostomy can be placed at the same setting to facilitate definitive chemotherapy.

Conclusion

Surgery of the esophagus for malignant disease continues to be challenging despite advances in surgical technique and perioperative management. Appropriate patient evaluation, selection, and optimization in the setting of multimodality therapy are critical to decreasing the overall morbidity and mortality of esophageal surgery for malignant disease.

References

1. Wouters MW, Wijnhoven BP, Karim-Kos HE, et al. High-volume versus low-volume for esophageal resections for cancer: the essential role of case-mix adjustments based on clinical data. Ann Surg Oncol. 2008;15(1):80–7. Accessed 19 Oct 2013.
2. Whooley BP, Law S, Murthy SC, Alexandrou A, Wong J. Analysis of reduced death and complication rates after esophageal resection. Ann Surg. 2001;233(3):338–44. Accessed 19 Oct 2013.
3. Ajani JA, Barthel JS, Bentrem DJ, et al. Esophageal and esophagogastric junction cancers. J Natl Compr Canc Netw. 2011;9(8):830–87. Accessed 1 Nov 2013.
4. Schröder W, Zähringer M, Stippel D, et al. Does celiac trunk stenosis correlate with anastomotic leakage of esophagogastrostomy after esophagectomy? Dis Esophagus. 2002;15(3):232–6. doi:10.1046/j.1442-2050.2002.00252.x. Accessed 24 Oct 2013.
5. Murthy SC, Law S, Whooley BP, Alexandrou A, Chu K, Wong J. Atrial fibrillation after esophagectomy is a marker for postoperative morbidity and mortality. J Thorac Cardiovasc Surg. 2003;126(4):1162–7. doi:10.1016/S0022-5223(03)00974-7. Accessed 14 Aug 2013.
6. Ojima T, Iwahashi M, Nakamori M, et al. Atrial fibrillation after esophageal cancer surgery: an analysis of 207 consecutive patients. Surg Today. 2014;44: 839–47. doi:10.1007/s00595-013-0616-3. Accessed 19 Oct 2013
7. Rao VP, Addae-Boateng E, Barua A, Martin-Ucar AE, Duffy JP. Age and neo-adjuvant chemotherapy increase the risk of atrial fibrillation following oesophagectomy. Eur J Cardiothorac Surg. 2012;42(3):438–43. doi:10.1093/ejcts/ezs085. Accessed 19 Oct 2013.
8. Ma J, Wang Y, Zhao Y, et al. Atrial fibrillation after surgery for esophageal carcinoma: clinical and prognostic significance. World J Gastroenterol. 2006;12(3): 449–52. Accessed 19 Oct 2013.
9. Tisdale JE, Wroblewski HA, Wall DS, et al. A randomized, controlled study of amiodarone for prevention of atrial fibrillation after transthoracic esophagectomy.

J Thorac Cardiovasc Surg. 2010;140(1):45–51. doi:10.1016/j.jtcvs.2010.01.026. Accessed 19 Oct 2013.

10. Fleisher LA, Beckman JA, Brown KA, et al. ACC/AHA 2007 guidelines on perioperative cardiovascular evaluation and care for noncardiac surgery: executive summary – a report of the American College of Cardiology/American Heart Association task force on practice guidelines (Writing Committee to revise the 2002 guidelines on perioperative cardiovascular evaluation for noncardiac surgery). Circulation. 2007;116(17):1971–96. doi:10.1161/CIRCULATIONAHA.107.185700. Accessed 26 Oct 2013.

11. Forshaw MJ, Strauss DC, Davies AR, et al. Is cardiopulmonary exercise testing a useful test before esophagectomy? Ann Thorac Surg. 2008;85(1):294–9. Accessed 19 Oct 2013.

12. London MJ, Hur K, Schwartz GG, Henderson WG. Association of perioperative ß-blockade with mortality and cardiovascular morbidity following major noncardiac surgery. JAMA. 2013;309(16):1704–13. doi:10.1001/jama.2013.4135. Accessed 19 Oct 2013.

13. Chopra V, Wesorick DH, Sussman JB, et al. Effect of perioperative statins on death, myocardial infarction, atrial fibrillation, and length of stay: a systematic review and meta-analysis. Arch Surg. 2012;147(2):181–9. Accessed 19 Oct 2013.

14. Kuwano H, Sumiyoshi K, Sonoda K, et al. Relationship between preoperative assessment of organ function and postoperative morbidity in patients with oesophageal cancer. Eur J Surg. 1998;164(8):581–6. doi:10.1080/110241598750005679. Accessed 14 Aug 2013.

15. Agrelli TF, De Carvalho Ramos M, Guglielminetti R, Silva AA, Crema E. Preoperative ambulatory inspiratory muscle training in patients undergoing esophagectomy. A pilot study. Int Surg. 2012;97(3):198–202. doi:10.9738/CC136.1. Accessed 19 Oct 2013.

16. Inoue J, Ono R, Makiura D, et al. Prevention of postoperative pulmonary complications through intensive preoperative respiratory rehabilitation in patients with esophageal cancer. Dis Esophagus. 2013;26(1):68–74. doi:10.1111/j.1442-2050.2012.01336.x. Accessed 24 Oct 2013.

17. Akutsu Y, Matsubara H. Perioperative management for the prevention of postoperative pneumonia with esophageal surgery. Ann Thorac Cardiovasc Surg. 2009;15(5):280–5. Accessed 26 Oct 2013.

18. Biere SS, Van Berge Henegouwen MI, Maas KW, et al. Minimally invasive versus open oesophagectomy for patients with oesophageal cancer: a multicentre, open-label, randomised controlled trial. Lancet. 2012;379(9829):1887–92. doi:10.1016/S0140-6736(12)60516-9. Accessed 21 Aug 2013.

19. Lu M, Liu Y, Wu Y, Kao C, Liu H, Hsieh M. Is it safe to perform esophagectomy in esophageal cancer patients combined with liver cirrhosis? Interact Cardiovasc Thorac Surg. 2005;4(5):423–5. Accessed 19 Oct 2013.

20. Tachibana M, Kotoh T, Kinugasa S, et al. Esophageal cancer with cirrhosis of the liver: results of

esophagectomy in 18 consecutive patients. Ann Surg Oncol. 2000;7(10):758–63. Accessed 22 Oct 2013.

21. Orringer MB. Editorial: Age does not preclude an esophagectomy··· if only it were that simple. Ann Surg Oncol. 2010;17(6):1487–9. doi:10.1245/s10434-010-0989-0. Accessed 20 Aug 2013.

22. Pultrum BB, Bosch DJ, Nijsten MW, et al. Extended esophagectomy in elderly patients with esophageal cancer: minor effect of age alone in determining the postoperative course and survival. Ann Surg Oncol. 2010;17(6):1572–80. doi:10.1245/s10434-010-0966-7. Accessed 20 Aug 2013.

23. Markar SR, Karthikesalingam A, Thrumurthy S, Ho A, Muallem G, Low DE. Systematic review and pooled analysis assessing the association between elderly age and outcome following surgical resection of esophageal malignancy. Dis Esophagus. 2013;26(3):250–62. doi:10.1111/j.1442-2050.2012.01353.x. Accessed 2 Nov 2013.

24. Partridge JSL, Harari D, Dhesi JK. Frailty in the older surgical patient: a review. Age Ageing. 2012;41(2):142–7. doi:10.1093/ageing/afr182. Accessed 2 Nov 2013.

25. Revenig LM, Canter DJ, Taylor MD, et al. Too frail for surgery? Initial results of a large multidisciplinary prospective study examining preoperative variables predictive of poor surgical outcomes. J Am Coll Surg. 2013;217(4):665–70.e1. doi:10.1016/j.jamcollsurg.2013.06.012. Accessed 4 Nov 2013.

26. Hodari A, Hammoud ZT, Borgi JF, Tsiouris A, Rubinfeld IS. Assessment of morbidity and mortality after esophagectomy using a modified frailty index. Ann Thorac Surg. 2013;96:1240–5. doi:10.1016/j.athoracsur.2013.05.051. Accessed 17 Oct 2013.

27. Owers CE, Abbas Y, Ackroyd R, Barron N, Khan M. Perioperative optimization of patients undergoing bariatric surgery. J Obes. 2012;2012:781546. doi:10.1155/2012/781546. Accessed 4 Nov 2013.

28. Donohoe CL, Feeney C, Carey MF, Reynolds JV. Perioperative evaluation of the obese patient. J Clin Anesth. 2011;23(7):575–86. doi:10.1016/j.jclinane.2011.06.005. Accessed 12 Nov 2013.

29. Underwood P, Askari R, Hurwitz S, Chamarthi B, Garg R. Preoperative A1C and clinical outcomes in patients with diabetes mellitus undergoing major noncardiac surgical procedures. Diabetes Care. 2014;37(3):611–6. doi:10.2337/dc13-1929.

30. Mullen JT, Davenport DL, Hutter MM, et al. Impact of body mass index on perioperative outcomes in patients undergoing major intra-abdominal cancer surgery. Ann Surg Oncol. 2008;15(8):2164–72. doi:10.1245/s10434-008-9990-2. Accessed 11 Oct 2013.

31. Kassis ES, Kosinski AS, Ross Jr P, Koppes KE, Donahue JM, Daniel VC. Predictors of anastomotic leak after esophagectomy: an analysis of the society of thoracic surgeons general thoracic database. Ann Thorac Surg. 2013. doi:10.1016/j.athoracsur.2013.07.119. Accessed 27 Oct 2013.

32. Bhayani NH, Gupta A, Dunst CM, Kurian AA, Halpin VJ, Swanström LL. Does morbid obesity worsen outcomes after esophagectomy? Ann Thorac Surg. 2013;95(5):

1756–61. doi:10.1016/j.athoracsur.2013.01.015. Accessed 27 Oct 2013.

33. Kayani B, Okabayashi K, Ashrafian H, et al. Does obesity affect outcomes in patients undergoing esophagectomy for cancer? A meta-analysis. World J Surg. 2012;36(8):1785–95. doi:10.1007/s00268-012-1582-4. Accessed 27 Oct 2013.

34. Melis M, Weber J, Shridhar R, et al. Body mass index and perioperative complications after oesophagectomy for adenocarcinoma: a systematic database review. BMJ Open. 2013;3(5). doi: 10.1136/bmjopen-2012-001336. Accessed 11 Oct 2013.

35. Scarpa M, Cagol M, Bettini S, et al. Overweight patients operated on for cancer of the esophagus survive longer than normal-weight patients. J Gastrointest Surg. 2013;17(2):218–27. doi:10.1007/s11605-012-2023-2. Accessed 27 Oct 2013.

36. Kilic A, Schuchert MJ, Pennathur A, et al. Impact of obesity on perioperative outcomes of minimally invasive esophagectomy. Ann Thorac Surg. 2009;87(2):412–5. doi:10.1016/j.athoracsur.2008.10.072. Accessed 11 Oct 2013.

37. Verhage RJJ, Van Der Horst S, Van Der Sluis PC, Lolkema MP, Van Hillegersberg R. Risk of thromboembolic events after perioperative chemotherapy versus surgery alone for esophageal adenocarcinoma. Ann Surg Oncol. 2012;19(2):684–92. doi:10.1245/s10434-011-2005-8. Accessed 20 Aug 2013.

38. Teman NR, Silski L, Zhao L, et al. Thromboembolic events before esophagectomy for esophageal cancer do not result in worse outcomes. Ann Thorac Surg. 2012;94(4):1118–25. doi:10.1016/j.athoracsur.2012.05.109. Accessed 20 Aug 2013.

39. Bakshi P, Partridge J. Indications for and use of inferior vena cava filters in the preoperative phase. BMJ (Online). 2013;347(7928). doi: 10.1136/bmj.f5807. Accessed 4 Nov 2013.

40. Chang AC, Lee JS, Sawicki KT, Pickens A, Orringer MB. Outcomes after esophagectomy in patients with prior antireflux or hiatal hernia surgery. Ann Thorac Surg. 2010;89(4):1015–23. doi:10.1016/j.athoracsur.2009.10.052. Accessed 20 Aug 2013.

41. Carter YM, Bond CD, Benjamin S, Marshall MB. Minimally invasive transhiatal esophagectomy after thoracotomy. Ann Thorac Surg. 2013;95(2):e41–3. doi:10.1016/j.athoracsur.2012.07.084. Accessed 21 Aug 2013.

42. Rossidis G, Browning R, Hochwald SN, Abbas H, Kim T, Ben-David K. Minimally invasive esophagectomy is safe in patients with previous gastric bypass. Surg Obes Relat Dis. 2014;10(1):95–100. doi:10.1016/j.soard.2013.03.015. Accessed 11 Oct 2013.

43. Bower MR, Martin II RC. Nutritional management during neoadjuvant therapy for esophageal cancer. J Surg Oncol. 2009;100(1):82–7. doi:10.1002/jso.21289. Accessed 15 Aug 2013.

44. Nitenberg G, Raynard B. Nutritional support of the cancer patient: issues and dilemmas. Crit Rev Oncol Hematol. 2000;34(3):137–68. doi:10.1016/S1040-8428(00)00048-2. Accessed 12 Nov 2013.

45. Perioperative total parenteral nutrition in surgical patients. N Engl J Med. 1991;325(8):525–32. Accessed 2 Nov 2013.

46. Sultan J, Griffin SM, Di Franco F, et al. Randomized clinical trial of omega-3 fatty acid-supplemented enteral nutrition versus standard enteral nutrition in patients undergoing oesophagogastric cancer surgery. Br J Surg. 2012;99(3):346–55. doi:10.1002/bjs.7799. Accessed 26 Oct 2013.

47. Zhang Y, Gu Y, Guo T, Li Y, Cai H. Perioperative immunonutrition for gastrointestinal cancer: a systematic review of randomized controlled trials. Surg Oncol. 2012;21(2):e87–95. doi:10.1016/j.suronc.2012.01.002. Accessed 26 Oct 2013.

48. Nespoli L, Coppola S, Gianotti L. The role of the enteral route and the composition of feeds in the nutritional support of malnourished surgical patients. Nutrients. 2012;4(9):1230–6. doi:10.3390/nu4091230. Accessed 26 Oct 2013.

49. Abunnaja S, Cuviello A, Sanchez JA. Enteral and parenteral nutrition in the perioperative period: state of the art. Nutrients. 2013;5(2):608–23. doi:10.3390/nu5020608 Accessed 26 Oct 2013.

50. Miyata H, Yano M, Yasuda T, et al. Randomized study of clinical effect of enteral nutrition support during neoadjuvant chemotherapy on chemotherapy-related toxicity in patients with esophageal cancer. Clin Nutr. 2012;31(3):330–6. doi:10.1016/j.clnu.2011.11.002. Accessed 12 Nov 2013.

51. Schattner M. Enteral nutritional support of the patient with cancer: route and role. J Clin Gastroenterol. 2003;36(4):297–302. doi:10.1097/00004836-200304000-00004. Accessed 12 Nov 2013.

52. Margolis M, Alexander P, Trachiotis GD, et al. Percutaneous endoscopic gastrostomy before multimodality therapy in patients with esophageal cancer. Ann Thorac Surg. 2003;76(5):1694–8. doi:10.1016/S0003-4975(02)04890-7. Accessed 14 Aug 2013.

53. Ellrichmann M, Sergeev P, Bethge J, et al. Prospective evaluation of malignant cell seeding after percutaneous endoscopic gastrostomy in patients with oropharyngeal/esophageal cancers. Endoscopy. 2013;45(7):526–31. doi:10.1055/s-0033-1344023. Accessed 27 Oct 2013.

54. Tessier W, Piessen G, Briez N, Boschetto A, Sergent G, Mariette C. Percutaneous radiological gastrostomy in esophageal cancer patients: a feasible and safe access for nutritional support during multimodal therapy. Surg Endosc. 2013;27(2):633–41. doi:10.1007/s00464-012-2506-y. Accessed 4 Oct 2013.

55. Van Overhagen H, Schipper J. Percutaneous jejunostomy. Semin Intervent Radiol. 2004;21(3):199–204. doi:10.1055/s-2004-860878. Accessed 5 Nov 2013.

56. Ben-David K, Kim T, Caban AM, Rossidis G, Rodriguez SS, Hochwald SN. Pre-therapy laparoscopic feeding jejunostomy is safe and effective in patients undergoing minimally invasive esophagectomy for cancer. J Gastrointest Surg. 2013;17(8):1352–8. doi:10.1007/s11605-013-2231-4. Accessed 27 Oct 2013.

57. Krokidis M, Burke C, Spiliopoulos S, et al. The use of biodegradable stents in malignant oesophageal strictures

for the treatment of dysphagia before neoadjuvant treatment or radical radiotherapy: a feasibility study. Cardiovasc Intervent Radiol. 2013;36(4):1047–54. doi:10.1007/s00270-012-0503-0. Accessed 27 Oct 2013.

58. Pellen MG, Sabri S, Razack A, Gilani SQ, Jain PK. Safety and efficacy of self-expanding removable metal esophageal stents during neoadjuvant chemotherapy for resectable esophageal cancer. Dis Esophagus. 2012;25(1):48–53. doi:10.1111/j.1442-2050.2011.01206.x. Accessed 4 Oct 2013.

59. Webb M, Griffin SM, Shenfine J. Self-expanding esophageal stents and neoadjuvant therapy. Ann Surg Oncol. 2011;18(1):286. doi:10.1245/s10434-010-1096-y. Accessed 5 Oct 2013.

60. Siddiqui AA, Sarkar A, Beltz S, et al. Placement of fully covered self-expandable metal stents in patients with locally advanced esophageal cancer before neoadjuvant therapy. Gastrointest Endosc. 2012;76(1):44–51. doi:10.1016/j.gie.2012.02.036. Accessed 15 Aug 2013.

Pathogenesis of Gastric Cancer

Fátima Carneiro and Heike I. Grabsch

Introduction

The vast majority of malignant neoplasms of the stomach are adenocarcinomas. Non-epithelial tumors of the stomach include lymphomas, neuroendocrine and soft tissue tumors. In this chapter, we will focus on gastric (adeno)carcinoma (GC).

GC represents a morphological, biologically and genetically heterogeneous group of tumors with multifactorial etiologies [1].

Most GCs are sporadic. However, familial clustering is observed in about 10 % of sporadic GC. Hereditary GC accounts for 1–3 % of cases and two hereditary syndromes have been described – hereditary diffuse type gastric cancer (HDGC) and gastric adenocarcinoma and proximal polyposis of the stomach (GAPPS).

Epidemiology

Despite a steady decline in GC incidence at a rate of approximately 5 % per year since the 1950s [2], GC is still the fifth most common cancer worldwide. In 2012, almost three quarters of new GCs occurred in Asia, and more than two fifths occurred in China [3]. Age-standardized GC incidence rates are twice as high in males compared to females and show prominent geographical variation ranging from 3.9 in Northern Africa to 42.4 in Eastern Asia per 100,000 males [4].

Over the past 50 years, incidence and mortality rates of the non-cardia GC have been decreasing in almost all countries, whereas incidence rates of GC at the cardia have been stable or increasing [3].

Etiology and Risk Factors of Gastric Adenocarcinoma

Helicobacter pylori (*H. pylori*) infection plays a major role in contributing to an increased risk of GC. Most non-cardia GCs develop from a background of *H. pylori* infected mucosa [5]. Factors associated with the pathogenicity of *H. pylori* include virulence factors such as cagA in the cag pathogenicity island and vacA, the vacuolating cytotoxin [6]. Interestingly, strains producing the cagA protein are associated with a greater risk of developing cancer of the distal stomach [7, 6]. Although the risk of GC has been related to the presence of a vacA genotype in some European countries and North America, such a relationship has not been observed in East Asia suggesting that consequences of the vacA genotype may be dependent on the geographical region.

F. Carneiro, MD, PhD (✉)
Department of Pathology, IPATIMUP and Medical Faculty, Centro Hospitalar de São João,
Rua Dr. Roberto Frias S/N, Porto 4200-465, Portugal
e-mail: fcarneiro@ipatimup.pt

H.I. Grabsch, MD, PhD, FRCPath (*)
Department of Pathology, Maastricht University Medical Center, P. Debyelaan 25, 6202 AZ Maastricht, The Netherlands
e-mail: Heike.Grabsch@mumc.nl

S.N. Hochwald, M. Kukar (eds.), *Minimally Invasive Foregut Surgery for Malignancy: Principles and Practice*,
DOI 10.1007/978-3-319-09342-0_6, © Springer International Publishing Switzerland 2015

The development of GC after *H. pylori* infection has been considered a multistep process progressing from chronic active pangastritis or corpus-predominant gastritis to increasing loss of gastric glands (atrophy), replacement of the normal mucosa by intestinal metaplasia, and malignant transformation [8]. However, corpus-predominant gastritis with multifocal gastric atrophy and hypochlorhydria or achlorhydria is only seen in approximately 1 % of subjects infected with *H. pylori*, and most *H. pylori* infected individuals will remain asymptomatic. Only 1–5 % of the *H. pylori* infected population will develop GC indicating a role for other causative agents and/or host factors. Individual genetic GC susceptibility appears to involve a relatively large number of different genes including those involved in the protection of the gastric mucosa against damaging agents and in inflammatory response, such as polymorphisms of the interleukin-1β (IL1B) gene [9, 10].

It has been estimated that 10 % of GC are associated with Epstein Barr virus (EBV) infection [11]. Considering the worldwide GC incidence, EBV-associated GC is the largest group of carcinomas within all EBV-associated malignancies.

Certain dietary habits have been associated with an increased risk of GC [12]. These include high intakes of salt-preserved and/or smoked foods as well as low intakes of fresh fruits and vegetables. A recent meta-analysis suggested a potential 50 % higher risk of GC associated with intake of pickled vegetables but interestingly indicated a potential stronger association between GC and intake of pickled vegetables for patients in Korea and China [13]. Meat consumption, specifically red meat and processed meat, has been associated with an increased risk of GC in the distal stomach, whereas a high consumption of fruits, vegetables, cereals, nuts and seeds, seafood, and olive oil was shown to be associated with a significant reduction in the risk of developing GC. There is currently no conclusive evidence for an association between alcohol consumption and GC.

Smoking has also been associated with an increased risk of GC depending on the number of cigarettes and the duration of smoking; the epidemiological association is not explicable by bias or confounding factors [14]. Smoking also appears to potentiate the carcinogenic effect of infection with cagA-positive *H. pylori*.

Other clinicopathological conditions which have been associated with an increased risk of GC are autoimmune gastritis, peptic ulcer disease, hypertrophic gastropathies, gastric stump (operated stomach), and gastric polyps.

Precursor Lesions of Gastric Carcinoma

Gastric dysplasia (synonym: intraepithelial neoplasia (IEN)) is considered the precursor lesion of the so-called intestinal type of gastric carcinoma and can have a flat, slightly depressed, or polypoid growth pattern. The prevalence of gastric dysplasia varies between 20 % in high-risk areas and 4 % in Western countries where gastric carcinoma is less common [15]. Dysplasia is more frequent in males, patients over 70 years of age and most commonly affects the lesser curve and the antrum.

Gastric dysplasia is characterized by cellular atypia and disorganized glandular architecture. Recognition of gastric dysplasia and determination of its grade is critical because it predicts both, the risk of malignant transformation and the risk of metachronous gastric cancer.

In an attempt to standardize the terminology used to describe the grade of dysplasia and distinguish it from adenocarcinoma, several proposals including the Padova and Vienna classifications have been made [16–18].

According to the most recent WHO classification [1], dysplasia is graded as high or low grade. Low-grade dysplasia/IEN shows minimal architectural disarray and only mild to moderate cytological atypia. The nuclei are elongated and basally located, and mitotic activity is mild to moderate (Fig. 6.1a). High-grade dysplasia/IEN shows pronounced architectural disarray and severe cytological atypia with numerous mitoses, which can be atypical (Fig. 6.1b). The cell nuclei in high-grade dysplasia are typically no longer basally located and may contain prominent nucleoli.

Low-grade dysplasia progresses to adenocarcinoma in up 23 % of cases within 10 months to

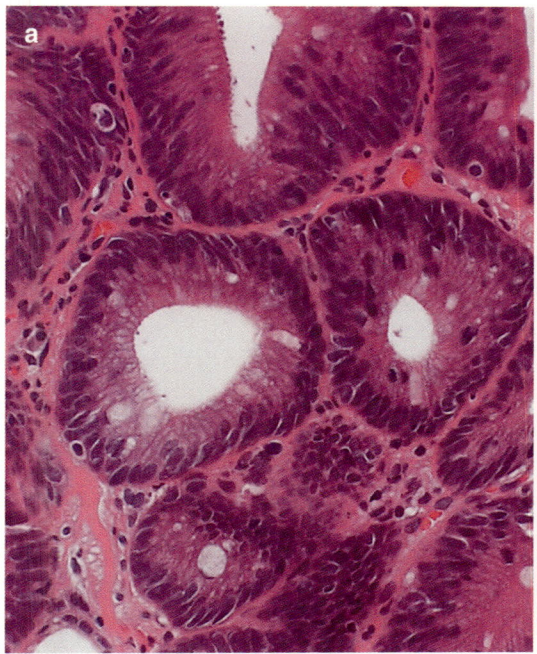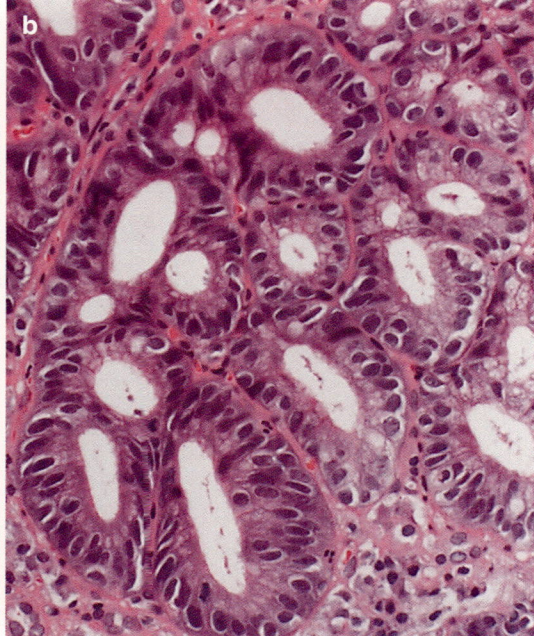

Fig. 6.1 Precursor lesion of intestinal type gastric cancer – dysplasia. (**a**) Low-grade dysplasia. Pseudostratification of nuclei. Nuclei are elongated and mostly basally orientated. Few mitotic figures. (**b**) High-grade dysplasia. Crowding of nuclei. Nuclei are larger and rounder and vary more in size and shape. Loss of basal orientation of nuclei in many cells. Basal membrane around individual glands still intact

4 years, whereas malignant transformation of high-grade dysplasia has been reported to occur in 60–80 % of cases.

It is noteworthy that precursor lesions of diffuse type GC are not well characterized, except for hereditary diffuse type GC (see below under the section on genetic predisposition and hereditary syndromes).

Pathology of Gastric Adenocarcinoma

Macroscopy

GC can present at an early or advanced disease stage. "Early gastric carcinoma" (EGC) is defined as a carcinoma which has infiltrated the mucosa or submucosa regardless of the presence or absence of lymph node metastases [19, 20]. Conversely, GCs infiltrating into the muscularis propria and beyond are defined as "advanced."

EGCs are classified into three types based on the endoscopic appearance according to the Paris classification: type I (protruded), polypoid growth (subcategorized into Ip (pedunculated) and Is (sessile)); type II (superficial), non-polypoid growth (subcategorized into type IIa (slightly elevated), type IIb (flat), and type IIc (slightly depressed)); and type III, excavated growth [21] (Figs. 6.2 and 6.3).

The macroscopic appearance of advanced GC is classified using the Borrmann classification [22] which divides GC into four distinct types: type I, polypoid type; type II, fungating; type III, ulcerated; and type IV, diffusely infiltrative (Fig. 6.4).

Microscopy

While the macroscopic appearances are different between early and advanced GC, the histological appearances are similar. Two major histological

Fig. 6.2 Paris classification of early gastric cancer: type I (protruding), *Ip* pedunculated and *Is* sessile; type II (superficial), *IIa* elevated, *IIb* flat, and *IIc* slightly depressed; type III (ulcerated)

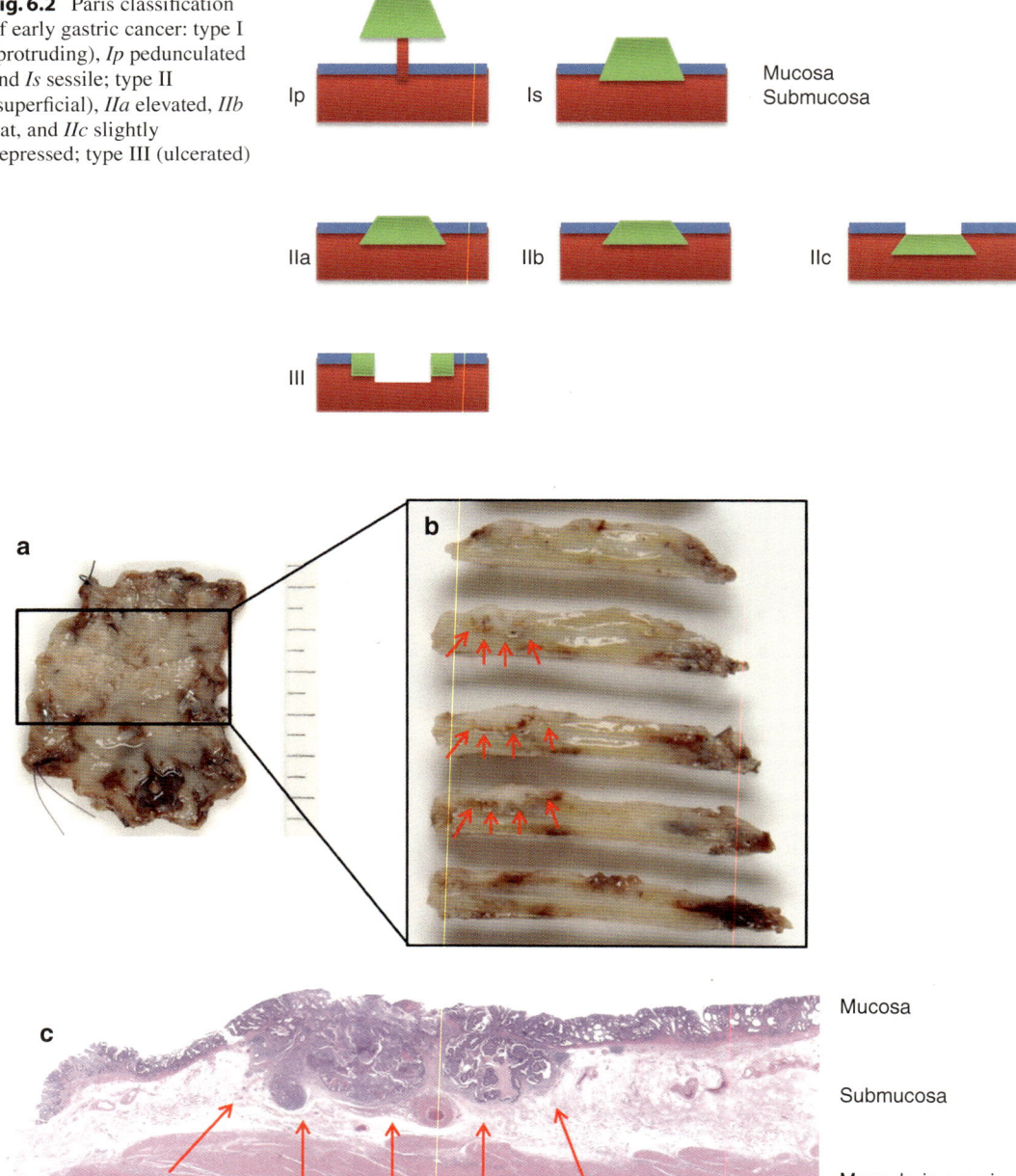

Fig. 6.3 Endoscopic resection (ESD) of a well-differentiated early gastric cancer. (**a**) Macroscopy of the endoscopic resection specimen after fixation with a superficially elevated lesion (Paris type IIa). (**b**) Macroscopy of the serial cross sections through the lesion showing a tumor which is infiltrating the submucosa (*red arrows*). Deep resection margin located in the muscularis propria ensuring complete (curative) resection of the tumor. (**c**) Microscopy of the well-differentiated adenocarcinoma infiltrating the submucosa (pT1b, *red arrow*) and adjacent intramucosal adenocarcinoma (Images courtesy of Dr. T. Arai, Tokyo)

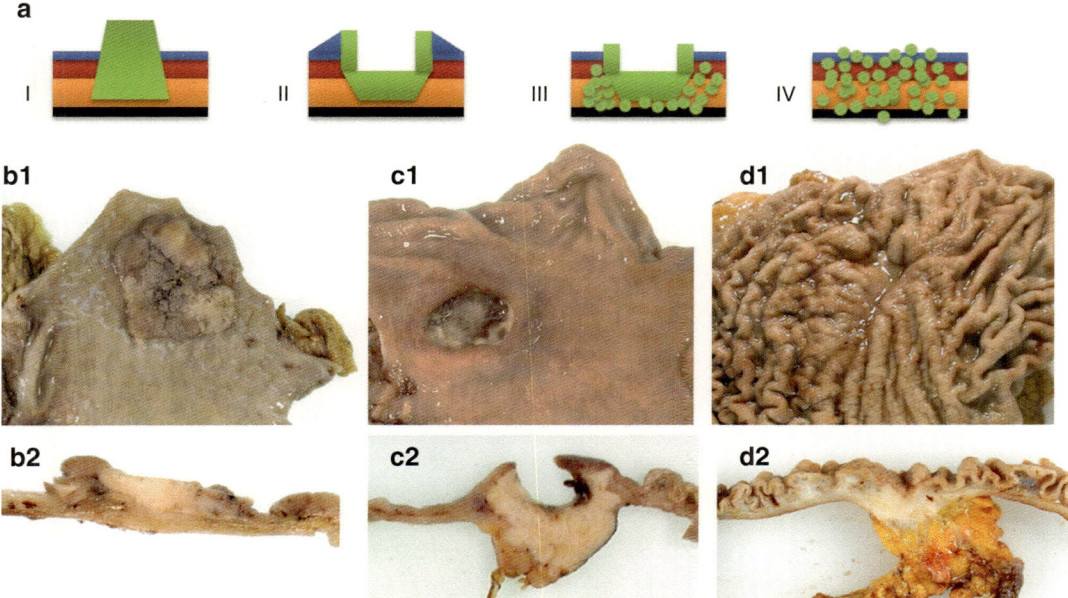

Fig. 6.4 Macroscopy of advanced gastric cancer. (**a**) Borrmann classification. *I* polypoid type, *II* fungating type, *III* ulcerated type, and *IV* diffusely infiltrative. (**b**) Polypoid gastric cancer (type I) – (**b1**) macroscopy of the mucosal surface showing a large polypoid lesion and (**b2**) cross section showing tumor infiltrating into the superficial layer of the muscularis propria. (**c**) Ulcerated gastric cancer (type III) – (**c1**) deep ulceration visible macroscopically from the mucosal surface and (**c2**) infiltration into the attached lesser omentum visible macroscopically on cross sectioning. (**d**) Diffusely infiltrative gastric cancer (type IV) – (**d1**) diffuse thickening of the gastric folds visible on macroscopy of the mucosal surface and (**d2**) diffuse infiltration of the whole depth of the wall into the perigastric fat on cross section

GC subtypes (intestinal type GC and diffuse type GC) have been described by Laurén [23] which have different clinicopathological profiles and molecular pathogenesis and often occur in distinct epidemiologic settings.

According to the World Health Organization (WHO) [1], GCs are classified as tubular, papillary, mucinous, poorly cohesive (with or without signet ring cells), and mixed (Fig. 6.5). Tubular and papillary carcinomas roughly correspond to the intestinal type and poorly cohesive carcinomas correspond to the diffuse type according to Laurén's classification (Table 6.1). The Laurén and WHO classifications are the ones most commonly used outside of Japan. In Japan, the recommended histological typing is similar but not 100 % identical to the WHO classification [24].

Nakamura's classification into differentiated and undifferentiated subtype is used together with the size of the lesion and presence or absence of ulceration to decide whether a lesion can be treated endoscopically [25, 26]. Apart from the classifications based on tumor morphology, GC can be classified on the basis of the presence or absence of cell differentiation markers – MUC5AC and trefoil peptide TFF1 (markers of surface gastric epithelium (foveolar cells)), MUC6 and trefoil peptide TFF2 (markers of mucus neck cell, pyloric gland, and Brunner's gland cells), and MUC2, CDX-2, and CD10 (markers of intestinal goblet cells) – into four phenotypes: (1) gastric, (2) mixed gastric and intestinal, (3) intestinal, and (4) unclassifiable or null phenotype which does not express any of these markers [27–29].

Staging and Prognosis of Advanced Gastric Cancer

Staging

The staging for carcinoma of the stomach was substantially modified in 2009 as detailed in Table 6.2. Major changes included the

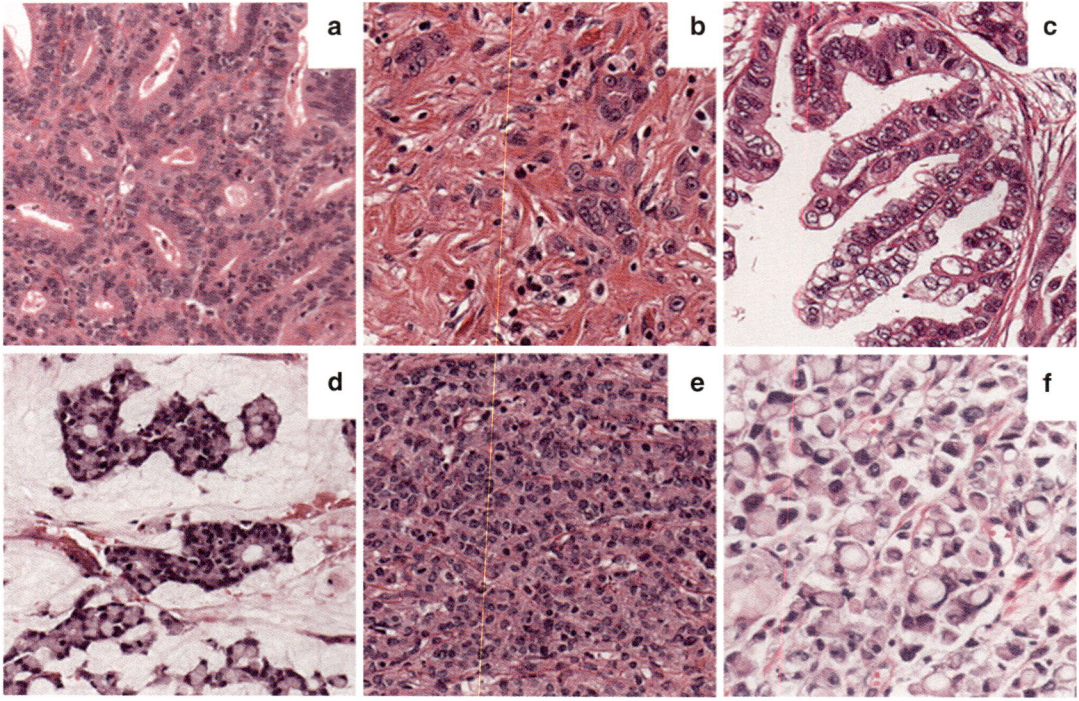

Fig. 6.5 Histological subtypes of gastric cancer. (**a**) Tubular type (moderately differentiated); (**b**) diffuse type; (**c**) papillary type; (**d**) mucinous type; (**e**) undifferentiated, solid type; and (**f**) poorly cohesive type with signet ring cells

Table 6.1 Classification of GC

Laurén classification	World Health Organization 2010	Japanese classification 2011	Nakamura classification
Intestinal type	Papillary	Papillary	Differentiated type
	Tubular	Tubular 1	
		Tubular 2	
	Mucinous	Mucinous	
Diffuse type	Poorly cohesive, including signet ring cell carcinoma and other variants	Signet ring cell	Undifferentiated type
		Poorly differentiated, non-solid type	
Mixed (intestinal and diffuse type)	Mixed type (tubular/papillary and poorly cohesive/signet ring)	–	–
Indeterminate type	Undifferentiated	Poorly differentiated, solid type	
	Adenosquamous		
	Medullary		Undifferentiated type
	Hepatoid		

subdivision of T1 cancers into T1a (mucosa) and T1b (submucosa), the renaming of T2a (muscularis propria) as T2 and T2b (subserosa) as T3, and the subdivision of T4 (serosa) into T4a (penetrates serosa) and T4b (invades adjacent structures). Consequently, the categorization of the T (depth of invasion) is now uniform throughout the gastrointestinal tract, whereas differences remain for the categorization of the N (presence or absence of regional

Table 6.2 TNM classification of gastric carcinoma

T – Primary tumor

TX Primary tumor cannot be assessed

T0 No evidence of primary tumor

Tis Carcinoma in situ: intraepithelial tumor without invasion of the lamina propria, high-grade dysplasia

T1 Tumor invades lamina propria, muscularis mucosae, or submucosa

    T1a Tumor invades lamina propria or muscularis mucosae

    T1b Tumor invades submucosa

T2 Tumor invades muscularis propria

T3 Tumor invades subserosa

T4 Tumor perforates serosa or invades adjacent structures

    T4a Tumor perforates serosa

    T4b Tumor invades adjacent structures

N – Regional lymph nodes

NX Regional lymph nodes cannot be assessed

N0 No regional lymph node metastasis

N1 Metastasis in 1–2 regional lymph nodes

N2 Metastasis in 3–6 regional lymph nodes

N3 Metastasis in 7 or more regional lymph nodes

    N3a Metastasis in 7–15 regional lymph nodes

    N3b Metastasis in 16 or more regional lymph nodes

M – Distant metastasis

M0 No distant metastasis

M1 Distant metastasis

From Edge et al. [20] with permission

lymph node metastases). The N categories for GC are N0 (no regional lymph node metastasis), N1 (1 to 2 lymph node metastases), N2 (3 to 6 lymph node metastases), N3a (7 to 15 lymph node metastases), and N3b (metastases in 16 or more regional lymph nodes) [19, 20].

Spreading and Prognosis

Gastric carcinomas can spread by (i) direct extension to adjacent organs, (ii) lymphatic invasion, (iii) blood vessel invasion, and/or (iv) peritoneal dissemination. Intestinal type GCs preferentially metastasize hematogenously to the liver, whereas diffuse type GCs preferentially metastasize to peritoneal surfaces [1]. GCs with mixed histological phenotype exhibit the metastatic patterns of both types.

A recent meta-analysis comparing survival rates after gastrectomy between GC patients from the West and the East from patients recruited into large randomized controlled clinical trials showed an association between type of surgical resection performed in the East and improved survival [30]. The known difference in surgical techniques between the East and the West is one potential variable that may be responsible for discrepancy in outcomes. Noguchi et al. [31] reported a survival difference between high-volume centers in the USA and Japan which was no longer apparent after adjusting for tumor location. Verdecchia et al. [32] demonstrated that the survival of Italian GC patients was inferior to that of Japanese GC patients and that this survival difference disappeared after adjusting for stage. Bollschweiler et al. [33] compared the survival of Japanese and German GC patients and concluded that the country itself was a prognostic factor. Higher frequency of early stage GC and more accurate staging have also been associated with improved survival in Japan compared with Western nations [34].

Early and advanced GCs differ in prognosis. Japanese patients with EGC have an excellent prognosis with a 5-year survival rate exceeding 90 % after surgical treatment. Nevertheless, approximately 2 % of EGC recur after curative resection and lymph node metastases occur in 2–3 % of intramucosal carcinomas [35, 36] and 20–30 % of submucosal carcinomas [37]. Risk factors for lymph node metastasis in EGC include age at time of diagnosis (the younger, the more frequent the lymph node metastases), size greater 20 mm, depressed macroscopic type, grade of differentiation, presence of an ulcer or scar, lymphatic channel invasion, and submucosal invasion by more than 500 µm [35, 37].

Five-year survival rate of advanced GC, the most frequent type in the West, is around 23 % when treated by surgery alone and around 36 % when treatment includes perioperative chemotherapy [38]. For advanced GC, depth of infiltration into the wall (T category of the TNM classification), number of lymph node metastases (N category of the TNM classification), and presence of distant metastases (M category of the TNM classification) remain the strongest

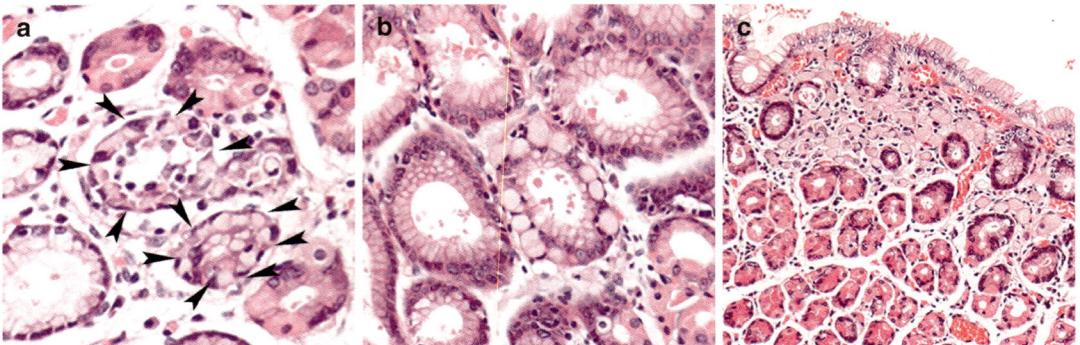

Fig. 6.6 Development model for diffuse type GC in *CDH1* germline mutation carriers encompassing: (**a**) in situ carcinoma, (**b**) pagetoid spread of signet ring cells, and (**c**) early intramucosal carcinoma. The *arrow heads* highlight a gland that shows *in situ* carcinoma

prognostic indicators [19, 20]. Lymphatic and venous invasion are also predictors of poor survival in GC. Perineural invasion correlates with T stage and tumor size and may serve as a marker of advanced disease [39].

Genetic Predisposition and Hereditary Syndromes

First-degree relatives of patients with GC are almost three times more likely to develop GC themselves compared to the general population which has been partially attributed to *H. pylori* infection and to the potential role of *IL-1* gene polymorphisms.

Genome-wide association studies have implicated the prostate stem cell antigen (PSCA) gene and the mucin 1 (MUC1) gene as GC susceptibility factors. Approximately 95 % of the Japanese population have at least one of the two risk genotypes, and approximately 56 % of the population have both risk genotypes [40]. Hereditary GC accounts for 1–3 % of GC, and two hereditary syndromes have been described – hereditary diffuse gastric cancer (HDGC) and gastric adenocarcinoma and proximal polyposis of the stomach (GAPPS).

Hereditary Diffuse Gastric Cancer (HDGC)

On the basis of clinical criteria, the International Gastric Cancer Linkage Consortium defined

families with HDGC syndrome as families meeting one of two criteria: (i) two or more documented cases of diffuse type GC in first- or second-degree relatives with at least one of them diagnosed before the age of 50 years or (ii) three or more documented cases of diffuse GC in first- or second-degree relatives independent of the age at diagnosis [41]. Women in these families have an elevated risk of lobular breast cancer. The criteria for genetic testing were updated in 2010 [42]. In several HDGC families, a higher incidence of orofacial clefts has been noted [43, 44].

Alterations of the *CDH1* gene, which encodes E-cadherin, constitute the genetic causal event in HDGC patients [45]. In clinically defined HDGC patients, *CDH1* germline mutations are detected in 30–40 % of cases [42]. Seventy-five to eighty percent of *CDH1* mutations are truncating mutations, and the remaining are missense mutations. In addition, large germline deletions have also been found in HDGC families which tested negative for point mutations [46].

Another rare but so far the only reported alternative to *CDH1* inactivation in HDGC is the presence of germline α-E-catenin mutations [47]. Since α-E-catenin functions in the same complex as E-cadherin, these results call attention to the broader signaling network surrounding these proteins in HDGC.

A development model has been proposed for diffuse type GC in *CDH1* germline mutation carriers encompassing foveolar hyperplasia, precursor (intraepithelial) lesions (*in situ* carcinoma and pagetoid spread of signet ring cells), early intramucosal carcinoma, and advanced cancer [48] (Fig. 6.6).

Genetic counseling is an essential component of the evaluation and management of HDGC patients and informed consent for genetic testing is required [49]. The recommended youngest age at which to offer testing to relatives at risk is not well established. Rare cases of clinically significant diffuse type GC have been reported in affected families before the age of 18, but the overall risk of diffuse type GC before the age of 20 is very low [49].

No therapies other than prophylactic total gastrectomy are currently available for HDGC patients. Since the penetrance of HDGC is >80 %, and analysis of gastrectomy specimens suggests that microscopic *foci* of signet ring cells are almost universally present in *CDH1* germline mutation carriers even if the endoscopic examination was unremarkable, prophylactic gastrectomy should be strongly considered [42].

Gastric Adenocarcinoma and Proximal Polyposis of the Stomach (GAPPS)

Recently, a new hereditary syndrome has been identified: gastric adenocarcinoma and proximal polyposis of the stomach, which is characterized by the autosomal dominant transmission of fundic gland polyposis including areas of dysplasia or intestinal type gastric adenocarcinoma restricted to the proximal stomach with no evidence of colorectal or duodenal polyposis or other heritable gastrointestinal cancer syndromes. This syndrome was originally identified in Australian and North American families [50] but has also been reported in Japanese families [51]. The genetic defect behind this syndrome has not yet been identified.

The clinical management of GAPPS families must balance the limitations of endoscopic surveillance, the patient-specific risk of morbidity associated with prophylactic surgery, and the risk of GC within the specific family. All first-degree relatives of affected patients should be advised to have an upper gastrointestinal endoscopy and colonoscopy [50].

Gastric Cancer in Other Hereditary Cancer Syndromes

The risk of GC is also increased in dominantly inherited cancer predisposition syndromes such as familial adenomatous polyposis and Lynch syndrome, as well as in patients with Li–Fraumeni syndrome with germline mutations of TP53 [52].

Molecular Pathology of Gastric Carcinoma

Like most cancers, GC is the result of accumulated genomic changes affecting a number of cellular functions essential for cancer development: self-sufficiency in growth signals, escape from anti-growth signals, resistance to apoptosis, sustained replicative potential, angiogenesis induction, and invasive or metastatic potential. These genomic changes arise through three major pathways: microsatellite instability, chromosomal instability, and a CpG island methylator phenotype.

Furthermore, genetic and epigenetic changes may affect oncogenes and tumor suppressor genes [53]. It seems that some oncogenes and some tumor suppressor genes are preferentially altered in a specific histological subtype of GC, such as *HER2*, *KRAS*, *APC*, and *DCC* in intestinal type GC and *BCL2*, *FGFR2* (formerly *K-SAM*), *CDH1*, and *RB1* in diffuse type GC. Other oncogenes and tumor suppressor genes such as *CTNNB1*, *MET*, *MYC*, *PTEN*, and *TP53* are altered in both histological subtypes (for a review, see Lauwers et al. 2010 [1]).

MicroRNA

Several miRNAs have been shown to be related to certain GC subtypes, GC progression, and potential treatment targets albeit with inconsistent results probably related to small sample sizes [54, 55].

Whole Genome Studies

Modern high-throughput molecular methods are being used with the aim to complement traditional histopathological diagnosis and prognosis prediction in GC and to contribute to a better understanding of the biology of GC at a molecular level.

Zang et al. found an average of 50 mutations/GC mostly affecting genes involved in cell adhesion and chromatin remodeling and identified two new putative tumor suppressor genes, *FAT4* and *ARID1A* [56].

Tan et al. investigated the gene expression profile in a large number of GC cell lines and identified two major genomic subtypes [57]. The genomic subtype classification was concordant with the phenotypic classification according to Laurén in 64 % of GC, suggesting that gene expression studies can lead to the identification of distinct GC subtypes which are not distinguishable based on histology.

Two very recent genome-wide copy number profiling studies using high-resolution SNP arrays have demonstrated the power of modern molecular technology in identifying new clinically relevant subtypes of GC [58, 59]. Both studies identified independently that up to 37 % of GC show high amplifications of genes encoding druggable tyrosine kinase receptor proteins such as *FGFR2*, *HER2*, *EGFR*, and *MET*. Furthermore, these gene amplifications were almost always exclusive emphasizing the molecular heterogeneity of GC and the need to select patient's treatment based on molecular profiles.

References

1. Lauwers GY, Carneiro F, Graham DY, Curado MP, Franceschi S, Montgomery E, Tatematsu M, Hattori T. Gastric carcinoma. In: Bosman FT, Carneiro F, Hruban RH, Theise ND, editors. WHO Classification of Tumours of the Digestive System. 4th ed. Lyon: IARC Press; 2010. p. 48–58.
2. Howson CP, Hiyama T, Wynder EL. The decline in gastric cancer: epidemiology of an unplanned triumph. Epidemiol Rev. 1986;8:1–27.
3. Carneiro F. Stomach cancer. In: Stewart BW, Wild CP, editors. World cancer report 2014. Lyon: IARC Press; 2014. p. 545–57.
4. Ferlay J, Shin HR, Bray F, et al. Estimates of worldwide burden of cancer in 2008: GLOBOCAN 2008. Int J Cancer. 2010;127:2893–917.
5. Fukase K, Kato M, Kikuchi S, et al. Effect of eradication of *Helicobacter pylori* on incidence of metachronous gastric carcinoma after endoscopic resection of early gastric cancer: an open-label, randomized controlled trial. Lancet. 2008;372:392–7.
6. Basso D, Zambon CF, Letley DP, et al. Clinical relevance of Helicobacter pylori cagA and vacA gene polymorphisms. Gastroenterology. 2008;135:91–9.
7. Figueiredo C, Machado JC, Pharoah P, et al. *Helicobacter pylori* and interleukin 1 genotyping: an opportunity to identify high-risk individuals for gastric carcinoma. J Natl Cancer Inst. 2002;94:1680–7.
8. Correa P. *Helicobacter pylori* and gastric carcinogenesis. Am J Surg Pathol. 1995;19 Suppl 1:S37–43.
9. El-Omar EM, Carrington M, Chow W-H, et al. Interleukin-1 polymorphisms associated with increased risk of gastric cancer. Nature. 2000;404:398–402.
10. Machado JC, Figueiredo C, Canedo P, et al. A proinflammatory genetic profile increases the risk for chronic atrophic gastritis and gastric carcinoma. Gastroenterology. 2003;125:364–71.
11. Fukayama M, Ushiku T. Epstein-Barr virus-associated gastric carcinoma. Pathol Res Pract. 2011;207:529–37.
12. World Cancer Research Fund/American Institute for Cancer Research. Food, nutrition, physical activity, and the prevention of cancer: a global perspective. Washington, DC: American Institute for Cancer Research; 2007.
13. Ren JS, Kamangar F, Forman D, Islami F. Pickled food and risk of gastric cancer – a systematic review and meta-analysis of English and Chinese literature. Cancer Epidemiol Biomarkers Prev. 2012;21:905–15.
14. Gonzalez CA, Pera G, Agudo A, et al. Smoking and the risk of gastric cancer in the European Prospective Investigation into Cancer and Nutrition (EPIC). Int J Cancer. 2003;107:629–34.
15. Farinati F, Rugge M, Di Mario F, et al. Early and advanced gastric cancer in the follow-up of moderate and severe gastric dysplasia patients. A prospective study. I.G.G.E.D.–Interdisciplinary Group on Gastric Epithelial Dysplasia. Endoscopy. 1993;25:261–4.
16. Rugge M, Correa P, Dixon MF, et al. Gastric dysplasia: the Padova international classification. Am J Surg Pathol. 2000;24:167–76.
17. Schlemper RJ, Riddell RH, Kato Y, et al. The Vienna classification of gastrointestinal epithelial neoplasia. Gut. 2000;47:251–5.
18. Dixon MF. Gastrointestinal epithelial neoplasia: Vienna revisited. Gut. 2002;51:130–1.
19. Sobin LH, Gospodarowicz MK, Wittekind C. TNM classification of malignant tumors. Oxford: Wiley-Blackwell; 2009.
20. Edge SB, Byrd DR, Compton CC, Fritz AG, Greene FL, Trotti A. AJCC cancer staging manual. New York: Springer; 2009.
21. The Paris endoscopic classification of superficial neoplastic lesions: esophagus, stomach, and colon: November 30 to December 1, 2002. Gastrointest Endosc. 2003;58:S3–43.

22. Borrmann R. Handbuch der speziellen pathologischen Anatomie und Histologie. In: von Henke F, Lubarch O, editors. IV/erster Teil. Berlin, Julius: Springer; 1926. p. 864–71.

23. Lauren P. The two histological main types of gastric carcinoma: diffuse and so-called intestinal-type carcinoma. An attempt at a histo-clinical classification. Acta Pathol Microbiol Scand. 1965;64:31–49.

24. JGCA. Japanese classification of gastric carcinoma, 3rd English edition. Gastric Cancer. 2011;14:101–12.

25. Nakamura K, Sugano H, Takagi K. Carcinoma of the stomach in incipient phase: its histogenesis and histological appearances. Gann. 1968;59:251–8.

26. Ono H. Early gastric cancer: diagnosis, pathology, treatment techniques and treatment outcomes. Eur J Gastroenterol Hepatol. 2006;18:863–6.

27. Machado JC, Nogueira AM, Carneiro F, Reis CA, Sobrinho-Simoes M. Gastric carcinoma exhibits distinct types of cell differentiation: an immunohistochemical study of trefoil peptides (TFF1 and TFF2) and mucins (MUC1, MUC2, MUC5AC, and MUC6). J Pathol. 2000;190:437–43.

28. Kushima R, Vieth M, Borchard F, Stolte M, Mukaisho K, Hattori T. Gastric-type well-differentiated adenocarcinoma and pyloric gland adenoma of the stomach. Gastric Cancer. 2006;9:177–84.

29. Shiroshita H, Watanabe H, Ajioka Y, Watanabe G, Nishikura K, Kitano S. Re-evaluation of mucin phenotypes of gastric minute well-differentiated-type adenocarcinomas using a series of HGM, MUC5AC, MUC6, M-GGMC, MUC2 and CD10 stains. Pathol Int. 2004;54:311–21.

30. Markar SR, Karthikesalingam A, Jackson D, Hanna GB. Long-term survival after gastrectomy for cancer in randomized, controlled oncological trials: comparison between West and East. Ann Surg Oncol. 2013;20:2328–38.

31. Noguchi Y, Yoshikawa T, Tsuburaya A, Motohashi H, Karpeh MS, Brennan MF. Is gastric carcinoma different between Japan and the United States? Cancer. 2000;89:2237–46.

32. Verdecchia A, Mariotto A, Gatta G, Bustamante-Teixeira MT, Ajiki W. Comparison of stomach cancer incidence and survival in four continents. Eur J Cancer. 2003;39:1603–9.

33. Bollschweiler E, Boettcher K, Hoelscher AH, Sasako M, Kinoshita T, Maruyama K, Siewert JR. Is the prognosis for Japanese and German patients with gastric cancer really different? Cancer. 1993;71:2918–25.

34. Reid-Lombardo KM, Gay G, Patel-Parekh L, Ajani JA, Donohue JH. Treatment of gastric adenocarcinoma may differ among hospital types in the United States, a report from the National Cancer Data Base. J Gastrointest Surg. 2007;11:410–20.

35. Yamao T, Shirao K, Ono H, et al. Risk factors for lymph node metastasis from intramucosal gastric carcinoma. Cancer. 1996;77:602–6.

36. Hirasawa T, Gotoda T, Miyata S, et al. Incidence of lymph node metastasis and the feasibility of endoscopic resection for undifferentiated-type early gastric cancer. Gastric Cancer. 2009;12:148–52.

37. Tajima Y, Murakami M, Yamazaki K, et al. Risk factors for lymph node metastasis from gastric cancers with submucosal invasion. Ann Surg Oncol. 2010;17:1597–604.

38. Cunningham D, Allum WH, Stenning SP, et al. Perioperative chemotherapy versus surgery alone for resectable gastroesophageal cancer. N Engl J Med. 2006;355:11–20.

39. Kooby D, Suriawinata A, Klimstra DS, et al. Biologic predictors of survival in node-negative gastric cancer. Ann Surg 2003;237:828–37.

40. Saeki N, Ono H, Sakamoto H, Yoshida T. Genetic factors related to gastric cancer susceptibility identified using a genome-wide association study. Cancer Sci. 2013;104:1–8.

41. Caldas C, Carneiro F, Lynch HT, et al. Familial gastric cancer: overview and guidelines for management. J Med Genet. 1999;36:873–80.

42. Fitzgerald RC, Hardwick R, Huntsman D, et al. International Gastric Cancer Linkage Consortium. Hereditary diffuse gastric cancer: updated consensus guidelines for clinical management and directions for future research. J Med Genet. 2010;47:436–44.

43. Frebourg T, Oliveira C, Hochain P, et al. Cleft lip/palate and CDH1/E-cadherin mutations in families with hereditary diffuse gastric cancer. J Med Genet. 2006;43:138–42.

44. Kluijt I, Siemerink EJ, Ausems MG, et al. CDH1-related hereditary diffuse gastric cancer syndrome: clinical variations and implications for counseling. Int J Cancer. 2012;131:367–76.

45. Guilford P, Hopkins J, Harraway J, et al. E-cadherin germline mutations in familial gastric cancer. Nature. 1998;392:402–5.

46. Oliveira C, Senz J, Kaurah P, et al. Germline CDH1 deletions in hereditary diffuse gastric cancer families. Hum Mol Genet. 2009;18:1545–55.

47. Majewski IJ, Kluijt I, Cats A, et al. An α-E-catenin (CTNNA1) mutation in hereditary diffuse gastric cancer. J Pathol. 2013;229:621–9.

48. Carneiro F, Huntsman DG, Smyrk TC, et al. Model of the early development of diffuse gastric cancer in E-cadherin mutation carriers and its implications for patient screening. J Pathol. 2004;203:681–7.

49. Oliveira C, Seruca R, Hoogerbrugge N, Ligtenberg M, Carneiro F. Clinical utility gene card for: Hereditary diffuse gastric cancer (HDGC). Eur J Hum Genet. 2013;21(8), doi:10.1038/ejhg.2012.247.

50. Worthley DL, Phillips KD, Wayte N, et al. Gastric adenocarcinoma and proximal polyposis of the stomach (GAPPS): a new autosomal dominant syndrome. Gut. 2012;61:774–9.

51. Yanaru-Fujisawa R, Nakamura S, Moriyama T, et al. Familial fundic gland polyposis with gastric cancer. Gut. 2012;61:1103–4.

52. Sereno M, Aguayo C, Guillén Ponce C, et al. Gastric tumours in hereditary cancer syndromes: clinical

features, molecular biology and strategies for prevention. Clin Transl Oncol. 2011;13:599–610.

53. Carneiro F, Oliveira C, Leite M, Seruca R. Molecular targets and biological modifiers in gastric cancer. Semin Diagn Pathol. 2008;25:274–87.

54. Wang F, Sun GP, Zou YF, Hao JQ, Zhong F, Ren WJ. MicroRNAs as promising biomarkers for gastric cancer. Cancer Biomark. 2012;11:259–67.

55. Yin Y, Li J, Chen S, Zhou T, Si J. MicroRNAs as diagnostic biomarkers in gastric cancer. Int J Mol Sci. 2012;13:12544–55.

56. Zang ZJ, Cutcutache I, Poon SL, et al. Exome sequencing of gastric adenocarcinoma identifies recurrent somatic mutations in cell adhesion and chromatin remodeling genes. Nat Genet. 2012;44:570–4.

57. Tan IB, Ivanova T, Lim KH, et al. Intrinsic subtypes of gastric cancer, based on gene expression pattern, predict survival and respond differently to chemotherapy. Gastroenterology. 2011;141:476–85. 485. e1–11.

58. Deng N, Goh LK, Wang H, et al. A comprehensive survey of genomic alterations in gastric cancer reveals systematic patterns of molecular exclusivity and co-occurrence among distinct therapeutic targets. Gut. 2012;61:673–84.

59. Dulak AM, Schumacher S, van Lieshout J, et al. Gastrointestinal adenocarcinomas of the esophagus, stomach and colon exhibit distinct patterns of genome instability and oncogenesis. Cancer Res. 2012.72: 4383–93.

Standards for Surgical Therapy of Gastric Cancer

Roderich E. Schwarz

Gastric cancer (GC) continues to represent a formidable health challenge worldwide based on its unaltered high incidence in certain geographic areas such as East Asia or South America, its commonly advanced stage at diagnosis, and its limited curability for disease in intermediate and advanced stages [1]. Even in the United States, where gastric adenocarcinoma mortality has gradually decreased from the most common form of cancer-related deaths in the 1940s and gastric cancer incidence is among the lowest in the world, curability remains a significant problem [2]. Before the onset of surgical therapy, gastric cancer was incurable. Since the first groundbreaking accomplishments with partial gastrectomy by Billroth in 1881, Y-jejunostomy reconstruction by Roux in 1893, and total gastrectomy by Schlatter in 1897, operative therapy of gastric malignancy has gone through more than a century of continued refinement and ever-improving accomplishments (Table 7.1) [3]. This chapter intends to highlight the critical objectives, indications, and standard techniques for operative procedures in gastric cancer treatment and to describe the position of surgical therapy within the context of multidisciplinary approaches for mid-stage and metastatic stomach malignancy.

R.E. Schwarz, MD, PhD, FACS (✉)
Department of Surgical Oncology, Indiana University
Health Goshen Center for Cancer Care,
200 High Park Ave, Goshen, IN 46526, USA
e-mail: Rschwarz@iuhealth.org

Surgical Objectives

General objectives of operative therapy for gastric cancer are more easily compiled than successfully accomplished on a consistent basis in clinical practice [4]. They include surgical removal of tumor tissue, the provision of local and regional disease control, the optimization of curative potential, the provision of intraoperative and pathologic staging information which occasionally includes the confirmation of a gastric cancer diagnosis, the restoration of function lost or limited through a resection such as reestablishing gastrointestinal continuity after gastrectomy, and minimizing any resulting postoperative morbidity. The latter objective, for example, would include strategies to avoid splenectomy or distal pancreatectomy if possible to reduce infectious morbidity or to furbish gastric rather than esophageal anastomoses when feasible to minimize anastomotic leaks. While all listed objectives appear equally valid in a minimally invasive surgery (MIS) context, improved recovery potential and minimized morbidity obviously carry special appeal for a MIS rationale and approach to gastric cancer treatment.

Operative Intent

The intent to conduct an operation for gastric cancer can be highly variable. In most cases, a procedure is justified to cure the underlying

Table 7.1 Important steps in the historic development of operative gastric cancer therapy

Surgeon(s)	Year of procedure or publication	Operative accomplishment
Pean	1879	Unsuccessful pyloric resection
Rydygier	1880	Unsuccessful pyloric resection
Billroth	1881	First successful pyloric resection (Billroth I)
Kocher	1893	Posterior gastroduodenostomy
Billroth	1885	Antrectomy after loop gastrojejunostomy (2-stage, Billroth II)
Krönlein	1887	End-to-side gastrojejunostomy
Woelfler	1881	Y-gastroenterostomy
Roux	1893	Retrocolic Y-gastrojejunostomy
Connor	1884	Unsuccessful total gastrectomy
Schlatter	1897	First successful total gastrectomy
Brigham, Richardson	1898	Three successful total gastrectomies
Hoffmeister	1908	Greater curvature gastrojejunostomy
Reichel–Polya	1911	Full length gastrojejunostomy
McNeer	1951	Radical gastrectomy, extended lymphadenectomy
Appleby	1953	Radical en bloc gastrectomy with resection of celiac artery
Hunt	1952	Pouch esophagojejunostomy reconstruction
Merendino	1955	Small bowel interposition reconstruction
Kitano	1992	Laparoscopically assisted distal gastrectomy
Azagra	1996	Laparoscopic total gastrectomy

malignancy. Curability criteria for surgical therapy depend on the underlying disease extent and biologic behavior and are set by the relatively limited scope of local and regional tumor control

a resection is able to accomplish [5]. In any circumstance, a curative outcome after resection cannot be expected unless all known locoregional disease is completely removed, usually en bloc, and is generally not possible if diffuse extraregional metastatic disease does exist. Even if the complete removal of all gross disease with negative margins (R0 resection) has been performed, subsequent recurrence remains common for gastric cancers of mid-stage due to the presence of nonvisualized micrometastases at the time of operation [6]. This mechanism and the fact that previously undetected metastatic disease is identified intraoperatively are the most common reasons if a preoperative curative intent cannot be achieved [4]. Macroscopically visible residual disease and positive peritoneal cytology are virtual guarantees for symptomatic disease recurrence to develop [7]. Microscopic positive margins (R1 status) impart an increased local recurrence risk, but are in addition a surrogate for higher-risk disease and a greater failure rate in extraregional sites [8]. In addition to the curative intentions, a diagnostic component or the provision of tumor tissue for specific purposes can provide the rationale to operate on a patient with gastric cancer, specifically if the diagnosis is suspected but remains unconfirmed through endoscopic biopsy means, or if more advanced intra-abdominal disease extent is suspected but not confirmed through imaging modalities. Another common preoperative intent is the palliation of symptoms that cannot be alleviated through lesser invasive means such as endoscopy or interventional radiologic techniques [9]. Examples for this approach are obstruction symptoms not relieved through stent placement or resection needs for tumor-related bleeding not amenable to palliative radiation or interventional vascular manipulation. In this context it is important not to confuse the terms "palliative" and "noncurative"; a noncurative operative procedure is hardly ever justifiable in a patient who does not suffer from symptoms that require a specific surgical intervention, while an operation with palliative intent is primarily driven by the patient's symptoms irrespective of whether potential curability is still given or not [10]. Therefore,

Table 7.2 Preoperative intents to provide operative therapy for gastric cancer

Intent	Examples	Comments on requirements or conditions
Diagnostic	Diagnostic laparoscopy	Enhances clinical staging either prior to induction therapy or at beginning of planned resection; rarely required to prove and treat suspected gastric cancer that failed endoscopic biopsy confirmation attempts
Curative	Gastrectomy with D2 lymphadenectomy	Requires absence of extraregional metastases; all multimodality options considered; goal not achieved through R2 and most R1 resections; need for symptom control may affect timing of resection
Palliative	Intestinal bypass for malignant peritoneal bowel obstruction, gastrojejunostomy bypass	Nonoperative or less invasive options always preferred if feasible; possible benefits to resection of tumor reported only in low tumor burden settings; although most often in noncurative setting, palliative-intent gastrectomy can result in curative procedure if disease extent is smaller than expected
Noncurative	Gastrectomy for asymptomatic stage IV tumor	Cannot be supported or justified without other compelling intents documented
Preemptive	Resection of gastric tumor to prevent obstruction in setting of metastatic disease	Hardly ever indicated; should not prompt a separate planned operation
Supportive	Surgical feeding jejunostomy tube placement prior to preoperative therapy	Nonoperative or less invasive means preferred if possible
Tissue provision	Resection of gastric cancer tissue for on-protocol vaccine generation	Hardly ever indicated; less invasive nonoperative means preferred

preoperative intents for operative therapy for gastric cancer can exist in single or in combined form (Table 7.2). The surgeon is advised to clearly define preoperative intents, for guidance of the informed consenting process with patient and family members, for appropriate positioning of the operative step within the sequence of multidisciplinary treatment options, as well as for enabling correct interpretation of outcomes. Preoperatively clearly defined palliative or diagnostic intents for operations have a greater chance to be successfully achieved compared to procedures performed with curative intent [4].

Operative Therapy as Part of a Multidisciplinary Strategy

Due to the high risk for recurrence after resection of mid-stage GC, additional treatment options have been increasingly applied. In numerous phase 3 randomized controlled trials, adjuvant therapy has been demonstrated to lead to superior overall survival (OS) compared to gastrectomy alone [11]. Adjuvant therapy options with OS benefits and particular relevance to practice within the United States include postoperative chemotherapy with chemoradiation according to the Intergroup 0116 trial [12], perioperative chemotherapy analogous to the MAGIC or ACCORD07 trials [13, 14], or preoperative chemoradiation analogous to the CROSS trial [15]. Details on these multimodality treatment options exceed the scope of this chapter. As there is currently no single, evidence-based approach to multimodal GC therapy, various regimens are in use based on local centers' expertise and preference. In general, preoperative (neoadjuvant) approaches are preferred, as tolerance to treatment is greater, delivery is more likely complete, and as clinical or pathologic response to such treatment may represent an important prognostic surrogate for disease behavior and future recurrence risk [16, 17]. Perioperative chemotherapy appears to be most useful for mid- and distal third gastric tumors, while preoperative chemoradiation may be preferred for proximal gastric or GE junction lesions. Importantly, any operation plans would have to be balanced against these important strategies, especially for curative goals, and formal multidisciplinary evaluation of appropriate treatment options prior to initiation of therapy should be mandatory. "Surgical" therapy of GC therefore includes knowledge of and support for multimodality treatment and the insight to adapt to effects of other treatments, especially regarding assessment of tumor response to preoperative therapy and delineation of an appropriate resection extent.

Preoperative Aspects

Most patients will present to the surgeon with biopsy-proven adenocarcinoma through endoscopic means. Accurate clinical staging includes computed tomography imaging and endoscopic ultrasound (EUS) evaluation. It is important to have precise documentation in regard to primary tumor location and extent prior to initiation of preoperative therapy, as responses to this treatment may render intraoperative localization attempts difficult. PET scans do not appear mandatory for GC staging, but may have a more reliable role in proximal or GE junction primaries or to guide preoperative chemotherapy on protocol; diffuse-type GCs tend to be less well imaged on PET scans [18, 19]. Resectable tumors are best approached in terms of resection extent based on their pretreatment extent and stage, irrespective of restaging findings. Even major clinical responses are often incomplete on pathologic examination, supporting this more "radical" approach [20, 21]. An exception would be the rare scenario of an unresectable tumor being rendered resectable due to a response to initial chemotherapy or radiation. The intraoperative specifics are thus best delineated preoperatively, including planned operative approach (open versus laparoscopic), placement of incision(s), resection extent, and preferred reconstruction. Staging laparoscopy is strongly recommended as an operative complement to preoperative imaging, as it is most sensitive in detecting small-volume peritoneal or visceral surface metastases [22, 23]; laparoscopic ultrasound may slightly increase metastasis detection rates [24]. In addition, peritoneal washing cytology may be considered if subsequent treatment steps are affected by positive results [25]. Timing or frequency of staging laparoscopy around preoperative therapy is being debated [26]. Patients with persisting positive washing cytology findings invariably have poor OS outlook, while those with positive peritoneal cytology status that turned negative have shown longer survival [7].

Standards for Curative Mid-Stage Gastric Cancer Operative Therapy

Technical Aspects of Resection

State-of-the-art curative-intent gastrectomy requires R0 resection and should be accompanied by an extended lymphadenectomy (D2 dissection) [27, 28]. Whether open or minimally invasive surgical (MIS) techniques are utilized appears to be of lesser consequence oncologically, as long as principles of complete local resection and regional dissection are adhered to [29–32]. The following operative components are based on open gastrectomy standards, but seem to be equally relevant for a MIS approach. For early GC (T1N0), endoscopic mucosal resection (EMR) or submucosal dissection (ESD) may suffice as definitive therapy [33]; both require proper specialty skills and currently appear to be limited to few centers within the United States with appropriate technical and clinical expertise. EMR and ESD techniques will not be described in further detail within this chapter. For all more advanced stages of nonmetastatic gastric adenocarcinoma, complete locoregional resection is the central component for curative-intent therapy. In the operating room, general endotracheal anesthesia is introduced, and the patient is usually placed in a supine position for a planed open celiotomy; planned laparoscopic resection may favor different positions based on the operating surgeon's preference. It may be helpful to consider a short repeat upper gastrointestinal endoscopy after induction of anesthesia prior to resection or later for anastomotic assessment [34]; the author has used this liberally to verify tumor location and extent and to assess the mucosal appearance of gastric or esophageal components to be used in the reconstruction or for anastomotic sites. In addition, laparoscopy should be performed now unless already done in a separate setting. In up to 20 % of cases, laparoscopic confirmation of intra-abdominal metastases will still provide the opportunity to avoid an otherwise noncurative gastrectomy in this setting.

A transabdominal approach will be sufficient for most complete resections, but incision placement for open gastrectomy is not standardized and follows personal preferences. While many surgeons choose upper midline incisions, the author prefers a bilateral subcostal margin incision approach. Rarely is there benefit to a combined left thoracoabdominal incision, but for high, large gastric tumors in obese patients, this can generate much superior exposure if needed. A routine thoracoabdominal approach for GC resection is not beneficial compared to the transabdominal-only access and thus not recommended [35, 36]. With proper exposure and resectability established, the main resective objectives are R0 resection and lymphadenectomy. Total gastrectomy out of principle is not necessary; lesser extent resections, especially for distally located tumors, have shown comparable survival results, with fewer morbidity and functional challenges [37, 38]. Appropriate macro- and microscopically negative margins should be obtained as feasible at duodenal and esophageal resection sites. In challenging scenarios of advanced disease burden, it can be acceptable to leave a positive margin at these sites, as long as parameters such as serosal involvement or significant nodal burden imply a minimal curative potential. Intragastric margins of 5 cm are traditionally recommended for subtotal gastrectomy, at least for intestinal-type disease [39, 40]; diffuse-type lesions may require wider margins. A healthy tissue esophageal margin length of 2 cm seems to be sufficient for resection of Siewert type II and III lesions treated with gastrectomy [41]. The choice of gastrectomy extent (and of lymphatic dissection extent) will not only depend on location and extent of the primary tumor but also on potential reconstruction needs and options (Fig. 7.1). In general, for distal lesions a subtotal gastrectomy is adequate. For lesions in the middle third of the stomach, the decision between total or near-total gastrectomy depends on the proximal margin status and considerations for possibly safer reconstruction (gastrojejunostomy leak rates have been described as occurring half as often as those after esophagojejunostomy [42]). Proximal third lesions will essentially always require either total gastrectomy or proximal gastrectomy with a special reconstruction such as small bowel interposition [43]. Proximal gastrectomy with subsequent esophagogastrostomy is not recommended, especially after pyloroplasty, for concerns of significant reflux. Avoiding any pyloromyotomy or pyloroplasty in this setting is recommended, but does not completely preempt reflux-related problems; distal gastric emptying problems that require endoscopic or even operative management may occur in 5–15 % of cases. Lesions at the GE junction require special operative planning based on the lesions' epicenter and, more importantly, the proximal disease extent. Siewert type I lesions require a transthoracic or transhiatal esophagectomy and should not be approached with an attempt to perform a gastrectomy [44]. Siewert type II lesions are located at the gastric cardia; these can either be approached via esophagogastrectomy with retrogastric LND analogous to type I lesions or through an extended gastrectomy as long as not more than 3 cm of distal esophageal involvement exists and proximal negative margins (of 2 cm or greater) can be obtained [45]. Siewert type III lesions are in biologic terms proximal gastric cancers, and a transabdominal approach should be fully sufficient as long as no more extensive submucosal esophageal involvement exists [44, 45]. It appears permissible to decide upon the best resection extent for proximal gastric cancers close to the GEJ intraoperatively through esophageal transection and frozen section analysis, as long as the surgeon is experienced with performing an esophagectomy in this setting and prepared to do so if necessary and as long as right gastric and gastroepiploic vasculature is initially preserved for a gastric tube reconstruction in case an esophageal resection becomes necessary.

Total or near-total omentectomy is frequently performed en bloc with a gastrectomy for cancer and represents a good way to initiate the dissection. Omental bursectomy has been widely applied as a means to accomplish more complete resection of posterior wall lesions; it includes removal of the anterior peritoneal leaf of the mesocolon in an attempt to not enter the lesser sac and completely remove this retrogastric structure. While it appears less sensible from an oncologic standpoint, especially for transmural tumors with serosal involvement and progression risks [46, 47], it nevertheless appears to be a useful technique to identify the relevant retroperitoneal plains above the pancreas for identifying lymph nodes at hepatic and splenic arteries. Careful attention is applied to not injure the

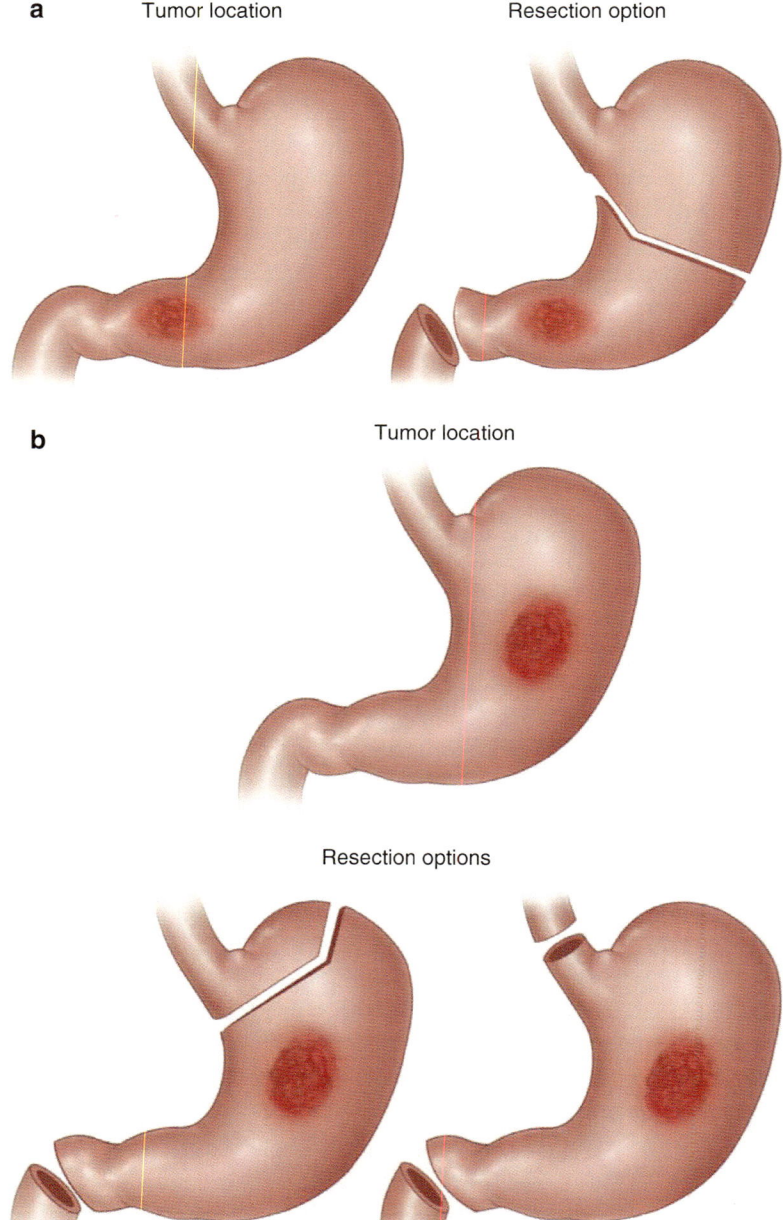

Fig. 7.1 Schematic representation of gastric resection extent based on the location of the primary adenocarcinoma. (**a**) Resection extent for distal third tumors; (**b**) resection extent options for middle third tumors; (**c**) resection extent options for proximal third tumors including Siewert type III lesions; (**d**) resection extent options for Siewert type II lesions

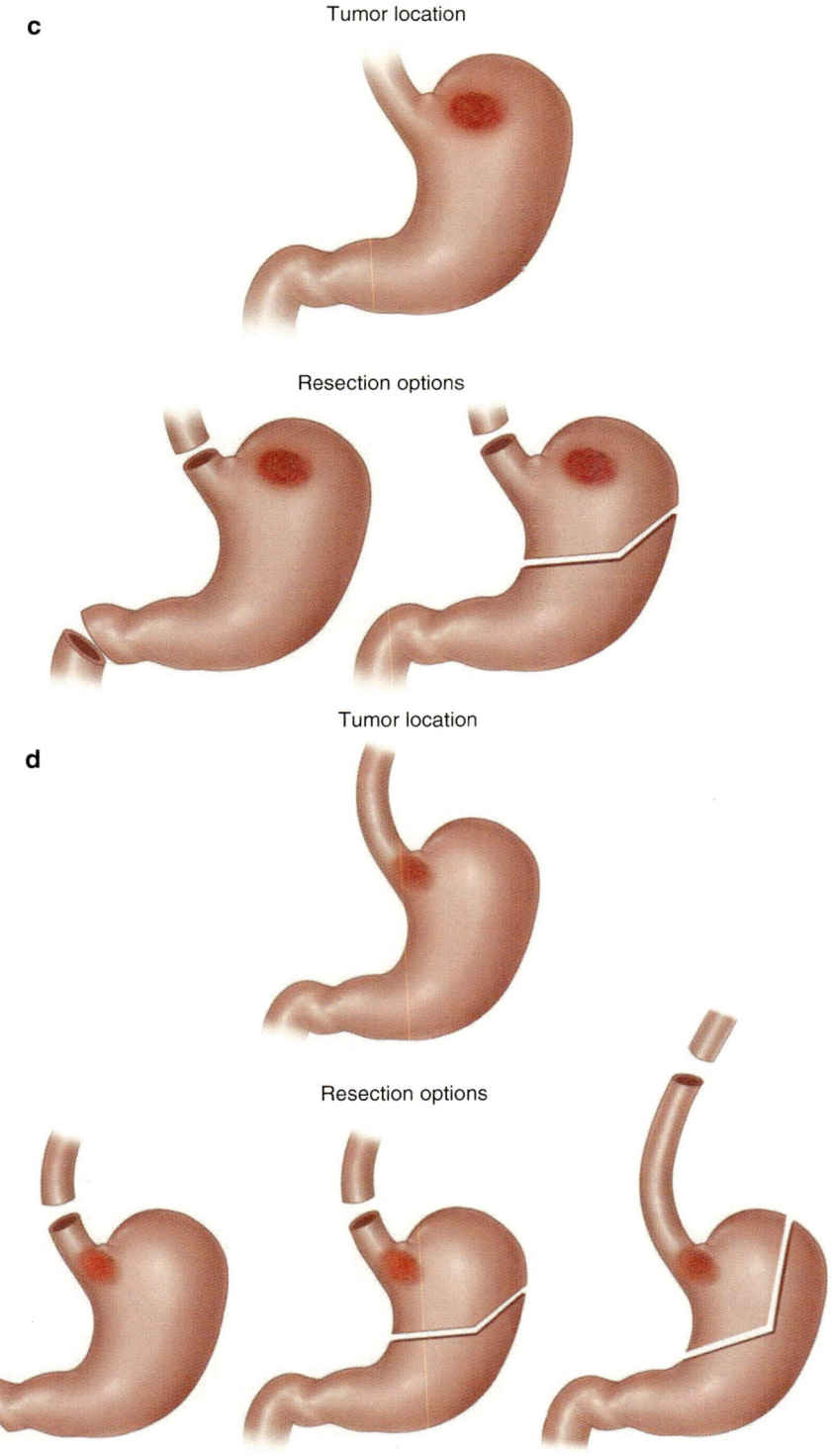

Fig. 7.1 (continued)

pancreas parenchyma in the process. For all gastric tumors except those close to the GE junction, the proximal duodenum is freed and prepared for transection; in this process, dissection of gastroepiploic LNs off the underlying pancreas and deep ligation and transection of gastroepiploic vessels will keep the inferior parapyloric and gastroepiploic (level 6) LNs on the specimen and will allow for easy access to the duodenum. The dissection is now carried from distal to proximal, with division of lesser omentum and mobilization of paragastric tissues at the lesser curvature up to the diaphragmatic crus. If the extended LND is to be performed en bloc, common hepatic artery LNs are now mobilized and kept with the specimen. The origin of the left gastric artery should always be identified and divided for cancer resections; splenic artery nodes are dissected away from pancreas and artery, and short gastric vessels are divided close to the spleen. The spleen can most frequently be preserved unless direct tumor involvement or a large hilar LN burden requires splenectomy. Splenic hilar LN involvement is rare for tumors not located at the fundus or proximal two thirds of the greater curvature. Even when splenic hilar dissection is desired in fundus or greater curvature primaries, spleen-preserving hilar LN dissection has been applied, since spleen preservation may have important benefits for reduced postoperative morbidity [48–51]. The proximal transection is now determined based on anticipated margin needs. This is either at the level of the distal esophagus or transgastric with preservation of the proximal stomach if feasible. In the latter scenario, the lesser curvature transection should extend close to the GE junction without narrowing the esophagogastric passage, primarily to support a complete left gastric artery LND, while more length can be preserved toward the greater curvature if possible. This then shall allow for an easier reconstruction, with a subsequent anastomosis close to the greater curvature transection site. Completion of the retroperitoneal dissection with celiac lymphadenectomy and clearance of tissues to the diaphragmatic crural tissue completes the gastrectomy. For locally advanced tumors, multivisceral resections are occasionally

necessary and indicated when resulting in a R0 resection that still offers curative potential. In this situation, the surgeon ought to be prepared to perform an en bloc segmental hepatectomy, diaphragmatic resection, pancreatosplenectomy, left adrenalectomy, or colectomy as required.

Additional Aspects of Lymph Node Dissection

The propensity of gastric adenocarcinomas to involve lymph nodes (LNs) is high. Although actively debated over the past decade, lymphadenectomy at the time of curative-intent gastrectomy has shown benefits to staging accuracy and to cancer control and has thus become standard of care [28, 52]. Resection of the appropriate paragastric and of second echelon (left gastric, common hepatic, splenic, celiac artery) LNs (D2 dissection) is generally sufficient; wider dissections have not shown superior results [35]. This procedure should yield at least 15 or more LNs for the pathologic evaluation, but greater total LN counts have been associated with better survival outcomes [53–55]. A long-term survival or disease-specific control benefit to extended LN dissection (ELND) has now been demonstrated in at least two randomized controlled trials, despite a greater early morbidity and mortality in the Dutch trial after D2 dissection [28, 52, 56]. These were related to an increased rate of pancreatosplenectomy with D2 dissection [57], but this survival hazard has been superseded by a long-term overall survival benefit due to greater disease control. As discussed earlier, splenectomy and distal pancreatectomy are strongly discouraged unless deemed necessary based on tumor involvement [58, 59].

ELND can be performed en bloc with the gastrectomy as described above, or in a separate specimen. The paragastric nodes (i.e., paracardial, lesser and greater curvature, right gastric artery, and gastroepiploic artery LNs) are always best removed with the adjacent stomach portion. Since the LN group to be removed is variable based on the tumor location, a good strategy is to remove any paragastric LNs adjacent to stomach that is also to be removed. Dissection of the

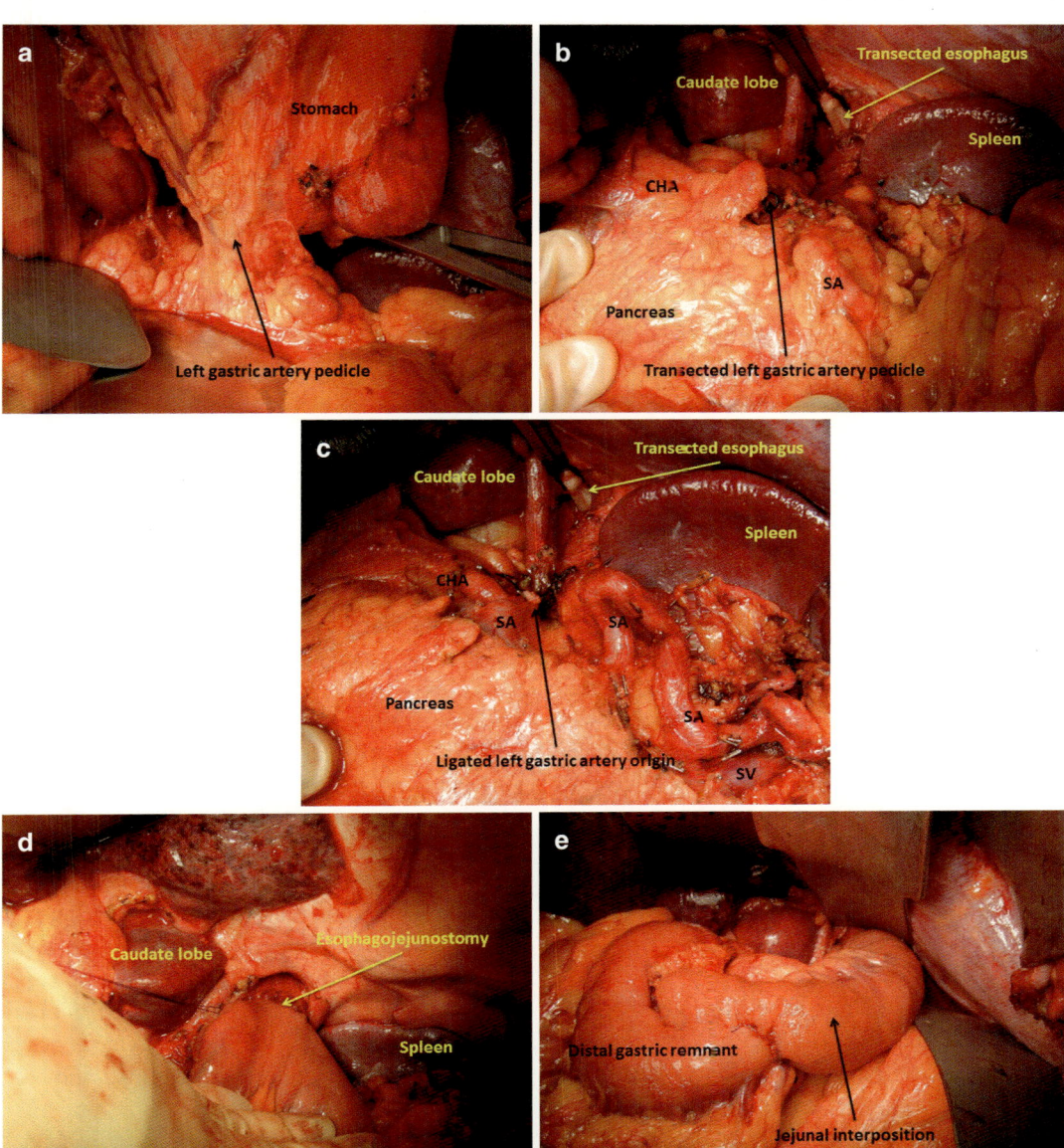

Fig. 7.2 Intraoperative images of a 2-step extended lymphadenectomy and subsequent reconstruction (**a**) Appearance of the left gastric artery pedicle during resection of a proximal gastric cancer; (**b**) Appearance after transection of the left gastric artery pedicle and proximal gastrectomy. *CHA* common hepatic artery, *SA* splenic artery; (**c**) Completion of retroperitoneal lymphadenectomy at celiac, hepatic, and splenic arteries. *CHA* common hepatic artery, *SA* splenic artery, *SV* splenic vein; (**d**) Completed esophagojejunostomy; (**e**) Completed jejunogastrostomy between small bowel (Merendino) interposition and distal remnant stomach

named artery LNs will then complete a sensible D2 dissection. If these left gastric, common hepatic, splenic, and celiac artery LNs do not appear grossly abnormal, the author has divided the left gastric artery pedicle to facilitate gastrectomy as initial step, to be followed by the retroperitoneal dissection of these structures as second step (Fig 7.2). This allows not only for better exposure but also improved pathologic identification of relevant retrogastric LN involvement. The left gastric artery should generally be divided in cancer resections, in part for better nodal clearance; occasionally, an accessory left hepatic artery is encountered that can be preserved, as LNs can be dissected around the proximal left gastric artery, and the gastric branch can be divided after separating from the hepatic branch. In most Western patients, it is not possible to identify all LNs of interest visually during the dissection. The goal is therefore to free the relevant and named arterial vasculature of all surrounding lympho-areolar and adipose tissue, rather than obtain specific LNs or a certain total number of LNs. LN counts are determined by the pathologist and do not only reflect radicality of dissection, but also quality of the specimen pathologic examination, and other clinicopathologic factors including preoperative therapy effects and nutritional implications. A median total LN count between 20 and 30 appears to be an acceptable standard [27, 53, 54]. In some Asian centers, limiting the LND in patients with low likelihood for LN involvement is being explored, such as through laparoscopic sentinel LN biopsy for early GCs [60, 61], but these techniques are not yet accepted as proven standards.

Technical Aspects of Reconstruction

Most gastric resections are followed by Roux-en-Y jejunal reconstruction, either as esophago-jejunostomy or gastrojejunostomy (Fig. 7.3). The jejunal limb is best created with a length of around 45 cm to achieve the lowest degree of both Roux-stasis and of dumping problems postoperatively [62]. Billroth 1 and 2 reconstructions have been described after distal gastrectomy, but appear acceptable regarding appropriate oncologic dissection extent and functional outcomes only for very distally located tumors [63, 64]. A potentially challenging scenario for either reconstruction technique is that of a small proximal gastric reservoir with uncontrolled access of biliary small bowel contents and the related bile reflux risk [65, 66]. Similarly, after proximal gastrectomy, a small distal reservoir too and biliary reflux have to be avoided. A Merendino small bowel interposition

between the esophagus and distal gastric reservoir and the avoidance of pyloric manipulation if possible present acceptable options, as shown in (Fig. 7.2) [43]. As a general important aspect, reconstruction preferences should not compromise the resection extent. Pouch reconstructions are rarely performed in the United States as there has been no convincing evidence of postoperative nutritional superiority; some reports describe a potential long-term quality of life benefit [67, 68].

Additional Intra- and Postoperative Considerations

Considerable variability and different preferences exist regarding technical details of operative aspects during gastrectomy. This applies to anastomotic techniques, duodenal stump closure, dissection techniques using sharp tools, traditional electrocoagulation, or newer energy devices and extends to details of incision closure and others. In general, no specific technique has demonstrated clear and universally accepted evidence of superiority over others, despite numerous trial or meta-analysis-based efforts. The author prefers hand-sewn inversion of the duodenal staple line closure, hand-sewn dual-layer anastomoses between the esophagus or stomach remnant and jejunum, and intraoperative integrity testing of proximal anastomoses through orogastric/orojejunal tube instillation of methylene blue-containing saline solution. After total gastrectomy, postoperative nasojejunal decompression is unnecessary [69, 70]; with a significant-size gastric remnant, temporary nasogastric decompression may be considered. There appears to be no benefit to routinely placed drains despite some divergent clinical results, but special indications for intraoperative drainage may exist such as after partial pancreatic resection or in case of a transhiatal high esophageal anastomosis in a setting of having entered the pleural space during the dissection [71–73]. Placement of feeding tubes for postoperative nutrition support is equally debatable [74, 75]. It is the author's practice to always provide jejunal feeding access to patients undergoing esophagectomy or total or near-total gastrectomy, but to use them selectively in the rare cases of distal gastrectomy based on the patient's nutritional risk status [76]. While most patients do not require postoperative enteral nutrition support, any failure of sufficient oral food intake within 1–2 weeks and severe preoperative malnutrition render the initiation of tube feeding unproblematic with a feeding tube available. Other means of standardized postoperative management including venous thromboembolic prophylaxis, incentive spirometry, early activation, cardioprotective therapy, etc. complete

the surgical planning for best postoperative recovery.

Surgical Palliation Aspects

Surgeons frequently are called upon to decide on the most appropriate way to palliate symptoms of GC. For mid-stage and potentially curable disease, obstructive symptoms caused by the primary tumor may influence the therapy sequence, with the resection performed up front to address

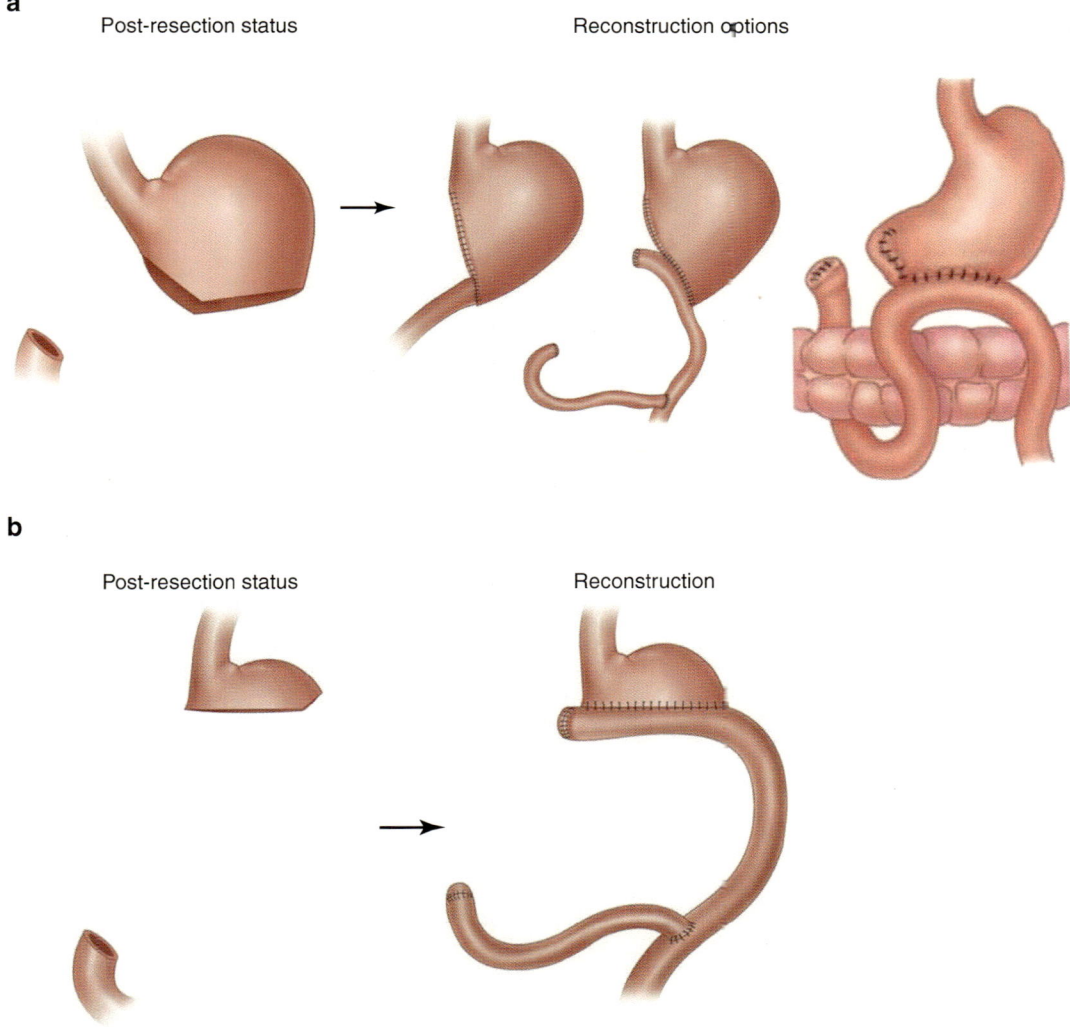

a

Post-resection status   Reconstruction options

b

Post-resection status   Reconstruction

Fig. 7.3 Reconstruction options after subtotal gastrectomy, total gastrectomy, or proximal gastrectomy. (**a**) Billroth II reconstruction options after distal gastrectomy; (**b**) reconstruction option after near-total gastrectomy; (**c**) preferred reconstruction option after total gastrectomy; (**d**) preferred reconstruction option after proximal gastrectomy; (**e**) gastric pull-up reconstruction after esophagogastrectomy

Fig. 7.3 (continued)

Post-resection status   Reconstruction

c

Post-resection status   Reconstruction

d

Post-resection status   Reconstruction

e

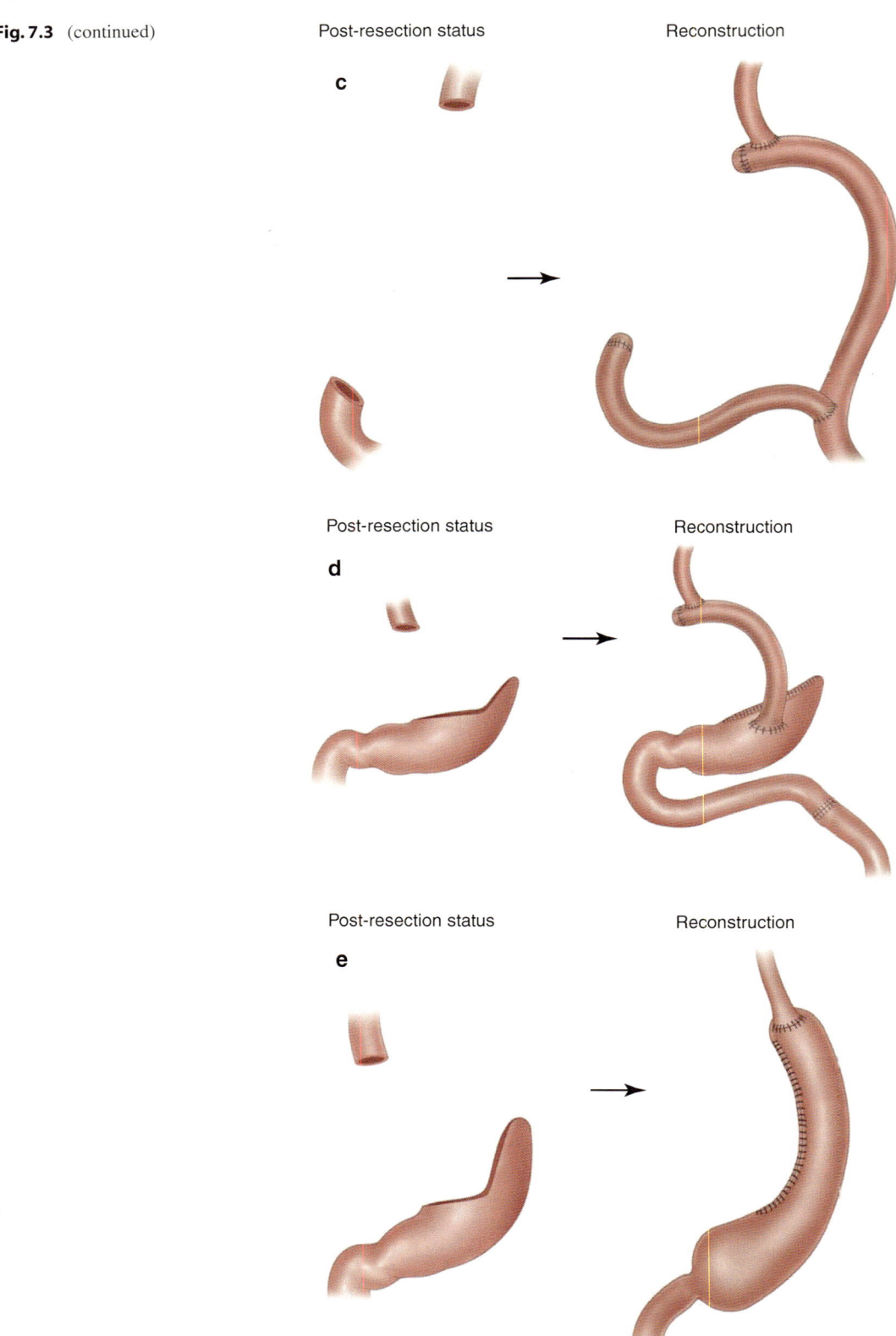

symptom control needs and complete resection. In cases of bleeding from the primary tumor, short course radiation has been an effective palliative option [77–79], and even chemotherapy may control the low continuous blood loss associated with larger, ulcerated tumors [80]. For symptom control in settings of incurable disease, operations should generally be avoided if possible. Nonoperative treatment can also improve mild symptoms, and specific nonoperative interventions such as endoscopic stenting, tumor reduction, or bleeding management may result in the desired control [81, 82]. Obstruction due to large intragastric tumor burden in the setting of metastatic disease provides great challenges. A palliative-intent gastrectomy under these circumstances may be indicated, but treatment goals are rarely reported well [9], outcomes are frequently disappointing, and benefits above available systemic and supportive therapies are unproven despite some retrospective reports of more effective palliation and longer survival in highly selected patients [83–85]. Success after palliative-intent gastrectomy also depends strongly on the overall disease burden and pattern [86]. In cases of distal gastric obstruction, gastrojejunostomy may succeed and allow for avoiding a more complex resection. Malignant bowel obstruction due to peritoneal carcinomatosis presents another scenario for which a palliative operation may be required, but where outcomes frequently fall short of the desired goal [87]. In this case, bypass or drainage procedures may be more feasible than resection.

Postoperative Outcomes

Postoperative morbidity after gastrectomy for GC remains formidable but manageable for most patients. Anastomotic leaks are linked to most deep site infections, and no specific reconstruction technique has emerged as superior in preventing leaks. Postoperative infections have been linked to inferior survival outcomes [88]. There are well-established volume-outcome relationships for postoperative mortality as well as overall long-term survival [89, 90]. Disease control

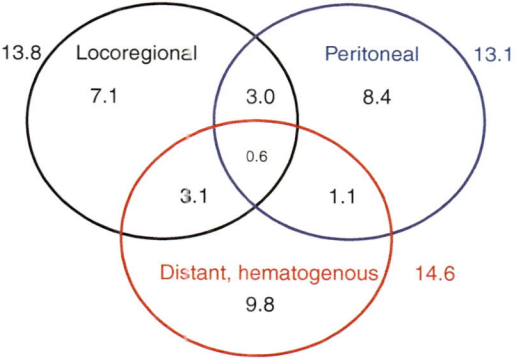

Fig. 7.4 Failure pattern after gastrectomy for gastric cancer. Graphic representation of failure patterns after gastrectomy and D2 dissection for gastric cancer, without routine use of adjuvant therapy. Data pooled from three series [91–93]. All numbers represent % values based on total patient $n = 2,753$; recurrences: $n = 909$ (33 %)

remains a significant challenge, as recurrence rates are high. Peritoneal recurrence is common among patients with T4 primaries, and significant LN involvement correlates with hematogenous metastasis and recurrence in distant sites [58]; isolated local recurrences appear rare (Fig. 7.4) [91, 92]. Overall survival after resections alone appears to be primarily dependent on whether serosal invasion of the primary tumor or nodal involvement is present (Fig. 7.5). Thus, TNM staging criteria remain the dominant prognostic components after gastrectomy alone within nomograms for disease-specific survival [94, 95]. However, response to preoperative therapy is another powerful prognostic parameter and likely a surrogate for favorable biologic behavior, as metabolic and pathologic responses are linked to best survival outcomes [16, 17]. It is possible that the recently observed improvement in postgastrectomy survival is due to increased use of adjuvant therapy options (Fig. 7.5b). Postoperative chemotherapy with radiation has led to a survival benefit [12], and contemporary perioperative chemotherapy such as in the MAGIC trial has improved long-term survival by roughly 10 % [13]. For proximal cancers including those of the GE junction, preoperative chemoradiation (as in the CROSS trial) has demonstrated survival benefits over surgical resection alone [15], with a significant reduction in locoregional and peritoneal

Fig. 7.5 Survival outcomes after gastrectomy for gastric cancer. (**a**) OS after curative-intent gastrectomy. MSKCC data from the era prior to widespread adjuvant therapy use, data from Schwarz et al. [58]. (**b**) OS after gastrectomy, by time period. SEER data (Courtesy of R. Nelson, Ph.D., 2014). (**c**) Survival outcomes in three key trials of adjuvant therapy (Adjuv.) in addition to surgical resection alone (Surg. only) of gastric or GE junction cancer. The bars represent 5-year overall survival data (in %) after gastrectomy with and without perioperative ECF chemotherapy from the MAGIC trial [13], 3-year recurrence-free survival (in %) after gastrectomy with and without postoperative 5FU-LV chemotherapy and chemoradiation from the Intergroup 0116 trial [12], and median overall survival (in months) after esophagogastrectomy with and without preoperative chemoradiation for GE junction and esophageal cancer from the CROSS trial [15]

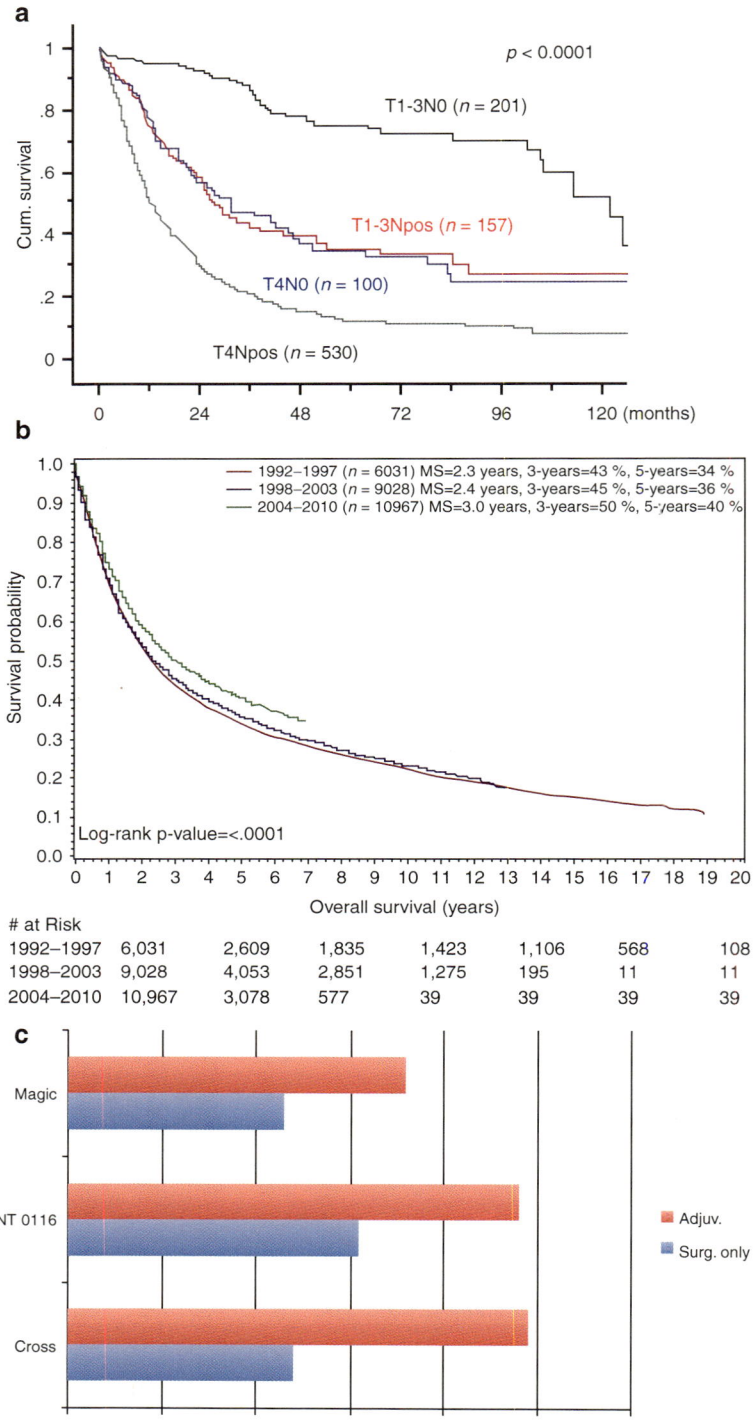

recurrences [96] (Fig. 7.5c). The only trial to compare preoperative chemoradiation with preoperative chemotherapy alone for resected GE junction cancers failed to show a statistically significant difference due to small numbers of enrolled patients, but also indicated a lower hazard ratio in favor of chemoradiation [97].

Prophylactic Gastrectomy

Hereditary diffuse-type GC based on germline CDH1 (E-cadherin) gene mutations can be effectively addressed through prophylactic gastrectomy prior to onset of invasive carcinoma [98]. Individuals from an affected kindred require genetic counseling and testing [99]. Total gastrectomy is the only sensible procedure and is usually performed during late adolescence or early adulthood, as endoscopic surveillance has shown challenges in identifying histologic alterations reliably [100]. Prophylactic gastrectomy specimens from gene carriers harbor occult microscopic cancer in as many as 80 % of cases. Long-term results after prophylactic gastrectomy show overall good functional recovery and adaptation [101]. Another autosomal dominant syndrome, in this case of intestinal-type gastric adenocarcinoma and proximal polyposis of the stomach (GAPPS), has recently been described [102].

Special Considerations for Gastrointestinal Stromal Tumors (GISTs)

GISTs are rare but well-defined mesenchymal tumors of the GI tract and most commonly occur in the stomach. They are characterized by unique biologic behavior and specific progression patterns and thus represent a small yet unique subset of "gastric cancers." Definitive therapy of GISTs greater than 2 cm in size is surgical resection, for which full-thickness local excision with negative margins is sufficient. Laparoscopic resection techniques are often applied. LN involvement is extremely rare, and ELND is not required. Cure rates are high for small, low-grade tumors, but recurrence rates are high for large lesions, high mitotic counts, and ruptured lesions or cases with intraoperative spillage of liquid contents. Modified NIH criteria have been validated to delineate well high- versus low-risk constellations [103]. Patients with resected high risk GISTs have been shown to benefit from postoperative targeted adjuvant therapy with the c-kit kinase inhibitor imatinib based on 2 RCTs [104, 105]. Longer therapy in this setting for 3 years or possibly more appears to have survival benefits compared to 1-year treatment.

References

1. Jemal A, Bray F, Center MM, Ferlay J, Ward E, Forman D. Global cancer statistics. CA Cancer J Clin. 2011;61(2):69–90.
2. Siegel R, Ma J, Zou Z, Jemal A. Cancer statistics, 2014. CA Cancer J Clin. 2014;64(1):9–29.
3. Robinson JO. The history of gastric surgery. Postgrad Med J. 1960;36:706–13.
4. Schwarz RE. Factors influencing change of preoperative treatment intent in a gastrointestinal cancer practice. World J Surg Oncol. 2007;5:32.
5. Karpeh Jr MS, Brennan MF. Gastric carcinoma. Ann Surg Oncol. 1998;5(7):650–6.
6. Karpeh MS, Leon L, Klimstra D, Brennan MF. Lymph node staging in gastric cancer: is location more important than Number? An analysis of 1,038 patients. Ann Surg. 2000;232(3):362–71.
7. Mezhir JJ, Shah MA, Jacks LM, Brennan MF, Coit DG, Strong VE. Positive peritoneal cytology in patients with gastric cancer: natural history and outcome of 291 patients. Ann Surg Oncol. 2010;17(12):3173–80.
8. Kim SH, Karpeh MS, Klimstra DS, Leung D, Brennan MF. Effect of microscopic resection line disease on gastric cancer survival. J Gastrointest Surg. 1999;3(1):24–33.
9. Miner TJ, Jaques DP, Karpeh MS, Brennan MF. Defining palliative surgery in patients receiving noncurative resections for gastric cancer. J Am Coll Surg. 2004;198(6):1013–21.
10. Schwarz RE. Defining palliation in patients undergoing gastrectomy for gastric cancer. J Am Coll Surg. 2004;199(6):1001–2.
11. Sehdev A, Catenacci DV. Perioperative therapy for locally advanced gastroesophageal cancer: current controversies and consensus of care. J Hematol Oncol. 2013;6:66.
12. Smalley SR, Benedetti JK, Haller DG, et al. Updated analysis of SWOG-directed intergroup study 0116: a phase III trial of adjuvant radiochemotherapy versus observation after curative gastric cancer resection. J Clin Oncol. 2012;30(19):2327–33.

13. Cunningham D, Allum WH, Stenning SP, et al. Perioperative chemotherapy versus surgery alone for resectable gastroesophageal cancer. N Engl J Med. 2006;355(1):11–20.

14. Ychou M, Boige V, Pignon JP, et al. Perioperative chemotherapy compared with surgery alone for resectable gastroesophageal adenocarcinoma: an FNCLCC and FFCD multicenter phase III trial. J Clin Oncol. 2011;29(13):1715–21.

15. van Hagen P, Hulshof MC, van Lanschot JJ, et al. Preoperative chemoradiotherapy for esophageal or junctional cancer. N Engl J Med. 2012;366(22): 2074–84.

16. Lowy AM, Mansfield PF, Leach SD, Pazdur R, Dumas P, Ajani JA. Response to neoadjuvant chemotherapy best predicts survival after curative resection of gastric cancer. Ann Surg. 1999;229(3):303–8.

17. Lordick F, Ott K, Krause BJ, et al. PET to assess early metabolic response and to guide treatment of adenocarcinoma of the oesophagogastric junction: the MUNICON phase II trial. Lancet Oncol. 2007;8(9): 797–805.

18. Ott K, Fink U, Becker K, et al. Prediction of response to preoperative chemotherapy in gastric carcinoma by metabolic imaging: results of a prospective trial. J Clin Oncol. 2003;21(24):4604–10.

19. Ott K, Herrmann K, Lordick F, et al. Early metabolic response evaluation by fluorine-18 fluorodeoxyglucose positron emission tomography allows in vivo testing of chemosensitivity in gastric cancer: long-term results of a prospective study. Clin Cancer Res. 2008;14(7):2012–8.

20. Cheedella NK, Suzuki A, Xiao L, et al. Association between clinical complete response and pathological complete response after preoperative chemoradiation in patients with gastroesophageal cancer: analysis in a large cohort. Ann Oncol. 2013;24(5):1262–6.

21. Yoshikawa T, Tanabe K, Nishikawa K, et al. Accuracy of CT staging of locally advanced gastric cancer after neoadjuvant chemotherapy: cohort evaluation within a randomized phase II study. Ann Surg Oncol. 2014;21: S385–9.

22. Conlon KC, Karpeh Jr MS. Laparoscopy and laparoscopic ultrasound in the staging of gastric cancer. Semin Oncol. 1996;23(3):347–51.

23. Badgwell B, Cormier JN, Krishnan S, et al. Does neoadjuvant treatment for gastric cancer patients with positive peritoneal cytology at staging laparoscopy improve survival? Ann Surg Oncol. 2008;15(10):2684–91.

24. Samee A, Moorthy K, Jaipersad T, et al. Evaluation of the role of laparoscopic ultrasonography in the staging of oesophagogastric cancers. Surg Endosc. 2009; 23(9):2061–5.

25. Lorenzen S, Panzram B, Rosenberg R, et al. Prognostic significance of free peritoneal tumor cells in the peritoneal cavity before and after neoadjuvant chemotherapy in patients with gastric carcinoma undergoing potentially curative resection. Ann Surg Oncol. 2010; 17(10):2733–9.

26. Cardona K, Zhou Q, Gonen M, et al. Role of repeat staging laparoscopy in locoregionally advanced gastric or gastroesophageal cancer after neoadjuvant therapy. Ann Surg Oncol. 2013;20(2):548–54.

27. Siewert JR, Bottcher K, Stein HJ, Roder JD. Relevant prognostic factors in gastric cancer: ten-year results of the German Gastric Cancer Study. Ann Surg. 1998; 228(4):449–61.

28. Songun I, Putter H, Kranenbarg EM, Sasako M, van de Velde CJ. Surgical treatment of gastric cancer: 15-year follow-up results of the randomised nationwide Dutch D1D2 trial. Lancet Oncol. 2010;11(5): 439–49.

29. Vinuela EF, Gonen M, Brennan MF, Coit DG, Strong VE. Laparoscopic versus open distal gastrectomy for gastric cancer: a meta-analysis of randomized controlled trials and high-quality nonrandomized studies. Ann Surg. 2012;255(3):446–56.

30. Choi YY, Bae JM, An JY, Hyung WJ, Noh SH. Laparoscopic gastrectomy for advanced gastric cancer: are the long-term results comparable with conventional open gastrectomy? A systematic review and meta-analysis. J Surg Oncol. 2013;108(8):550–6.

31. Kim HH, Han SU, Kim MC, et al. Long-term results of laparoscopic gastrectomy for gastric cancer: a large-scale case–control and case-matched Korean multicenter study. J Clin Oncol. 2014;32(7):627–33.

32. Oh SY, Kwon S, Lee KG, et al. Outcomes of minimally invasive surgery for early gastric cancer are comparable with those for open surgery: analysis of 1,013 minimally invasive surgeries at a single institution. Surg Endosc. 2014;28(3):789–95.

33. Tanabe S, Ishido K, Higuchi K, et al. Long-term outcomes of endoscopic submucosal dissection for early gastric cancer: a retrospective comparison with conventional endoscopic resection in a single center. Gastric Cancer. 2014;17(1):130–6.

34. Nishikawa K, Yanaga K, Kashiwagi H, Hanyuu N, Iwabuchi S. Significance of intraoperative endoscopy in total gastrectomy for gastric cancer. Surg Endosc. 2010;24(10):2633–6.

35. Sasako M, Sano T, Yamamoto S, et al. D2 lymphadenectomy alone or with para-aortic nodal dissection for gastric cancer. N Engl J Med. 2008;359(5):453–62.

36. Kurokawa Y, Sasako M, Sano T, et al. Functional outcomes after extended surgery for gastric cancer. Br J Surg. 2011;98(2):239–45.

37. Gouzi JL, Huguier M, Fagniez PL, et al. Total versus subtotal gastrectomy for adenocarcinoma of the gastric antrum. A French prospective controlled study. Ann Surg. 1989;209(2):162–6.

38. Bozzetti F, Marubini E, Bonfanti G, Miceli R, Piano C, Gennari L. Subtotal versus total gastrectomy for gastric cancer: five-year survival rates in a multicenter randomized Italian trial. Italian Gastrointestinal Tumor Study Group. Ann Surg. 1999;230(2):170–8.

39. Pugliese R, Maggioni D, Sansonna F, et al. Subtotal gastrectomy with D2 dissection by minimally invasive surgery for distal adenocarcinoma of the stomach:

results and 5-year survival. Surg Endosc. 2010;24(10): 2594–602.

40. Shin D, Park SS. Clinical importance and surgical decision-making regarding proximal resection margin for gastric cancer. World J Gastrointest Oncol. 2013; 5(1):4–11.

41. Mine S, Sano T, Hiki N, et al. Proximal margin length with transhiatal gastrectomy for Siewert type II and III adenocarcinomas of the oesophagogastric junction. Br J Surg. 2013;100(8):1050–4.

42. Bozzetti F, Marubini E, Bonfanti G, et al. Total versus subtotal gastrectomy: surgical morbidity and mortality rates in a multicenter Italian randomized trial. The Italian Gastrointestinal Tumor Study Group. Ann Surg. 1997;226(5):613–20.

43. Stein HJ, Feith M, Mueller J, Werner M, Siewert JR. Limited resection for early adenocarcinoma in Barrett's esophagus. Ann Surg. 2000;232(6):733–42.

44. Siewert JR, Stein HJ. Classification of adenocarcinoma of the oesophagogastric junction. Br J Surg. 1998;85(11):1457–9.

45. Siewert JR, Feith M, Werner M, Stein HJ. Adenocarcinoma of the esophagogastric junction: results of surgical therapy based on anatomical/topographic classification in 1,002 consecutive patients. Ann Surg. 2000;232(3):353–61.

46. Yoshikawa T, Tsuburaya A, Kobayashi O, et al. Is bursectomy necessary for patients with gastric cancer invading the serosa? Hepatogastroenterology. 2004; 51(59):1524–6.

47. Yamamura Y, Ito S, Mochizuki Y, Nakanishi H, Tatematsu M, Kodera Y. Distribution of free cancer cells in the abdominal cavity suggests limitations of bursectomy as an essential component of radical surgery for gastric carcinoma. Gastric Cancer. 2007; 10(1):24–8.

48. Schwarz RE. Spleen-preserving splenic hilar lymphadenectomy at the time of gastrectomy for cancer: technical feasibility and early results. J Surg Oncol. 2002;79(1):73–6.

49. Schwarz RE, Zagala-Nevarez K. Gastrectomy circumstances that influence early postoperative outcome. Hepatogastroenterology. 2002;49(48):1742–6.

50. Hyung WJ, Lim JS, Song J, Choi SH, Noh SH. Laparoscopic spleen-preserving splenic hilar lymph node dissection during total gastrectomy for gastric cancer. J Am Coll Surg. 2008;207(2):e6–11.

51. Huang CM, Chen QY, Lin JX, et al. Laparoscopic spleen-preserving no. 10 lymph node dissection for advanced proximal gastric cancer using a left approach. Ann Surg Oncol. 2014;21:2051.

52. Wu CW, Hsiung CA, Lo SS, et al. Nodal dissection for patients with gastric cancer: a randomised controlled trial. Lancet Oncol. 2006;7(4):309–15.

53. Smith DD, Schwarz RR, Schwarz RE. Impact of total lymph node count on staging and survival after gastrectomy for gastric cancer: data from a large US-population database. J Clin Oncol. 2005;23(28): 7114–24.

54. Schwarz RE, Smith DD. Clinical impact of lymphadenectomy extent in resectable gastric cancer of advanced stage. Ann Surg Oncol. 2007;14(2):317–28.

55. Smith DD, Nelson RA, Schwarz RE. A comparison of five competing lymph node staging schemes in a cohort of resectable gastric cancer patients. Ann Surg Oncol. 2014;21(3):875–82.

56. Bonenkamp JJ, Hermans J, Sasako M, et al. Extended lymph-node dissection for gastric cancer. N Engl J Med. 1999;340(12):908–14.

57. Hartgrink HH, Van De Velde CJ, Putter H, et al. Extended lymph node dissection for gastric cancer: who may benefit? Final results of the randomized Dutch gastric cancer group trial. J Clin Oncol. 2004; 22(11):2069–77.

58. Schwarz RE, Karpeh MS, Brennan MF. Surgical management of gastric cancer: the Western experience. In: Daly JM, Hennessy TPJ, Reynolds JV, editors. Management of upper gastrointestinal cancer. London: W.B. Saunders; 1999. p. 83–106.

59. Kodera Y, Schwarz RE, Nakao A. Extended lymph node dissection in gastric carcinoma: where do we stand after the Dutch and British randomized trials? J Am Coll Surg. 2002; 95(6):855–64.

60. Kitagawa Y, Takeuchi H, Takagi Y, et al. Sentinel node mapping for gastric cancer: a prospective multicenter trial in Japan. J Clin Oncol. 2013;31(29):3704–10.

61. Mayanagi S, Takeuchi H, Kamiya S, et al. Suitability of sentinel node mapping as an index of metastasis in early gastric cancer following endoscopic resection. Ann Surg Oncol. 2014;21:2987–93.

62. Behrns KE, Sarr MG. Diagnosis and management of gastric emptying disorders. Adv Surg. 1994;27:233–55.

63. Zong L, Chen P. Billroth I. vs. Billroth II vs. Roux-en-Y following distal gastrectomy: a meta-analysis based on 15 studies. Hepatogastroenterology. 2011;58(109): 1413–24.

64. Hirao M, Takiguchi S, Imamura H, et al. Comparison of Billroth I and Roux-en-Y reconstruction after distal gastrectomy for gastric cancer: one-year postoperative effects assessed by a multi-institutional RCT. Ann Surg Oncol. 2013;20(5):1591–7.

65. Ishikawa M, Kitayama J, Kaizaki S, et al. Prospective randomized trial comparing Billroth I and Roux-en-Y procedures after distal gastrectomy for gastric carcinoma. World J Surg. 2005;29(11):1415–20; discussion 1421.

66. Kojima K, Yamada H, Inokuchi M, Kawano T, Sugihara K. A comparison of Roux-en-Y and Billroth-I reconstruction after laparoscopy-assisted distal gastrectomy. Ann Surg. 2008;247(6):962–7.

67. Fein M, Fuchs KH, Thalheimer A, Freys SM, Heimbucher J, Thiede A. Long-term benefits of Roux-en-Y pouch reconstruction after total gastrectomy: a randomized trial. Ann Surg. 2008;247(5):759–65.

68. Zong L, Chen P, Chen Y, Shi G. Pouch Roux-en-Y vs No Pouch Roux-en-Y following total gastrectomy: a meta-analysis based on 12 studies. J Biomed Res. 2011;25(2):90–9.

69. Carrere N, Seulin P, Julio CH, Bloom E, Gouzi JL, Pradere B. Is nasogastric or nasojejunal decompression necessary after gastrectomy? A prospective randomized trial. World J Surg. 2007;31(1):122–7.

70. Pacelli F, Rosa F, Marrelli D, et al. Naso-gastric or naso-jejunal decompression after partial distal gastrectomy for gastric cancer. Final results of a multicenter prospective randomized trial. Gastric Cancer 2013. [Epub ahead of print].

71. Petrowsky H, Demartines N, Rousson V, Clavien PA. Evidence-based value of prophylactic drainage in gastrointestinal surgery: a systematic review and meta-analyses. Ann Surg. 2004;240(6):1074–84; discussion 1084–1075.

72. Kumar M, Yang SB, Jaiswal VK, Shah JN, Shreshtha M, Gongal R. Is prophylactic placement of drains necessary after subtotal gastrectomy? World J Gastroenterol. 2007;13(27):3738–41.

73. Ishikawa K, Matsumata T, Kishihara F, Fukuyama Y, Masuda H. Laparoscopy-assisted distal gastrectomy for early gastric cancer with versus without prophylactic drainage. Surg Today. 2011;41(8):1049–53.

74. McCarter MD, Gomez ME, Daly JM. Early postoperative enteral feeding following major upper gastrointestinal surgery. J Gastrointest Surg. 1997;1(3):278–85; discussion 285.

75. Patel SH, Kooby DA, Staley 3rd CA, Maithel SK. An assessment of feeding jejunostomy tube placement at the time of resection for gastric adenocarcinoma. J Surg Oncol. 2013;107(7):728–34.

76. Schwarz RE. Simple feeding jejunostomy technique for postoperative nutrition after major upper gastrointestinal resections. J Surg Oncol. 2002;79(2):126–30.

77. Kim MM, Rana V, Janjan NA, et al. Clinical benefit of palliative radiation therapy in advanced gastric cancer. Acta Oncol. 2008;47(3):421–7.

78. Hashimoto K, Mayahara H, Takashima A, et al. Palliative radiation therapy for hemorrhage of unresectable gastric cancer: a single institute experience. J Cancer Res Clin Oncol. 2009;135(8):1117–23.

79. Chaw CL, Niblock PG, Chaw CS, Adamson DJ. The role of palliative radiotherapy for haemostasis in unresectable gastric cancer: a single-institution experience. Ecancermedicalscience. 2014;8:384.

80. Koucky K, Wein A, Konturek PC, et al. Palliative first-line therapy with weekly high-dose 5-fluorouracil and sodium folinic acid as a 24-hour infusion (AIO regimen) combined with weekly irinotecan in patients with metastatic adenocarcinoma of the stomach or esophagogastric junction followed by secondary metastatic resection after downsizing. Med Sci Monit. 2011;17(5):CR248–58.

81. Boskoski I, Tringali A, Familiari P, Mutignani M, Costamagna G. Self-expandable metallic stents for malignant gastric outlet obstruction. Adv Ther. 2010; 27(10):691–703.

82. Mahar AL, Coburn NG, Karanicolas PJ, Viola R, Helyer LK. Effective palliation and quality of life outcomes in studies of surgery for advanced, non-curative

gastric cancer: a systematic review. Gastric Cancer. 2012;15 Suppl 1:S138–45.

83. Chang YR, Han DS, Kong SH, et al. The value of palliative gastrectomy in gastric cancer with distant metastasis. Ann Surg Oncol. 2012;19(4):1231–9.

84. Kokkola A, Louhimo J, Puolakkainen P. Does non-curative gastrectomy improve survival in patients with metastatic gastric cancer? J Surg Oncol. 2012;106(2):193–6.

85. Karpeh Jr MS. Palliative treatment and the role of surgical resection in gastric cancer. Dig Surg. 2013;30(2): 174–80.

86. Bonenkamp JJ, Sasako M, Hermans J, van de Velde CJ. Tumor load and surgical palliation in gastric cancer. Hepatogastroenterology. 2001;48(41):1219–21.

87. Blair SL, Chu DZ, Schwarz RE. Outcome of palliative operations for malignant bowel obstruction in patients with peritoneal carcinomatosis from nongynecological cancer. Ann Surg Oncol. 2001;8(8):632–7.

88. Tokunaga M, Tanizawa Y, Bando E, Kawamura T, Terashima M. Poor survival rate in patients with postoperative intra-abdominal infectious complications following curative gastrectomy for gastric cancer. Ann Surg Oncol. 2013;20(5):1575–83.

89. Birkmeyer JD, Sun Y, Goldfaden A, Birkmeyer NJ, Stukel TA. Volume and process of care in high-risk cancer surgery. Cancer. 2006;106(11):2476–81.

90. Birkmeyer JD, Sun Y, Wong SL, Stukel TA. Hospital volume and late survival after cancer surgery. Ann Surg. 2007;245(5):777–83.

91. Schwarz RE, Zagala-Nevarez K. Recurrence patterns after radical gastrectomy for gastric cancer: prognostic factors and implications for postoperative adjuvant therapy. Ann Surg Oncol. 2002;9(4):394–400.

92. D'Angelica M, Gonen M, Brennan MF, Turnbull AD, Bains M, Karpeh MS. Patterns of initial recurrence in completely resected gastric adenocarcinoma. Ann Surg. 2004;240(5):808–16.

93. Yoo CH, Noh SH, Shin DW, Choi SH, Min JS. Recurrence following curative resection for gastric carcinoma. Br J Surg. 2000;87(2):236–42.

94. Dikken JL, Baser RE, Gonen M, et al. Conditional probability of survival nomogram for 1-, 2-, and 3-year survivors after an R0 resection for gastric cancer. Ann Surg Oncol. 2013;20(5):1623–30.

95. Hirabayashi S, Kosugi S, Isobe Y, et al. Development and external validation of a nomogram for overall survival after curative resection in serosa-negative, locally advanced gastric cancer. Ann Oncol. 2014;25:1179–84.

96. Oppedijk V, van der Gaast A, van Lanschot JJ, et al. Patterns of recurrence after surgery alone versus preoperative chemoradiotherapy and surgery in the CROSS trials. J Clin Oncol. 2014;32(5):385–91.

97. Stahl M, Walz MK, Stuschke M, et al. Phase III comparison of preoperative chemotherapy compared with chemoradiotherapy in patients with locally advanced adenocarcinoma of the esophagogastric junction. J Clin Oncol. 2009;27(6):851–6.

98. Chen Y, Kingham K, Ford JM, et al. A prospective study of total gastrectomy for CDH1-positive heredi-

tary diffuse gastric cancer. Ann Surg Oncol. 2011; 18(9):2594–8.

99. Seevaratnam R, Coburn N, Cardoso R, Dixon M, Bocicariu A, Helyer L. A systematic review of the indications for genetic testing and prophylactic gastrectomy among patients with hereditary diffuse gastric cancer. Gastric Cancer. 2012;15 Suppl 1:S153–63.

100. Fujita H, Lennerz JK, Chung DC, et al. Endoscopic surveillance of patients with hereditary diffuse gastric cancer: biopsy recommendations after topographic distribution of cancer foci in a series of 10 CDH1-mutated gastrectomies. Am J Surg Pathol. 2012;36(11):1709–17.

101. Worster E, Liu X, Richardson S, et al. The impact of prophylactic total gastrectomy on health-related quality of life: a prospective cohort study. Ann Surg. 2014;260:87–93.

102. Worthley DL, Phillips KD, Wayte N, et al. Gastric adenocarcinoma and proximal polyposis of the stomach (GAPPS): a new autosomal dominant syndrome. Gut 2012;61(5):774–9.

103. Joensuu H, Vehtari A, Riihimaki J, et al. Risk of recurrence of gastrointestinal stromal tumour after surgery: an analysis of pooled population-based cohorts. Lancet Oncol. 2012;13(3):265–74.

104. Dematteo RP, Ballman KV, Antonescu CR, et al. Adjuvant imatinib mesylate after resection of localised, primary gastrointestinal stromal tumour: a randomised, double-blind, placebo-controlled trial. Lancet. 2009;373(9669):1097–104.

105. Joensuu H, Eriksson M, Sundby Hall K, et al. One vs three years of adjuvant imatinib for operable gastrointestinal stromal tumor: a randomized trial. JAMA. 2012;307(12):1265–72.

Endoscopic Submucosal Dissection for Gastric Cancer: Its Indication, Technique, and Our Experience

8

Hiroki Sato and Haruhiro Inoue

Introduction

Implementation of screening and surveillance upper GI endoscopy and the availability of endoscopes allowed for the identification and diagnosis of early gastric carcinoma (EGC) which can still be resected endoscopically.

EGCs are defined as those in which invasion is limited to either the mucosa or submucosa irrespective of lymph node involvement [1]. In those lesions, at present, widely accepted techniques for endoscopic resection (ER), particularly endoscopic mucosal resection (EMR), are indicated only for differentiated adenocarcinoma smaller than 2 cm and confined to the mucosa [2, 3] so as to assure en bloc resection of the tumor. EMR is an endoscopic resection technique which utilizes snare wire [4, 5]. In 1993, Cap-EMR method was developed, which allows easy resection of mucosal lesions [6]. This technique is currently modified and further popularized as EMR-C.

Compared to these techniques, however, advancements in the technique of endoscopic submucosal dissection (ESD) expanded the criteria to include tumors more than 2 cm with or without ulcers to be successfully removed endoscopically in an en bloc fashion [7, 8]. As an extended indication, submucosal invasion (sm1, infiltration depth less than 500 µm with no vessel permeation) is also accepted. Several retrospective studies in EGC tumors with a low risk of lymph node metastasis further support the extension of the indication for ESD [3, 9].

Moreover, patients with EGC who are poor surgical candidates due to underlying comorbidities may be managed safely and less invasively through ESD [10, 11].

In this chapter, we present the principles and practice of ESD for EGC and describe our experience and clinical outcomes.

Indication for Cure Rates with Endoscopic Resection

The Japanese EMR/ESD guidelines have been described [2, 12].

Indication for Endoscopic Resection

Contrary to the conventional criteria for ER which limits EMR/ESD to differentiated-type

H. Sato, MD (✉) • H. Inoue, MD, PhD
Digestive Disease Center, Showa University,
Northern Yokohama Hospital,
35-1 Chigasakichuo, Tsuzuki-ku,
Yokohoma 224-8503, Japan
e-mail: pyloki.sato@gmail.com

S.N. Hochwald, M. Kukar (eds.), *Minimally Invasive Foregut Surgery for Malignancy: Principles and Practice*,
DOI 10.1007/978-3-319-09342-0_8, © Springer International Publishing Switzerland 2015

adenocarcinomas without ulcerative findings (UL(−)), of which the depth of invasion is clinically diagnosed as T1a and the diameter is ≤2 cm, the expanded criteria for ESD encompass tumors clinically diagnosed as T1a which includes the following:

(i) Differentiated type, UL(−), but >2 cm in diameter

(ii) Differentiated type, UL(+), and ≤3 cm in diameter

(iii) Undifferentiated type, UL(−), and ≤2 cm in diameter

Data regarding the "therapeutic efficacy" of ESD when applying the expanded criteria is limited; hence, the decision to do ESD should be on a case-to-case basis and the procedure offered with caution (Fig. 8.1).

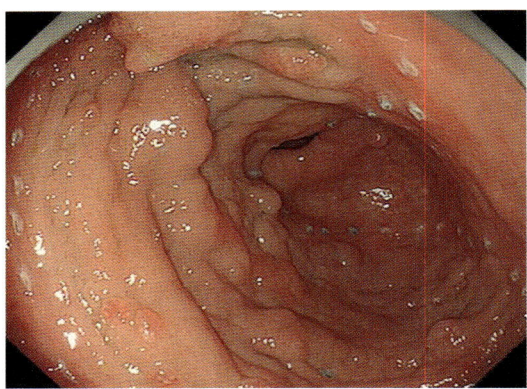

Fig. 8.1 This is a case of a 93-year-old female who was referred to our hospital for the treatment of a gastric tumor that by biopsy was group 3. Conventional endoscopy revealed a circumferential, slightly elevated lesion in the gastric antrum, which was resected by ESD as an expanded indication. Pathological diagnosis was 110×65 mm, type 0–IIa, adenocarcinoma, T1a, ly0, v0, HM0, and VM0

Therapeutic Efficacy of Endoscopic Resection

The resected specimen should be handled according to the rules described in the Japanese classification [2] (Table 8.1).

Curative tumor resection was previously defined as en bloc resection of a differentiated-type tumor, ≤2 cm in size, pT1a, negative horizontal margin (HM0), negative vertical margin (VM0), and no lymphovascular infiltration (ly(−), v(−)).

Following the expanded criteria for ESD in EGC, resection is considered curative when all of the following conditions are fulfilled:

- En bloc resection, HM0, VM0, ly(−), v(−)
  (a) Tumor size ≥2 cm, histologically of a differentiated type, pT1a, UL(−)
  (b) Tumor size ≤3 cm, histologically of a differentiated type, pT1a, UL(+)
  (c) Tumor size ≤2 cm, histologically of undifferentiated type, pT1a, UL(−)
  (d) Tumor size ≤3 cm, histologically of differentiated type, pT1b (SM1,<500 μm from the muscularis mucosae)

Follow-up abdominal ultrasonography or computed tomography (CT) scan and annual or biannual endoscopy are still recommended in all cases of curative resection meeting the expanded criteria.

Summary

The expanded criteria for ESD are now being employed as more endoscopists become skillful in performing ESD. As the procedure is offered

Table 8.1 Indication for ESD: current and expanded indications

	T1a				T1b	
	UL(−)		UL(+)		≦ SM1	SM1<
	≦ 20 mm	20 mm<	≦ 30 mm	30 mm<	≦ 30 mm	Any size
Differentiated-type						
Undifferentiated-type						

■ :current indication

■ :expanded indication

Table 8.2 High-frequency knives for ESD

Needle Knife type	Flush knife (DK2618JB/DK2618JN, Fujifilm Co.)
	Flex knife (KD-630 L, Olympus Co.)
	Triangle Tip Knife (KD-640 L, Olympus Co)
	Dual Knife (KD-650 L/KD-650Q, Olympus Co)
	Hook Knife (KD-620LR/KD-620QR, Olympus Co.)
IT-knife type	IT-knife, IT-knife-2, IT-knife-nano (KD-610 L/KD-611 L/KD-612, Olympus Co.)
Non-IT-knife type	Mucosectom (DP-2518, PENTAX Co.)
	SAFE knife (DK2518DV1, Fujifilm Co.)
	Swanblade (DC-D2618, PENTAX, Tokyo)
Scissors forceps type	Clutch Cutter (DP2618DT, Fujifilm Co.)
	SB knife and SB knife Jr. (MD-47706/MD-47704 and MD-47703, Sumitomo Bakelite Co.)

to more patients, further studies on clinical efficacy and safety following the expanded criteria are warranted [13].

Device for ESD [14–16]

Knives for ESD

Knives used for ESD have been conventionally classified into needle type or insulated tip type based on the design, shape, and method of use. At present, various knives are available including those designed for use in areas in which the approach is difficult or knives which increase the safety intraoperatively. However, use of this wide range of knives requires an adequate understanding of the properties of each to allow their application under appropriate conditions.

The ESD knives currently available in Japan are described and classified below into (1) needle type, (2) IT-knife type (insulation-tipped type), (3) non-IT-knife type, and (4) scissors forceps type (Table 8.2, Fig. 8.2).

Needle Type

Short needle is the representative type in this category (although Needle Knife (Olympus Co.,

Tokyo Japan), which has a long sharp non-covered needle, was originally used for ESD). This knife enables the endoscopist to perform ESD with direct visualization of the area to be cut. Both incision and dissection can be done using this device. Among the short-needle type, Flush knife (Fujifilm Co., Tokyo, Japan) is used routinely in our hospital. The Flush knife has a water-jet function that makes additional submucosal injection possible. It also has two kinds of tip types (needle or ball-chip), and four kinds of knife lengths are available at 5 mm intervals (1.0–3.0 mm). The endoscopist should take into consideration both which organ (i.e., esophagus, stomach, colon) and the location of the lesion in choosing the suitable tip type and protruding length to be used for treatment. In our hospital, the Flush knife with a needle type tip, 2.0 mm in length, is employed for gastric ESD.

The other category is the hook type, represented by the Hook Knife (Olympus Co., Tokyo, Japan). The distal L-shaped hook has a rotatory function allowing for incision and dissection in longitudinal and lateral directions. This is done by simply turning the handle to point the tip of the hook in the desired direction. Moreover, the Hook Knife also enables the operator to "hook" tissue and pull away from the muscle layer, as its name suggests. This method minimizes the risk of perforation especially in cases of severe fibrosis as cutting is done away from the muscle layer. The drawback of using this knife, however, is that the amount of tissue that can be hooked at a time is limited prolonging procedure time.

IT-Knife Type

IT-knife and IT-knife-2 (Olympus Co., Tokyo, Japan) are the main knives used for gastric ESD. The ceramic insulator attached at the tip of the needle-shaped knife does not conduct electricity thereby minimizing invasiveness and reduces the risk of perforation. It allows lateral cutting from a vertical approach. To perform steady submucosal dissection, the ceramic globule and the sheath should be positioned properly on the surface of the incision or area to be dissected. It is said that procedure time is shorter when using IT-knife effectively because the

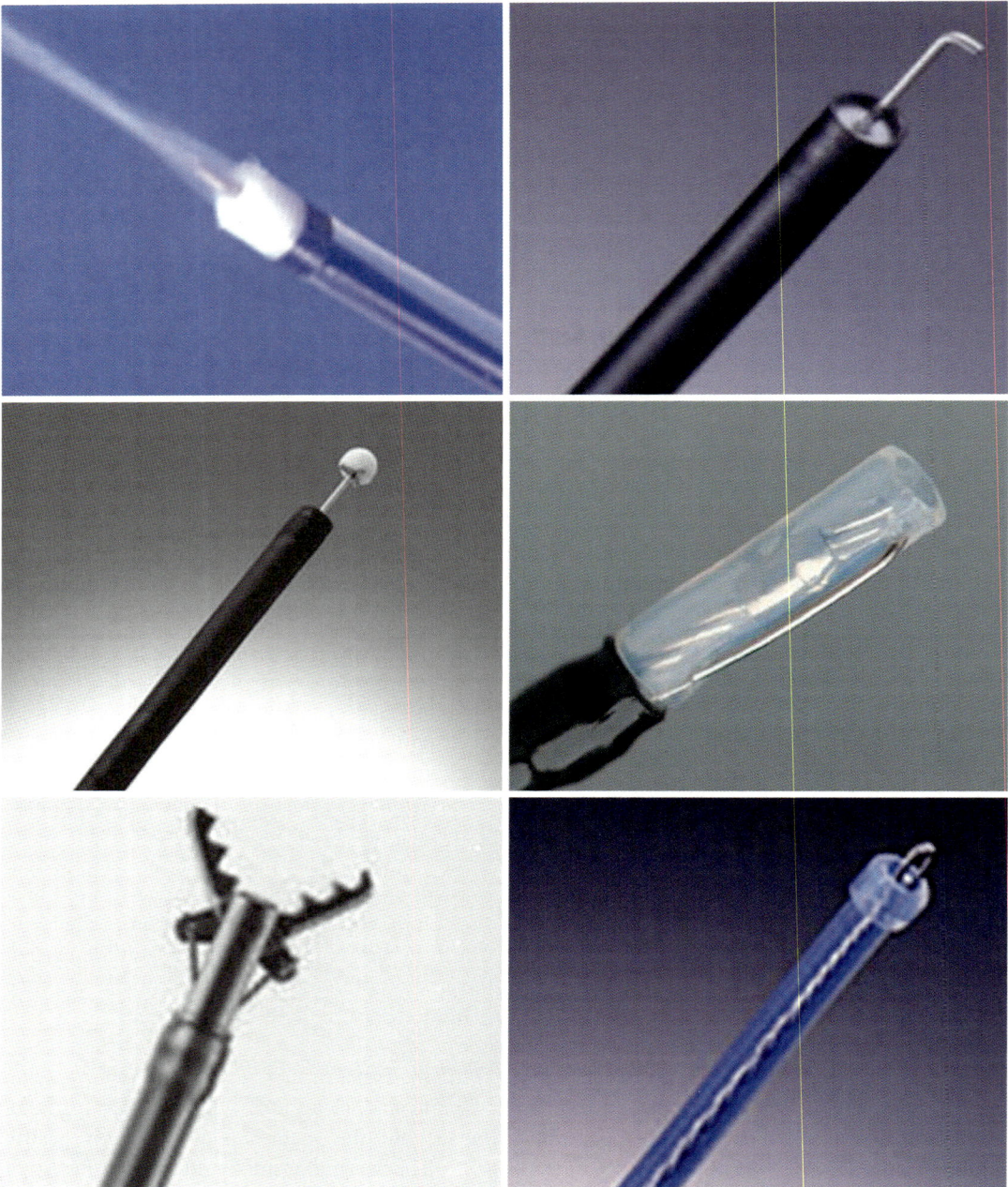

Fig. 8.2 Knives for ESD. *Upper left*, Flush knife; *Upper right*, Hook Knife; *Center left*, IT-knife-2; *Center right*, Mucosectom; *Lower left*, Clutch Cutter; *Lower right*, Flex knife

contact area between the blade and surface is increased due to "line" touch (understandably, needle type attach in a point), and tension can be applied during the dissection due to non-electrical conductivity of the tip. The downside of this knife is its high coagulation capacity causing tissue carbonization or charring which eventually prevents proper tissue contact and adequate depth dissection (see below "high-frequency generator").

Recently, the IT-knife-nano was developed, with a compact ceramic tip and small disklike structure of the backside electrical blade. It is expected to work effectively in difficult cases particularly with severe fibrosis.

Non-IT-Knife Type (Insulator Processing)

Mucosectom (HOYA PENTAX Co., Tokyo, Japan) is a knife wherein the tip and the lateral sides are covered by an insulator. In addition, the blade has a rotatable function enabling adjustments in the direction of dissection. This knife can be used as a secondary knife rather than a primary knife, reserving its use in cases where the position of the knife is perpendicular to the muscle layer and area of dissection especially in cases of severe fibrosis.

Scissors Forceps Type

This device was developed combining the design concepts of the conventional knife like Needle Knife and IT-knife type. The Clutch Cutter (Fujifilm Co., Tokyo, Japan) is representative of this category. These knives have the capability to grasp and cut tissue in direct view. Moreover the Clutch Cutter can also be used to perform hemostasis.

A large variety of ESD devices have now been developed and launched by several companies. Each knife has some unique characteristics in terms of sharpness for incision/dissection and capacity to do hemostasis. Therefore, the endoscopist should be cognizant of the knife features which will guide choosing the tool or device to be used in a particular situation.

Endoscope

The endoscope for ESD should have the following:
1. Flush function

    The water-jet function is important to clear the mucus from the lesion or to find the bleeding point. Clear water with small amount of dimethicone is used in our hospital.
2. Channel (size, number)

    The internal diameter of scope is a minimum of 2.8 mm considering the external diameter of each device. For the purpose of removing the smoke or mucus during the procedure, a 3.2 mm diameter channel is more desirable. A two-channel scope enables us to perform efficient suction (one channel for the device, another for suction) and effective dissection (one channel for the device, another for injection).
3. Flexure point

    The maximum angle of the scope is an important factor in approaching the lesion.

    The multi-bending function means that the second flexure point is set at the posterior side of the first, which enables an approach to any lesion.
4. Outside diameter

    In general, big external diameter means multi-function (water-jet function, 2-channel, etc.). However, for lightening patients' pain, using the small scope is better.

    Small scope also has a small turning circle, which is useful when dissection is performed by handling the endoscopic arm, particularly in the curve.

    In our hospital, a 9.9 mm endoscope with water-jet function (Olympus GIF Q260J) is used as our standard. Then if a close approach is difficult, the multi-bending scope (Olympus GIF 2TQ260M) is used.

Distal Attachment

A transparent tip hood is necessary for manipulation in ESD. It exerts tension on the submucosal layer and aids in easy entry into the submucosa. In addition, stable knife operation is possible during the procedure with good visibility even under conditions of body motion, breath movement, and heartbeat by holding down the front mucosa or holding up the lesion.

During the procedure with distal attachment, frequent use of an anti-fouling composition is important. Particularly when ST hood is used, because of its narrow vision, it is effective.

In our hospital, cylindrical hood (Olympus Co D-201-11804) and ST hood (Fujifilm Co

DH-15GR)/Short ST hood (Fujifilm Co DH-15GR) are used depending on the situation.

High-Frequency Generator (HFG)

A high-frequency generator (HFG) is an appliance designed for incision or coagulation of tissue. It uses heat-generated high-frequency electrical current applied to the tissue. Incision results from a vapor explosion of cellular membrane caused by continuous delivery of low-voltage current resulting in rapid generation of heat, whereas coagulation results from shrinkage of tissue and evaporation of moisture using intermittent, high-voltage current.

The details with regard to the energy setting of the HFG were discussed previously [14, 17]; however, in general, the configuration mode should be arranged per organ (i.e., esophagus, stomach, colon) and per knife or forceps devices.

Regarding the current density, if it is high, large amount of heat is made, and the incision capacity increases. If it is low, coagulation capacity increases. Meanwhile, current density is influenced by contact area. For example, a point attach (Flush knife, Flex knife) has high current density; on the contrary, a line attach (IT-knife) has low current density. Therefore, if the same output waveforms are used, the needle type point has more incision capacity, and IT-knife has more coagulation capacity (the tissue carbonizes easily). Thus, if the same device is used, current density would also change depending on the method of attaching the tissue.

In our hospital, the HFG VIO 300D (ERBE Elektromedizin GmbH, Tübingen, Germany) is being used during ESD. The following are the HFG settings we use for gastric ESD during the different procedural steps: mucosal marking, forced coagulation mode, 30 w, and effect 4; mucosal incision, Endocut I mode, cut duration 3, cut interval 2, and effect 2; and submucosal dissection, forced coagulation mode, 45 w, and effect 4.

In the next section, among the expanded indications, ESD for EGC with gastric ulcer and for undifferentiated adenocarcinoma is described.

Endoscopic Resection for EGC with Gastric Ulcer

Before Endoscopic Resection

In principle, open gastric ulcer with EGC should be cured by antisecretory medication such as proton pump inhibitor (PPI) or H_2 receptor antagonist (H2 blocker) if ESD is kept in mind as the first choice. (In this sentence, open gastric ulcer is defined as active (A) and healing (H) stages, not including the scar (S) stage according to the classification proposed by Sakita and Fukutomi [18].) One of the reasons is, particularly in the acute phase, it is difficult, almost impossible to assess the details of tumors (invasion depth, the extent, etc.) because of modifying factors like inflammatory reaction and edema. Another reason is that the specimen is easily torn by submucosal dissection because the tissue connection is too weak, particularly in the acute ulcer phase. Antisecretory medication is also effective to prevent ulcer relapse of EGC with scar.

In cases of gastric ESD at Northern Yokohama Hospital from July 2007 through March 2013, 38 differentiated adenocarcinomas had endoscopic ulcer findings on the first endoscopy (recurrent cancers were excluded). Thirteen carcinomas were found with the open ulcer. Every patient received medication therapy of PPI or H2 blocker and follow-up endoscopy was performed to assess the ulcer stage (improvement/no change/exacerbation). Regarding cases with open gastric ulcer ($n = 13$), as the median interval between the first and follow-up endoscopic examinations was 81.6 days (range 28–152), a change in ulcer stage was observed with improvement for 12 patients (92.3 %) and exacerbation for 1 patient (7.7 %). The case with unhealed ulcer is described separately below.

Additionally, regarding cases of scar stage, no exacerbation was found with a mean of 60.4 follow-up days (range 15–150) (Fig. 8.3).

ESD Procedure

(i) *Marking*

Marking should be performed 3–5 mm away from the margin of the tumor.

Fig. 8.3 Every patient who was diagnosed with a differentiated mucosal cancer with ulcer received antisecretory medication. Out of 13 cases with active ulcer, improvement was seen in 12 patients (92.3 %) and exacerbation in 1 patient (7.7 %). In cases with ulcer scarring (*n* = 25), no exacerbation was found. We may infer antisecretory medication is useful to prevent ulcer relapse

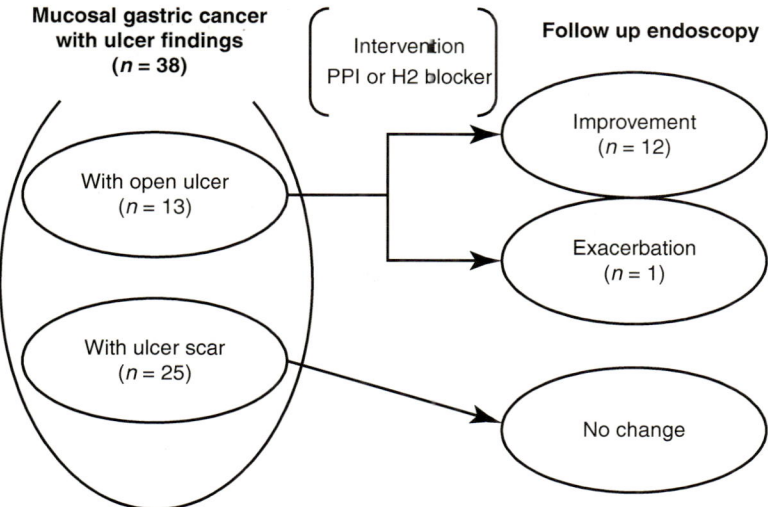

(ii) *Injection and incision*

Mucosal distention is accomplished by injection of a solution in to the submucosa through the mucosa. Injection is done prior to incision with the objective of lifting the mucosa away from the muscle layer. In cases where submucosal injection does not produce an adequate bleb, fibrosis should be suspected and the incision line reconsidered. In our hospital, glycerine (glycerol; Chugai Pharm Co., Tokyo, Japan) is routinely used as an injection solution. An alternative to this is normal saline with indigo carmine. In the presence of severe fibrosis, sodium hyaluronate solution (MucoUp; Johnson & Johnson Co., Tokyo, Japan) is effective to keep enough distance between the mucosal and muscle layer and prevent perforation.

Incision is made with reference to the location of the tumor and scar. In cases when the scar is located at the margins of the tumor, the incision should be made 1 cm away (Fig. 8.4) [19]. This allows creation of an adequate flap making dissection of the submucosal layer in the fibrotic area possible.

(iii) *Submucosal dissection*

EGC with ulceration has a very thin, clear layer of fibrotic submucosa separating the mucosa and muscle layer. Submucosal

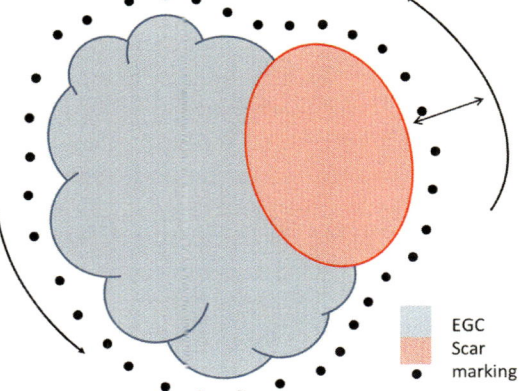

Fig. 8.4 If fibrosis is suspected in the marginal area of EGC, the incision line should be 1 cm away from the margin of the scar to make enough of a flap allowing access into the fibrotic submucosal layer

dissection is accomplished over the muscle layer with repeated injection.

In cases where the muscle layer and submucosal fibrosis are adherent, the clear layer is absent. Submucosal dissection is performed starting from the periphery going to the center of the lesion. Dissection is performed connecting bilateral submucosal layers paying careful attention not to damage the muscle layer.

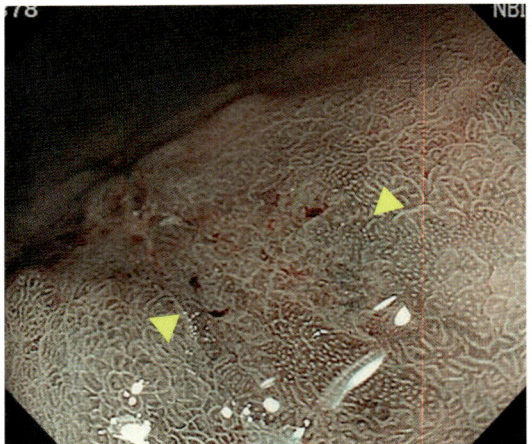

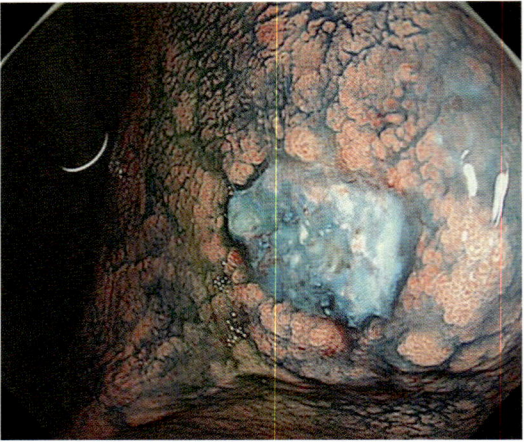

Fig. 8.5 ME with NBI shows fine-network superficial pattern indicative of well-differentiated adenocarcinoma. This allows identification of demarcation for cancer (*arrows* point to the demarcation line for cancer)

Fig. 8.6 Exacerbation of the gastric ulcer was seen despite PPI and *H. pylori* eradication therapy. However, the endoscopic appearance shows no evidence of invasion into the submucosa

In addition, CO_2 insufflation should be used throughout the procedure in case a perforation occurs.

A Case of Severe Fibrosis with Ulcer

This is a case of a 65-year-old male with history of unstable angina. He had coronary angioplasty and was maintained on antiplatelet medications.

Six months prior to ESD, he presented at our institution with 2-week history of abdominal pain. Endoscopic examination revealed a 2 cm ulcer at the posterior wall of the gastric angle. The patient was prescribed PPI and triple therapy for *H. pylori* eradication because of the positive serologic test. A repeat endoscopy was performed at a later date with a week of antiplatelet cessation and biopsies were taken from margin of the ulcer. The histopathologic results were indefinite for neoplasia; hence endoscopically, no cancer was identified.

A follow-up endoscopy 3 months after initial endoscopy showed a healing ulcer; however, magnifying endoscopy with narrow band imaging (ME-NBI) showed a fine-network pattern with demarcation line suggesting a well-differentiated adenocarcinoma [20] (Fig. 8.5). Thus, ESD was contemplated for diagnostic and therapeutic purposes.

Figure 8.6 shows the state of the gastric ulcer before treatment. Unfortunately at this time, the endoscopic appearance of the ulcer was worse compared to its condition on the previous endoscopy. However, a decision was made to perform ESD due to the following reasons as follows: (1) for definitive diagnosis (biopsy has a high bleeding risk due to antiplatelet therapy and not a reliable enough diagnostic tool, so in this case, resection biopsy was chosen) and (2) according to the endoscopic appearance, the depth of the relapsed ulcer was estimated as less deep than the layer dissected by the ESD technique; hence en bloc resection is possible.

Submucosal dissection was started from the periphery (1 cm away from the scar) going to the center of the lesion taking all the precautions by assessing dissection depth. Then, as anticipated, dissection was technically difficult because of paucity of submucosal space and much fibrosis below the ulcer (Fig. 8.7). With repeated injection, as the safe layer on each side was connected, submucosal dissection was performed. Nonetheless, a minor perforation was encountered at the bottom of the ulcer, which was successfully closed by placing endoscopic clips (Olympus Co., Tokyo, Japan). However, after dissection was further advanced before clipping because instant clipping interferes with dissection. Finally, ESD was accomplished in an en bloc fashion.

The patient was started on clear liquids 24 h post procedure and diet was progressed subsequently without untoward events.

Histological examination of the resected specimen showed well-differentiated adenocarcinoma, pT1a-M, 30×19 mm, UL(+), ly0, v0, pHM0, and pVM0, satisfying the currently expanded indication for endoscopic treatment (Fig. 8.8). Although careful follow-up is needed, ESD was considered to have accomplished the same objective as radical therapy.

This case shows that ulcerations in EGC may relapse even after PPI treatment due to its

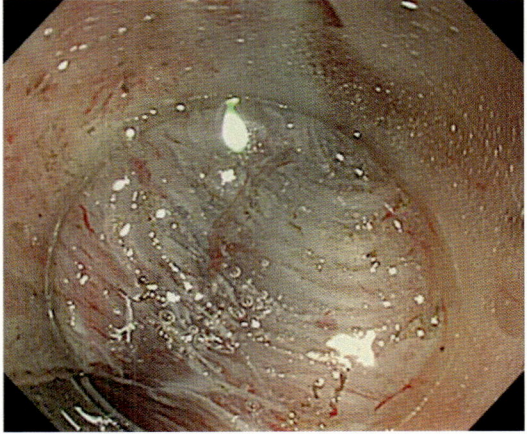

Fig. 8.7 Severe fibrosis was encountered below the ulcer which made identification and dissection of the submucosa difficult

malignant nature. Malignant ulceration usually arises at the margin of cancer in the presence of acid and pepsin. The repetitive cycle of inflammation and repair in the epithelial cells triggers the formation of fibrosis. Ultimately, cancer cells spread superficially or malignant invasion may occur along the fibrosis [18].

Jong Pil Im et al. reported that the use of antisecretory medication in mucosal cancer and a longer interval between the first and follow-up endoscopy were independently associated with healing of malignant ulcers [21]. Cancer should be resected at the most appropriate time when the ulcer is healed.

It has been recognized that ESD for EGC should be delayed until after ulcer healing has occurred; however, it is difficult to ascertain the time interval when this would occur even with PPI therapy. Ulcers in EGC behave in a different manner as peptic ulcer and healing is dependent on factors such as ulcer size and depth. Moreover, documentation of healing on endoscopy does not guarantee that the ulcer will not recur. A malignant ulcer may relapse as the cancer cells invade into the submucosa due to the malignant cycle [22].

Jae IK Lee reported that endoscopic resection should be restricted to cases showing significant improvement in the size and depth of ulcer at follow-up endoscopy [7]. Although this proposition is ideal, the fact that it is difficult to determine when significant improvement in ulcer size and depth occurs makes this problematic. In the untoward event of perforation, endoscopic closure

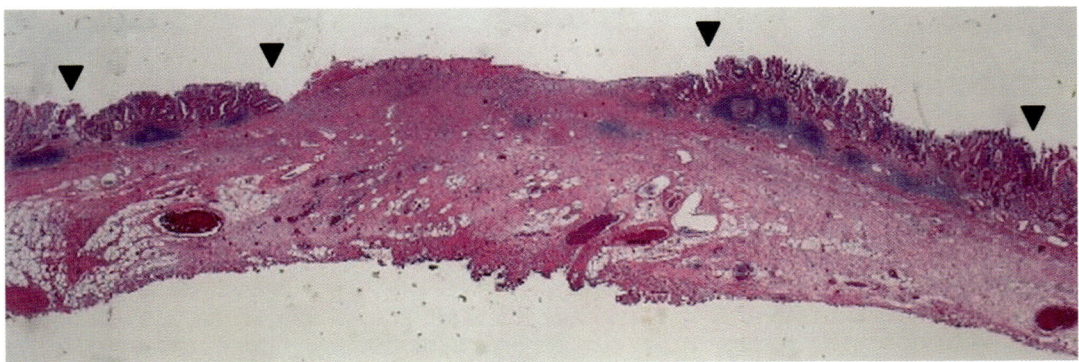

Fig. 8.8 Pathological diagnosis was well-differentiated adenocarcinoma, pT1a-M, 30×19 mm, UL(+), ly0, v0, pHM0, and pVM0, satisfying the criteria for expanded indication for ESD, *Arrow* demarcation line of mucosal cancer

using clips is effective [23]. An experienced endoscopist can successfully remove EGCs limited to the mucosa with non-healing ulcers via ESD and also manage its complications (i.e., perforation) endoscopically when it occurs. Of course, such high-quality ESD should be performed only by an experienced endoscopist.

In our opinion, it is of utmost importance to ascertain tumor depth prior to ESD. The presence of gastric ulcer makes endoscopic and even pathological diagnosis by biopsy challenging due to factors like inflammation, edema, and superficial regenerated epithelial cell infiltration [24–27]. Biopsy and ME-NBI are complementary diagnostic tools. In circumstances when biopsy is contraindicated or inconclusive, ME-NBI proves to be a useful tool to aid in the assessment of invasion depth and extent of cancer and also determine pathologic type based on the examination of surface patterns [20, 28–33].

ESD for Undifferentiated Adenocarcinoma

Principle

Undifferentiated intramucosal EGC demonstrates a relatively higher probability of lymph node metastasis (LNM) (4.2 %) than differentiated

intramucosal EGC (0.4 %) [3]. Thus, the currently accepted definitive treatment worldwide is surgical resection.

However, in a study by Gotoda et al., none of the 141 undifferentiated lesions without ulceration, less than 20 mm in size, were associated with positive lymph nodes [3]. Recently, the Japanese Gastric Cancer Treatment Guidelines expanded the indication for ESD to include undifferentiated EGC without ulceration.

Procedure

Undifferentiated carcinomas sometimes have diffuse invasion; hence, submucosal dissection should be done in the deep submucosal layer to achieve adequate tumor-free vertical margins. In general, the technique used to perform ESD on undifferentiated carcinoma follows the same principles as in differentiated cancer.

Signet ring cell carcinoma usually expands superficially with 0–IIb or 0–IIc macroscopic type, with white color or same color of adjacent normal epithelium (Fig. 8.9). The non-exposed expanding subepithelium of the tumor margin is often very difficult to identify. A 1 cm tumor-free margin confirmed by biopsy in 4 directions around the lesion should be made in order to achieve complete resection (Fig. 8.10).

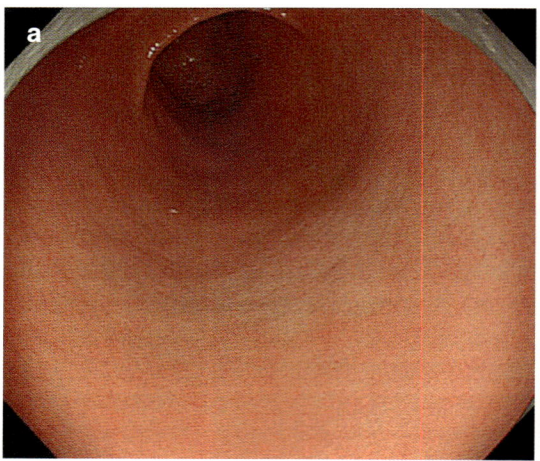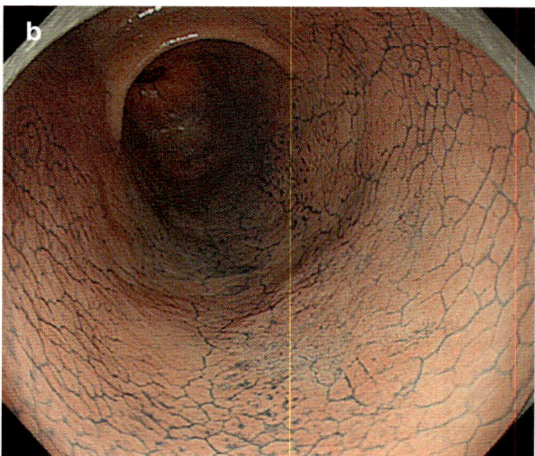

Fig. 8.9 Conventional endoscopy reveals a faded color, flat lesion in the gastric antrum (**a**), and gastric area has irregular pattern with indigo carmine stain (**b**). Under NBI, the area appears slightly brownish (**c**). With ME-NBI, microsurface architecture begins to disintegrate, and corkscrew-like vessels are observed (**d**)

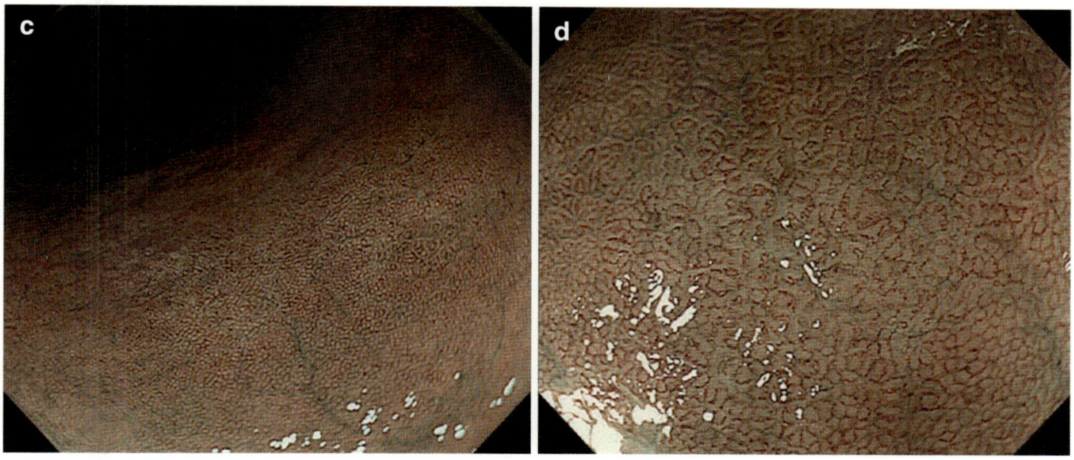

Fig. 8.9 (continued)

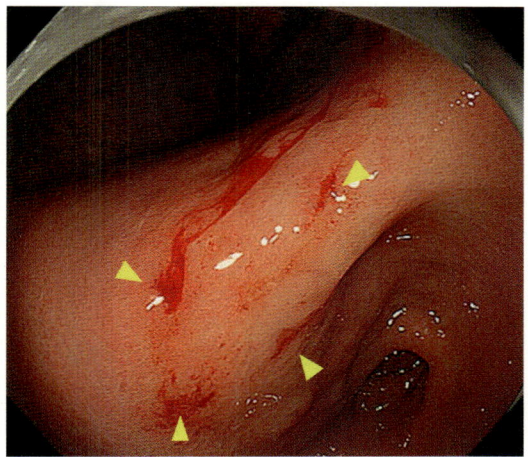

Fig. 8.10 Negative biopsies (4 points around the lesion) were performed to determine the margin histopathologically. ESD including the 4 negative biopsies is a good method for complete resection (*arrows* point to the biopsy points)

Conclusion

We summarized the technique used for ESD in EGC. With the improvements in equipment, technique, and endoscopic skills, the indication for ESD has now expanded to include undifferentiated cancers. However, due diligence is needed in determining which patients are good candidates for this procedure. Performing ER is only half of the equation in the treatment of EGC. We cannot overemphasize the importance of proper recognition of lesions and this can be achieved by ME-NBI. Identification of lesions amenable for endoscopic treatment and endoscopic skills is equally important to accomplish a safe and curative treatment.

The outcome of expanded criteria for ESD in EGC appears promising. However, data is limited and studies to validate the "new" criteria are warranted.

References

1. Japanese Research Society for Gastric Cancer. The general rules for the gastric cancer study in surgery and pathology. Jpn J Surg. 1981;11:127–39.
2. Japanese Gastric Cancer Association. Japanese gastric cancer treatment guidelines 2010 (ver. 3). Gastric Cancer. 2011;14:113–23.
3. Gotoda T, Yanagisawa A, Sasako M, et al. Incidence of lymph node metastasis from early gastric cancer: estimation with a large number of cases at two large centers. Gastric Cancer. 2000;3:219–25.

4. Tada M, Murakami A, Karita M, et al. Endoscopic resection of early gastric cancer. Endoscopy. 1993;25:445–50.

5. Deyhle P, Largiader F, Jenny S, et al. A method for endoscopic electroresection of sessile colonic polyps. Endoscopy. 1973;5:38–40.

6. Inoue H, Takeshita K, Hori H, et al. Endoscopic mucosal resection with a cap-fitted panendoscope for esophagus, stomach, and colon mucosal lesions. Gastrointest Endosc. 1993;39:58–62.

7. Lee JI, Kim JH, Choi BJ, et al. Indication for endoscopic treatment of ulcerative early gastric cancer according to depth of ulcer and morphological change. J Gastroenterol Hepatol. 2012;27:1718–25.

8. Gotoda T, Yamamoto H, Soetikno RM. Endoscopic submucosal dissection of early gastric cancer. J Gastroenterol. 2006;41:929–42.

9. Lee H, Yun WK, Min BH, et al. A feasibility study on the expanded indication for endoscopic submucosal dissection of early gastric cancer. Surg Endosc. 2011;25:1985–93.

10. Shimura T, Joh T, Sasaki M, et al. Endoscopic submucosal dissection is useful and safe for intramucosal gastric neoplasms in the elderly. Acta Gastroenterol Belg. 2007;70:323–30.

11. Isomoto H, Ohnita K, Yamaguchi N, et al. Clinical outcomes of endoscopic submucosal dissection in elderly patients with early gastric cancer. Eur J Gastroenterol Hepatol. 2010;22:311–7.

12. Ishikawa S, Togashi A, Inoue M, et al. Indications for EMR/ESD in cases of early gastric cancer: relationship between histological type, depth of wall invasion, and lymph node metastasis. Gastric Cancer. 2007;10:35–8.

13. Seiichiro A, Ichiro O, Haruhisa S, et al. Short- and long-term outcomes of endoscopic submucosal dissection for undifferentiated early gastric cancer. Endoscopy. 2013;45(09):703–7.

14. Matsui N, Akahoshi K, Nakamura K, et al. Endoscopic submucosal dissection for removal of superficial gastrointestinal neoplasms: a technical review. World J Gastrointest Endosc. 2012;4:123–36.

15. Oyama T. Basic technique of endoscopic submucosal dissection for esophageal and gastric tumor-knack, pit fall, and indications. Medical View Co., Ltd, Tokyo; 2007.

16. Kodashima S, Fujishiro M, Koike K. The features of the high-frequency Knives for ESD of colorectal neoplasms. Stomach Intestine. 2013;48:193–6.

17. Rey JF, Beilenhoff U, Neumann CS, et al. European Society of Gastrointestinal Endoscopy (ESGE) guideline: the use of electrosurgical units. Endoscopy. 2010;42:764–72.

18. Sakita T, Oguro Y, Takasu S, et al. Observations on the healing of ulcerations in early gastric cancer. The life cycle of the malignant ulcer. Gastroenterology. 1971;60:835–9. passim.

19. Takahashi A, Oyama O. ESD for early gastric cancer with ulcer scar. Stomach Intestine. 2013;48:63–71.

20. Yokoyama A, Inoue H, Minami H, et al. Novel narrow-band imaging magnifying endoscopic classification for early gastric cancer. Dig Liver Dis. 2010;42:704–8.

21. Im JP, Kim SG, Kim JS, et al. Time-dependent morphologic change in depressed-type early gastric cancer. Surg Endosc. 2009;23:2509–14.

22. Shimizu S, Tada M, Kawai K. Early gastric cancer: its surveillance and natural course. Endoscopy. 1995;27:27–31.

23. Minami S, Gotoda T, Ono H, et al. Complete endoscopic closure of gastric perforation induced by endoscopic resection of early gastric cancer using endoclips can prevent surgery (with video). Gastrointest Endosc. 2006;63:596–601.

24. Sano T, Okuyama Y, Kobori O, et al. Early gastric cancer. Endoscopic diagnosis of depth of invasion. Dig Dis Sci. 1990;35:1340–4.

25. Namieno T, Koito K, Hiigashi T, et al. Endoscopic prediction of tumor depth of gastric carcinoma for assessing the indication of its limited resection. Oncol Rep. 2000;7:57–61.

26. Lv SX, Gan JH, Ma XG, et al. Biopsy from the base and edge of gastric ulcer healing or complete healing may lead to detection of gastric cancer earlier: an 8 years endoscopic follow-up study. Hepatogastroenterology. 2012;59:947–50.

27. Banerjee S, Cash BD, Dominitz JA, et al. The role of endoscopy in the management of patients with peptic ulcer disease. Gastrointest Endosc. 2010;71:663–8.

28. Nagahama T, Yao K, Maki S, et al. Usefulness of magnifying endoscopy with narrow-band imaging for determining the horizontal extent of early gastric cancer when there is an unclear margin by chromoendoscopy (with video). Gastrointest Endosc. 2011;74:1259–67.

29. Kiyotoki S, Nishikawa J, Satake M, et al. Usefulness of magnifying endoscopy with narrow-band imaging for determining gastric tumor margin. J Gastroenterol Hepatol. 2010;25:1636–41.

30. Nakayoshi T, Tajiri H, Matsuda K, et al. Magnifying endoscopy combined with narrow band imaging system for early gastric cancer: correlation of vascular pattern with histopathology (including video). Endoscopy. 2004;36:1080–4.

31. Hayee B, Inoue H, Sato H, et al. Magnification narrow-band imaging for the diagnosis of early gastric cancer: a review of the Japanese literature for the Western endoscopist. Gastrointest Endosc. 2013;78:452–61.

32. Kobara H, Mori H, Fujihara S, et al. Prediction of invasion depth for submucosal differentiated gastric cancer by magnifying endoscopy with narrow-band imaging. Oncol Rep. 2012;28:841–7.

33. Kikuchi D, Iizuka T, Hoteya S, et al. Usefulness of magnifying endoscopy with narrow-band imaging for determining tumor invasion depth in early gastric cancer. Gastroenterol Res Pract. 2013;2013:217695.

Multimodality Therapy in Gastric Cancer

Usha Malhotra and Mei Ka Fong

Introduction

Gastric cancer is common worldwide with extensive variations between continents. Though the incidence of gastric cancer overall has been declining steadily since the 1970s, it still remains an enormous health issue. Also notable is the increase in proximal gastric cancer in the western hemisphere over the past few decades. Worldwide 989,600 new cases of gastric cancer were estimated in 2008 with 738,000 deaths accounting for 10 % of total cancer-related deaths [1]. In the United States, 21,600 new cases of gastric cancer were estimated in 2013 with 10,990 deaths [2]. Based on SEER data, 5-year survival rate still remains a dismal 25 % which is a marginal improvement over 14 % in 1970s.

For patients diagnosed with localized or locally advanced disease defined as disease confined to the stomach and/or regional lymph nodes, the intent of therapy is curative. Historically, for this subset of patients, the mainstay of treatment has been surgery. However, due to high failure rates with surgical resection alone, optimal management of locoregional gastric cancer involves utilization of chemotherapy and/or radiation in conjunction with surgery. For patients with surgically unresectable advanced stage or metastatic disease, treatment algorithms are palliative involving utilization of cytotoxic chemotherapy in combination with other modalities for symptomatic management.

In this chapter, pivotal studies supporting the role of chemotherapy and radiation in management of both localized and metastatic gastric cancer will be reviewed. Surgical approaches are described in detail in other sections.

Management of Localized and Locoregional Gastric Cancer

Based on patterns and risk of recurrence, the benefit of additional chemotherapy and/or radiation is most substantial in stages IB–III where the cancer is resectable and potentially curable but there is a high risk of recurrence. There is currently a wide variation in utilization of these modalities in the adjuvant (after surgical resection) and neoadjuvant (prior to surgical resection) settings with no established standard of care. This is due to a multitude of factors including postulated regional variations in tumor biology between eastern and western hemisphere dictating a preference for certain treatment paradigms

U. Malhotra, MD (✉)
Department of Medicine,
Roswell Park Cancer Institute,
Elm and Carlton Street, Buffalo, NY 41263, USA
e-mail: usha.malhotra@roswellpark.org

M.K. Fong, PharmD
Department of Pharmacy,
Roswell Park Cancer Institute, Buffalo, NY, USA

Table 9.1 Perioperative chemotherapy trials

Treatment arms		Primary end point	Secondary end points
MAGIC [3]			
Surgery alone	Epirubicin 50 mg/m² day 1	*5-year OS*	*5-year PFS*
	Cisplatin 60 mg/m² day 1	HR 0.75	HR 0.66
	5-FU 200 mg/m² daily	95 % CI 0.6–0.93	95 % CI 0.53–0.81
	Every 21 days ×3 cycles		*P*<0.001
	Surgery		*Rate of resection*
	Epirubicin 50 mg/m² day 1		79.3 % vs. 70.3 %
	Cisplatin 60 mg/m² day 1		(*p*=0.03)
	5-FU 200 mg/m² daily		
	Every 21 days ×3 cycles		
French FNCLCC/FFCD [5]			
Surgery alone	5-FU 800 mg/m² days 1–5	*5-year OS*	*Disease-free survival*
	Cisplatin 100 mg/m² day 1	38 % vs. 24 % (HR 0.69; 95 % CI 0.5–0.95; *p*=0.02)	34 % vs. 19 % (5-year rate: 34 % *v* 19 %; HR, 0.65; 95 % CI, 0.48–0.89; *P*=0.003)
	Every 28 days ×2–3 cycles		*R0 resection*
	Surgery		84 % vs. 73 %
	5-FU 800 mg/m² days 1–5		
	Cisplatin 100 mg/m² day 1 or 2		
	Every 28 days ×3–4 cycles		
EORTC 40954 [7]			
Surgery alone	Cisplatin 50 mg/m² on days 1, 15, 29	*OS*	*Rate of resection*
	5-FU 2,000 mg/m² continuous intravenous infusion over 24 h on days 1, 8, 15, 22, 29, 36	Trial terminated prematurely	81.9 % vs. 66.7 % (*p*=0.036)
	Leucovorin 500 mg/m² over 2 h every 48 days ×2 cycles		*PFS*
	Surgery		Trial terminated prematurely

including surgical techniques and change in classification of gastric and gastroesophageal junction (GEJ) cancers over time. For instance, in the most recent TNM classification, tumors arising in the gastric cardia that are within 5 cm of GEJ and extend to the GEJ are staged and treated as esophageal cancer rather than gastric cancer. Additionally, the majority of clinical trials have included broad-category patients with esophageal, GEJ, and gastric cancers, hence making the interpretation of data for any of the locations challenging. There is a lack of phase III trials addressing these controversies and hence lack of a consensus for establishing uniform guidelines worldwide.

Role of Chemotherapy

Perioperative Neoadjuvant Chemotherapy (Table 9.1)

A number of studies have evaluated the benefit of chemotherapy both in the neoadjuvant/perioperative as well as postoperative settings. The rationale behind adding chemotherapy in the neoadjuvant setting is potential downstaging of cancer by early exposure to chemotherapy in chemosensitive cases and improving patient selection by sparing surgery in patients that are at high risk of metastasis as micrometastatic disease may become evident after chemotherapy but prior to surgery. A possible disadvantage is delaying

Fig. 9.1 Kaplan-Meier curve showing overall survival from date of random assignment (From Ychou et al. [5] with permission)

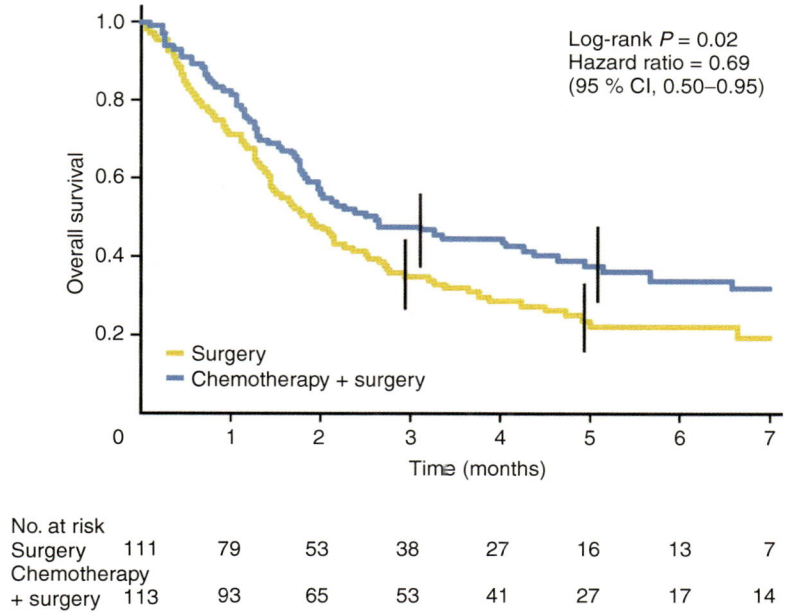

Log-rank $P = 0.02$
Hazard ratio = 0.69
(95 % CI, 0.50–0.95)

No. at risk								
Surgery	111	79	53	38	27	16	13	7
Chemotherapy + surgery	113	93	65	53	41	27	17	14

surgery and hence resectable disease may become unresectable in the interim.

A pivotal trial, MAGIC, conducted by Medical Research Council (MRC) in the United Kingdom, evaluated the role of perioperative chemotherapy in combination with surgery. A total of 503 patients were randomly assigned to either surgery alone or surgery with three preoperative and three postoperative 21-day cycles of chemotherapy consisting of epirubicin (50 mg/m^2 day 1), cisplatin (60 mg/m^2 day 1), and 5-fluorouracil, 5-FU (200 mg/m^2 daily) also known as ECF [3]. Eligibility criteria required the presence of T2 or more advanced biopsy-proven adenocarcinoma with good performance status. Seventy-four percent had gastric, 11 % distal esophageal, and 15 % had GEJ cancer. The trial demonstrated benefit of adding chemotherapy with significant improvement in 5-year survival (36 % vs. 23 % hazard ratio [4], 0.75; 95 % confidence interval (CI), 0.6–0.93 in favor of combined modality arm) as well as progression-free survival (HR 0.66, 95 % CI 0.53–0.81, $p < 0.001$ in favor of combined modality arm). Additionally, increased rate of curative resection was seen in the combined modality arm (79.3 % in combined modality arm and 70.3 % in surgery-only

arm, $p = 0.03$). Hematologic toxicity with grade 3 and 4 neutropenia was reported in 23 %, and the incidence of non-hematologic grade 3 and 4 toxicities was not very high (12 %) demonstrating an acceptable toxicity profile, but only 42 % of the patients assigned to the combined modality arm were able to complete all therapy. This highlights the decreased tolerance to chemotherapy in the postoperative setting. This trial established perioperative chemotherapy as standard of care for operable gastric cancer in Europe.

Another trial demonstrating the benefit of perioperative chemotherapy is the French FNLCC/FFCD multicenter trial [5]. A total of 224 patients were randomized to surgery alone or surgery with perioperative chemotherapy consisting of infusional 5-FU (800 mg/m daily for 5 days) and cisplatin (100 mg/m^2 on day 1 or 2) every 28 days with two or three cycles delivered preoperatively and three or four cycles given postoperatively for a total of six cycles. Of the 224 patients with stage II or higher resectable disease enrolled in this trial, 55 had gastric 144 GEJ and 25 had distal esophageal cancer. This trial also demonstrated an improvement in 5-year survival (38 % vs. 24 %, Fig. 9.1) and disease-free survival (34 % vs. 19 %) with the addition of chemotherapy. Additionally, the rate of R0 resection also improved with addition of perioperative chemotherapy (84 % vs. 73 %). Like the prior study, only 50 % of patients were able to receive therapy postoperatively.

In contrast, an EORTC randomized trial failed to show any benefit of adding preoperative chemotherapy to surgery. In the EORTC 40954 trial, a total of 144 of the planned 360 patients with stage III and IV gastric and GEJ adenocarcinoma were randomized to surgery or preoperative chemotherapy consisting of two 48-day cycles of cisplatin (50 mg/m^2 on days 1, 15, and 29) and leucovorin with FU (leucovorin 500 mg/m^2 over 2 h followed by FU 2,000 mg/m^2 continuous infusion over 24 h on days 1, 8, 15, 22, 29, and 36) [6, 7]. The trial was stopped early due to poor accrual and failed to show a survival benefit with the addition of chemotherapy. Analysis of the accrued patients demonstrated an improvement in the R0 resection rate (81.9 % vs. 66.7 %, $p = .036$) and a higher incidence of postoperative complications in the chemotherapy arm (27 % vs. 16 %).

Adjuvant Chemotherapy (Table 9.2)

A number of trials have been conducted to assess role of chemotherapy in the adjuvant setting for gastric cancer and have failed to show any survival benefit [6, 8–12]. Two large phase III studies, ACTS-GS and CLASSIC conducted in Japan and East Asia (South Korea, Taiwan and China), respectively, demonstrated a significant survival benefit with adjuvant chemotherapy establishing adjuvant chemotherapy after adequate surgery as standard of care in these regions. In the ACTS-GS trial, 1,059 patients with stage II and III gastric cancer were randomized to surgery (included a D2 lymphadenectomy in both arms) with and without adjuvant therapy with S1 administered at a dose of 80–120 mg daily for 4 out of 6 weeks for one year. S1 is an oral fluoropyrimidine that consists of three components: ftorafur (tegafur), gimeracil (5-chloro-2,4 dihydropyridine), and oteracil (potassium oxonate). The addition of adjuvant S1 led to an improvement in 5-year overall survival from 61 to 72 %. Relapse-free survival at 5 years was also found to be

Table 9.2 Adjuvant chemotherapy

Treatment arms		Primary end point	Secondary end points
ACTS-GS [16]			
Surgery alone	Surgery	*Overall survival* at 5 years: 72 % vs. 61 % (HR 0.68; 95 % CI 0.52–0.87; p=0.003)	*Relapse-free survival* at 5 years 65.4 % vs. 53.1 % (HR 0.653; 95 % CI 0.537–0.793)
	S1 80–120 mg daily for 4 weeks every 6 weeks for 1 year		
CLASSIC [13]			
Surgery alone	Surgery Capecitabine 1,000 mg/m^2 twice daily in days 1–14 Oxaliplatin 130 mg/m^2 on day 1 every 21 days for 8 cycles	*Disease-free survival, 3 years:* 74 % vs. 59 % (HR 0.56, 95 % CI 0.44–0.72, p<0.0001)	*Overall survival, 3 years:* 78 % vs. 69 %. HR 0.66, 95 % CI 0.51–0.85

significantly better at 65.4 % in the S1 group compared to 53.1 % in the surgery-only group (HR 0.653; 95 % CI, 0.537–0.793).

In the multicenter CLASSIC trial, the adjuvant chemotherapy regimen consisted of capecitabine (1,000 mg/m^2 twice daily in days 1–14) plus oxaliplatin (130 mg/m^2 on day 1) given every 21 days for 8 cycles. A total of 1,035 patients with stage II, IIIA, or IIIB gastric cancer patients were randomly assigned to surgery with D2 lymphadenectomy alone vs. surgery followed by adjuvant chemotherapy. At a median follow-up of 34 months, there was a significant improvement in 3-year disease-free survival in the chemotherapy arm (74 vs. 59 % in chemotherapy vs. surgery-alone arm, HR for death 0.56, 95 % CI 0.44–0.72, p<0.0001) as well as a marginally significant improvement in OS at the time of initial report in 2012 (83 vs. 78 %, HR 0.72, 95 % CI 0.52–1.00) with more robust improvement in OS with longer follow-up (78 vs. 69 %, HR for death 0.66 %, 95 % CI 0.51–0.85) [13, 14].

9 Multimodality Therapy in Gastric Cancer

109

On evaluation of tolerance and toxicity, grade 3 and 4 adverse events were reported in 56 % of patients in the combined modality group and in only 6 % of patients in the surgery-only group. Only 67 % of patients were able to complete all 8 planned cycles of chemotherapy with 90 % of patients requiring dose modifications.

High survival rates even in the surgery-alone arms in both these trials have led to a debate about the pertinence of this data to western population. Epidemiological and clinical variations in gastric cancer between eastern and western populations have led to a hypothesis that there is a difference in biology of gastric cancer and hence variable response to therapies in different parts of the world.

Additionally a recent meta-analysis also supported the role of adjuvant chemotherapy for resectable gastric cancer [15]. Based on these studies, adjuvant chemotherapy only is the standard of care in East Asia.

Role of Radiation

Radiation in most cancers has been shown to have a role in improving local disease control. Based on the natural history of gastric cancer, local recurrence has been reported in a high proportion of cases, which led evaluation of radiation with or without chemotherapy in addition to surgical resection for patients with potentially curable disease.

In one of the earlier studies conducted by the British Stomach Cancer Group (Table 9.3), patients were randomly assigned to surgery alone, surgery followed by 45–50 Gy of radiation, and surgery followed by chemotherapy consisting of eight courses of 5-FU, doxorubicin, and mitomycin [9]. This trial demonstrated an improvement in the local control rate with the addition of adjuvant radiation (27 % vs. 10 % in favor of radiation), but no significant difference was observed in OS between the three arms.

In another study conducted by the European Organization for Research and Treatment of Cancer (EORTC), 115 patients underwent surgery and then were randomly assigned to four different groups in the adjuvant setting [17]. The first group received 55.5 Gy of postoperative radiation only, while the other three groups received radiation in combination with short-term 5-FU, long-term 5-FU, and both short-term and long-term 5-FU. Unadjusted analysis showed a significant difference in OS between the four groups, but when other pertinent prognostic factors were added to the model, there was no significant difference in survival.

A number of trials have evaluated the role of radiation in combination with chemotherapy in the adjuvant setting. In the Intergroup 0116 study, 556 patients with stage IB through IV gastric or gastroesophageal cancer were randomized to observation vs. adjuvant chemoradiation after surgery [18]. Chemoradiation consisted of an initial 28-day cycle of 5-FU and leucovorin given on days 1–5, followed by 5-FU based concurrent chemoradiation for 5 weeks (radiation dosage was 45 Gy at 1.8 Gy per day, given 5 days per week along with 5-FU on first 4 and last 3 days of radiation), break for 1 month, and then two additional cycles of chemotherapy. At a 4-year median follow-up, there was a significant difference in median survival (36 vs. 27 months), 3-year disease-free survival (48 % vs. 31 %), OS (50 % vs. 41 %), and local failures (29 % vs. 19 %) in favor of the tri-modality therapy arm. With a longer 10-year median follow-up, OS continued to be significantly better in the combined modality arm (43 % vs. 28 %, HR 1.32, 95 % CI 1.10–1.60, $p=0.0046$) [19]. This study established the role of concurrent chemoradiation

Table 9.3 Postoperative radiation (RT)

British Stomach Cancer Group [9, 17]				
Surgery alone	Surgery 45–50 Gy RT	Surgery 5FU, doxorubicin, mitomycin ×8 cycles	*Overall survival* No difference in OS among the 3 treatment arms	*Local control* 17 % increase in improvement in local control with adjuvant RT

as an effective adjuvant regimen but has been a focus of considerable criticism as more than half of the patients enrolled in this study underwent inadequate D0 lymph node dissection and only 10 % underwent D2 lymph node dissection.

In a CALGB 80101 study, adjuvant combination chemotherapy with chemoradiation based on the INT 0116 regimen was compared with a more intense postoperative regimen consisting of one cycle of ECF followed by concurrent chemoradiation and 2 more cycles of dose-reduced ECF. The rationale was that more intensive systemic chemotherapy may translate to better OS. As reported in the American Society of Clinical Oncology meeting in 2011, there was no difference in survival between the two arms [20]. To evaluate an alternative chemotherapy backbone with concurrent radiation, a trial conducted at MD Anderson Cancer Center evaluated a neoadjuvant regimen consisting of induction chemotherapy for 2 cycles (5-FU 750 mg/m^2/day days 1–5, cisplatin 15 mg/m^2/days 1–5, and paclitaxel 200 mg/m^2 day 1) followed by concurrent chemoradiation (45 Gy over 5 weeks, 5-FU 300 mg/m^2/day 5 days/week, and paclitaxel 45 mg/m^2 on days 1, 8, 15, 22, and 29) and then surgery. Of the 41 patients enrolled, the majority had proximal gastric cancer (83 %), 40 patients underwent surgery, and 78 % had an R0 resection. Pathological complete and partial response (defined as less than 10 % residual cancer cells) was seen in 20 and 15 % of patients, respectively. At a median follow-up of 36 months, OS was found to be significantly associated with pathological response (both complete and partial, $p = 0.006$) in addition to R0 resection, postsurgical nodal positivity, N stage, and T stage [21].

In the Radiation Therapy Oncology Group (RTOG) 0114 randomized phase II study, two postoperative adjuvant regimens consisting of induction chemotherapy followed by concurrent chemoradiation were evaluated. A total of 87 patients were randomly assigned to receive two cycles of chemotherapy consisting of paclitaxel/cisplatin/5-FU (PCF) followed by concurrent chemoradiation with paclitaxel and 5-FU or paclitaxel/cisplatin (PC) for two cycles followed by concurrent chemoradiation with paclitaxel and cisplatin. The PCF arm was closed early due to excessive gastrointestinal toxicity and the trial failed to achieve its primary end point of improvement in 2-year DFS and, hence, further evaluation in a phase III study was not recommended [22].

A recent phase III ARTIST trial conducted in Korea provided a direct comparison of chemotherapy and chemoradiation in the adjuvant setting after surgery with D2 lymph node dissection [23]. Four hundred and fifty-eight patients were randomly assigned postoperatively to either chemotherapy arm consisting of capecitabine and cisplatin (capecitabine 2,000 mg/m^2/day 1–14 and cisplatin 60 mg/m^2 on day 1, repeated every 3 weeks) for 6 cycles or the chemoradiation arm consisting of two cycles of chemotherapy with capecitabine and cisplatin as above followed by concurrent chemoradiation for 5 weeks (capecitabine 1,650 mg/m^2/day with radiation, 1.8 Gy/day for 5 days/week for a total of 45 Gy) followed by two additional cycles of chemotherapy. Though DFS was not significantly prolonged with addition of radiation for the entire study group ($p = 0.0862$), a subgroup of patients with surgical pathological lymph node involvement experienced superior DFS in the chemoradiation arm ($p = 0.0365$). Based on these results a subsequent trial ARTIST II will evaluate the role of chemoradiation in node-positive disease.

Table 9.4 summarizes the abovementioned trials.

Management of Metastatic Gastric Cancer

Unlike localized and locoregional gastric cancer, the predominant method of treatment for metastatic gastric cancer is chemotherapy. Best supportive care for metastatic gastric cancer has a median survival of 3 months [24]. With the advent of newer chemotherapy treatment options in advanced gastric cancer, survival has improved by 60 % (HR 0.39) with minimal impact on quality of life [24].

Table 9.4 Postoperative chemoradiation

		Outcomes
Intergroup 0116 [19]		
Surgery only	Surgery	*4-year OS* 36 months vs. 27 months; *3-year DFS* 48 % vs. 31 %
5-FU plus leucovorin days 1–5 in a 28-day cycle ×1 cycle followed by RT 45 Gy given over 5 days per week for 5 weeks with 5-FU plus leucovorin on days 1–5 and days 28–32 followed by 1 month off treatment then 5-FU plus leucovorin days 1–5 in a 28-day cycle ×2 cycles		
EORTC [17]		
Surgery 55.5 Gy RT	Surgery 55.5 Gy RT + 5-FU short term	*10-year OS* 43 % vs. 28 % HR 1.32, 95 % CI 1.10–1.60, $p=0.0046$
Surgery 55.5 Gy RT + 5-FU short term	Surgery 55.5 Gy RT + 5-FU short term and long term	No difference in OS among the 4 arms after adjusting for appropriate prognostic factors
Surgery 55.5 Gy RT + 5-FU long term		
CALGB 80101 [20]		
Surgery	Surgery	No difference in OS
	ECF ×1 cycle followed by concurrent chemoradiation followed by reduced-dose ECF ×2 cycles	
RTOG 0114 [22]		
Paclitaxel/cisplatin/5-FU ×2 cycles	Paclitaxel/cisplatin ×2 cycles	*Disease-free survival, 2 years*
	Chemoradiation with paclitaxel and cisplatin ×2 cycles	Failed to reach 2-year disease-free survival; PCF arm terminated early due to toxicity
ARTIST [23]		
Capecitabine and cisplatin every 21 days ×6 cycles	Capecitabine and cisplatin ever 21 days ×2 cycles followed by chemoradiation 45 Gy over 5 days for 5 weeks	*Disease-free survival*; Not statistically significant; however DFS improved significantly in patients with pathological lymph node involvement

First-Line Treatment of Metastatic Gastric Cancer

First-line treatment of metastatic gastric cancer began with single-agent chemotherapy. Many different classes of chemotherapeutic agents have been used, including anthracyclines, platinums, taxanes, and fluoropyrimidines. However, single-agent chemotherapy had an overall response rate of approximately 20 %[25]. Wagner et al. conducted a meta-analysis regarding the effects of chemotherapy on advanced gastric cancer and showed that the combination of chemotherapy agents improved overall survival by 17 % [24]. The combination cisplatin and fluorouracil (CF) became the standard of comparison, with a median survival of approximately 7 months [26].

The combination fluorouracil and irinotecan, which had been used with success in metastatic colorectal cancer, was studied in the V306 noninferiority trial comparing it to CF [27]. The V306 study demonstrated noninferiority of fluorouracil and irinotecan, with a median overall survival of 9 months in the irinotecan arm vs. 8.7 months in the control arm. Similarly, the JCOG9912 supported the efficacy of irinotecan with fluorouracil in gastric cancer with a median overall survival of 12.3 months [16].

The doublet therapy with platinum and a pyrimidine analogue was then subsequently paired with other chemotherapy classes and studied for improved survival compared to that of the doublet therapy. The TAX325 trial studied the effect of docetaxel, cisplatin, and fluorouracil (DCF) compared to CF in untreated advanced gastric cancer [28]. Ninety-seven percent of the patients enrolled in this study had metastatic gastric cancer with the remaining population having locally advanced or recurrent gastric cancer. The study included patients who had received prior treatment with radiation, surgery, and chemotherapy. However, this study essentially assessed the effects of DCF in the chemotherapy-naïve population, as the percentage of patients who had received prior treatment with chemotherapy was 3 %. The study was powered to measure time to progression (TTP) with superiority of DCF as compared to CF in overall

survival and overall response rates as secondary outcomes. The DCF arm significantly improved TTP by 1.9 months compared to CF (5.6 months vs. 3.7 months, $p < 0.001$). In addition to TTP, overall survival significantly improved, from 8.6 months in the CF arm to 9.2 months in the DCF arm with a median follow-up of 23.4 months. The two-year survival was doubled in the DCF arm, from 9 to 18 %.

The frequency of neutropenia was higher in the DCF arm with 82 % developing grade 3/4 neutropenia and 29 % with reported febrile neutropenia or neutropenia infection. However, the incidence of febrile neutropenia or neutropenia infection was reduced by more than half (12 %) when secondary prophylaxis with granulocyte colony-stimulating growth factors was administered. The frequency of the non-hematologic toxicities was similar in both arms with the exception of diarrhea where DCF had a significantly higher incidence. The CF arm had a higher incidence of stomatitis, although this did not prove to be statistically significant. The frequency of dose reductions and treatment discontinuation was similar in both arms. In addition, follow-up study assessing quality of life was prospectively performed using a validated quality of life questionnaire [29]. The quality of life study showed time to 5 % definitive deterioration was significantly higher in the DCF arm at 6.5 months compared to 4.2 months in the CF arm, indicating that quality of life is preserved in patients receiving DCF.

Due to the high risk of neutropenia in the DCF arm, several modified versions of the DCF regimen were made and studied. A phase II study by Shah et al. [30] involving 60 patients had two arms that investigated the effects of a modification, using the results of the historical DCF regimen for comparison. The modified DCF regimen was as such: docetaxel 40 mg/m², fluorouracil 400 mg/m² bolus, leucovorin 400 mg/m², fluorouracil 1,000 mg/m² daily for 2 days starting on day 1, and followed by cisplatin 40 mg/m² on day 3 of a 14-day cycle. The second arm of the study kept the original DCF regimen (docetaxel 75 mg/m², cisplatin 75 mg/m², fluorouracil 1,000 mg/m² daily for 5 days starting on day 1 of a 28-day cycle) but with the addition of granulocyte colony-stimulating factor (GCSF). Thirty-eight percent of patients who received mDCF had grade 3/4 neutropenia, with 4 % developing febrile neutropenia. Forty-three percent of those who received standard DCF with GCSF had neutropenia, and there was incidence of 14 % febrile neutropenia. The 6-month PFS was 90 and 78 % in the mDCF and standard DCF arms, respectively. This small study demonstrates a reduction in neutropenia and febrile neutropenia with mDCF, without compromising on efficacy.

There are several toxicities and inconveniences associated with the CF regimen that could be improved upon. While cisplatin is shown to be active in gastric cancer, some of its toxicities such as neuropathy, nephropathy, and ototoxicity may limit the use of cisplatin after toxicities have set in. Oxaliplatin is a third-generation platinum with an oxalate leaving group, replacing the chlorine leaving groups that are found in cisplatin. The oxalate binding to the DNA adducts results in a bulky side group inhibiting DNA base excision [31]. This mechanism has proved to be effective in gastrointestinal malignancies, such as colorectal cancer [32].

Fluorouracil is administered as a continuous intravenous infusion, requiring patients to carry an infusion pump or hospital admission for chemotherapy. Capecitabine is an oral fluoropyrimidine that was shown to be noninferior to its intravenous counterpart in the treatment of colorectal cancer. The REAL-2 study evaluated the potential replacement of cisplatin with oxaliplatin and fluoropyrimidine with capecitabine through a two-by-two study design, powered to determine noninferiority [33]. In this study, patients were randomized to either epirubicin with cisplatin or oxaliplatin. Each group was then further randomized to receive either fluorouracil or capecitabine. The majority of the study participants had metastatic disease, but all participants were chemotherapy naïve. The median follow-up was similar among all groups, with a range of 17.5–19.3 months. The study found that both substitutions met their prespecified margin for noninferiority. The survival data for EOX showed an improvement over ECF by 1.3 months with a 9 % increase in 1-year survival. There was no significant difference in any of the arms regarding progression-free survival and overall response rate. Each regimen had its own unique set of toxicities. There was a higher incidence of grade 3/4 hand-foot syndrome and neutropenia in ECX, compared to ECF. Conversely, both the EOF and EOX arms held significantly lower rates of grade 3/4 neutropenia when compared to ECF. However, the frequency of febrile neutropenia was similar among all groups. Other grade 3/4 toxicities that were significantly higher in the EOF arm included anemia, diarrhea, stomatitis, and peripheral neuropathy when compared to ECF. EOX also had a significantly higher rate of grade 3/4 diarrhea, peripheral neuropathy, and lethargy. The REAL-2 study supports the use of capecitabine and oxaliplatin in triple therapy with epirubicin.

Targeted Therapies for Metastatic Disease

Targeted therapies have more recently made their way into cancer treatments. The first targeted therapy approved in metastatic gastric cancer was bevacizumab, a vascular endothelial growth factor (VEGF) inhibitor. At the time of the study, median survival for metastatic gastric cancer with cisplatin-based treatment capped at 10 months [34]. The phase II study of bevacizumab in gastric cancer in combination with cisplatin and irinotecan improved TTP to 8.3 months and showed an overall survival of 12.3 months [35]. VEGF inhibition-related toxicities were seen including grade 3 hypertension in 28 % of patients. Notably, 25 % of patients developed thromboembolism. Similarly, Shah et al. utilized bevacizumab in combination with modified DCF in a phase II trial showing improvement in median progression-free survival of 12 months [36].

The human epidermal growth factor receptor 2 (HER2) inhibitor, trastuzumab, was originally developed for HER2-positive breast cancer and has shown to improve outcomes in HER2 protein expressing gastric cancer. The ToGA trial randomized patients to receive cisplatin with a fluoropyrimidine with or without trastuzumab [37]. Participants in this study could not have received

Fig. 9.2 (**a**) Median
overall survival and
(**b**) progression-free
survival in the primary
analysis population.
HR hazard ratio
(From Bang et al. [37]
with permission)

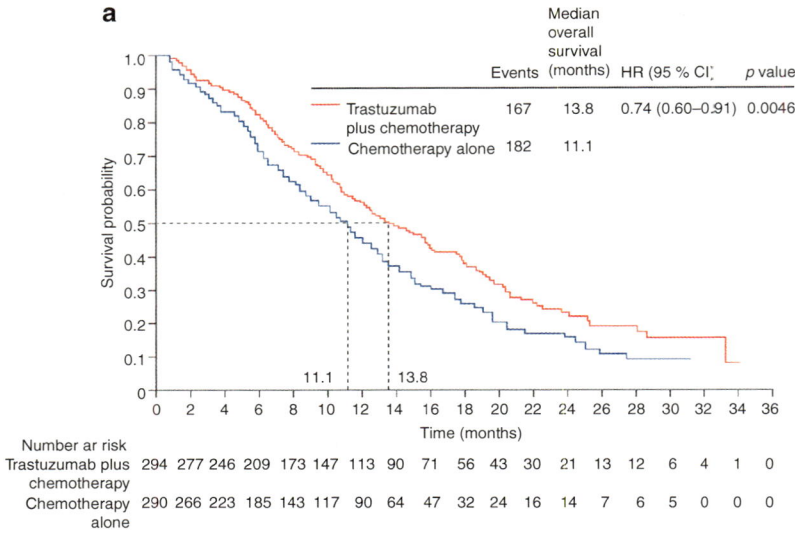

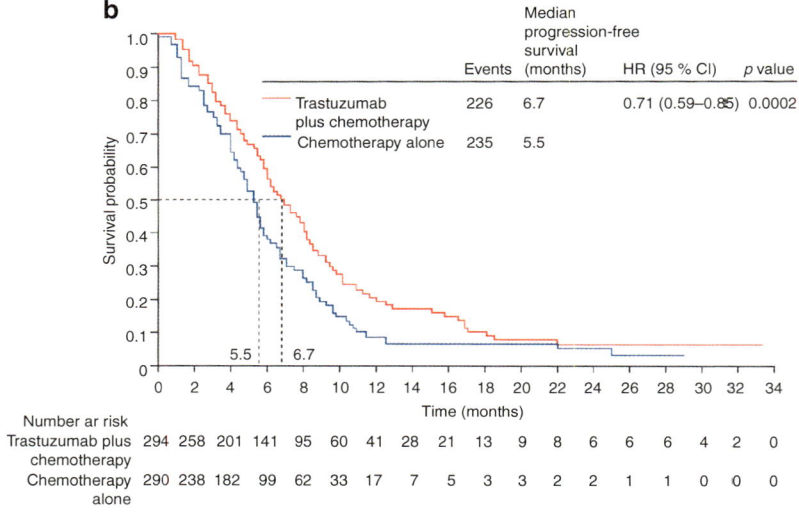

prior chemotherapy treatment for their metastatic disease and had to have adequate cardiac function, as measured by ejection fraction, blood pressure, and medical history. The study was primarily designed to detect overall survival with secondary measures of progression-free survival, TTP, and overall tumor response rate. Median overall survival in the trastuzumab arm was 13.8 months, compared to 11.1 months in the chemotherapy alone arm (Fig. 9.2). There were no significant differences in grade 3/4 toxicities with the exception of diarrhea, which was 5 % higher in the trastuzumab arm. Less than 1 % of

patients developed cardiac complications and there was no significant difference between the two arms.

Salvage Therapy in Metastatic Gastric Cancer

Several studies have been conducted regarding salvage therapy in metastatic gastric cancer. For the most part, all agents and combinations studied in first-line treatment may be successfully used as second-line treatment and salvage therapy.

However, residual side effects from previous treatments, such as neuropathy from cisplatin, may limit the effectiveness of future combination therapies employing similar agents. Kang et al. studied the benefits of salvage chemotherapy in patients with metastatic gastric cancer who failed first-line therapy [38]. Study participants were randomized in a 2:1 ratio of salvage chemotherapy to best supportive care. Salvage chemotherapy involved single-agent docetaxel 60 mg/m^2 every 3 weeks or single-agent irinotecan 150 mg/m^2 every 2 weeks. The study was powered to detect an improvement in overall survival. There was a 34 % reduced risk of death in the chemotherapy arms compared to best supportive care (HR 0.657, $p=0.007$); however, there was no difference between the two chemotherapy arms.

While there are no published studies regarding trastuzumab in the second-line setting, a newer agent was recently studied as second line in a phase III trial. Ramucirumab is a fully humanized IgG1 monoclonal antibody that targets the VEGF2 receptor [39]. The REGARD trial randomized patients with metastatic gastric cancer who failed first-line therapy to either ramucirumab 8 mg/kg every 14 days plus best supportive care or placebo plus best supportive care [40]. The primary objective was overall survival with secondary outcomes in progression-free survival, overall response rate, duration of response, and quality of life. The results of the study showed a median OS advantage of 1.4 months in the ramucirumab arm ($p=0.042$). As expected with VEGF inhibition, the frequency of hypertension was higher in the ramucirumab arm (16 % vs. 8 %), but with no other significant differences in toxicities between the two arms.

Conclusion

Poor overall survival and high recurrence rates after surgery for potentially curable localized and locoregional gastric cancer have supported the need for additional therapy. Based on pivotal phase III trials, perioperative chemotherapy, postoperative chemoradiation, and postoperative chemotherapy are acceptable options, but the choice of regimen varies widely based on institutional and regional practices around the world. In North America, postoperative chemoradiation remains popular based on INT 0116, perioperative chemotherapy based on MAGIC trial is preferred in Europe and also employed in North America, while in East Asia the trend is more toward postoperative chemotherapy after surgical resection with standard of care being D2 lymph node dissection. Role of targeted therapies in this setting is still under clinical evaluation and recommended only in the setting of a clinical trial.

While metastatic gastric cancer is chemotherapy sensitive, the relapse rate is high with a low 2-year survival. Over the years, combination chemotherapy has improved median OS with minimal added toxicities. The development of targeted therapies has improved the landscape of cancer treatment outcomes in general, but its role in gastric cancer is limited. With the success of targeted therapies such as trastuzumab and ramucirumab, there is great potential for further improvements in survival in patients with metastatic gastric cancer.

References

1. Jemal A, et al. Global cancer statistics. CA Cancer J Clin. 2011;61(2):69–90.
2. National Cancer Institute: PDQ® Gastric Cancer Treatment. Bethesda: National Cancer Institute. Date last modified 15 Feb 2013. Available at. http://cancer.gov/cancertopics/pdq/treatment/gastric/Health Professional. Accessed 20 Nov 2013.
3. Cunningham D, et al. Perioperative chemotherapy versus surgery alone for resectable gastroesophageal cancer. N Engl J Med. 2006;355(1):11–20.
4. du Bois A, et al. Addition of epirubicin as a third drug to carboplatin-paclitaxel in first-line treatment of advanced ovarian cancer: a prospectively randomized gynecologic cancer intergroup trial by the Arbeitsgemeinschaft Gynaekologische Onkologie Ovarian Cancer Study Group and the Groupe d'Investigateurs Nationaux pour l'Etude des Cancers Ovariens. J Clin Oncol. 2006;24(7):1127–35.
5. Ychou M, et al. Perioperative chemotherapy compared with surgery alone for resectable gastroesophageal adenocarcinoma: an FNCLCC and FFCD multicenter phase III trial. J Clin Oncol. 2011;29(13):1715–21.
6. Adjuvant treatments following curative resection for gastric cancer. The Italian Gastrointestinal Tumor Study Group. Br J Surg. 1988;75(11):1100–4.

7. Schuhmacher C, et al. Neoadjuvant chemotherapy compared with surgery alone for locally advanced cancer of the stomach and cardia: European Organisation for Research and Treatment of Cancer randomized trial 40954. J Clin Oncol. 2010;28(35):5210–8.

8. Engstrom PF, et al. Postoperative adjuvant 5-fluorouracil plus methyl-CCNU therapy for gastric cancer patients. Eastern Cooperative Oncology Group study (EST 3275). Cancer. 1985;55(9):1868–73.

9. Hallissey MT, et al. The second British Stomach Cancer Group trial of adjuvant radiotherapy or chemotherapy in resectable gastric cancer: five-year follow-up. Lancet. 1994;343(8909):1309–12.

10. Coombes RC, et al. A randomized trial comparing adjuvant fluorouracil, doxorubicin, and mitomycin with no treatment in operable gastric cancer. International Collaborative Cancer Group. J Clin Oncol. 1990;8(8):1362–9.

11. Nitti D, et al. Randomized phase III trials of adjuvant FAMTX or FEMTX compared with surgery alone in resected gastric cancer. A combined analysis of the EORTC GI Group and the ICCG. Ann Oncol. 2006;17(2):262–9.

12. De Vita F, et al. Adjuvant chemotherapy with epirubicin, leucovorin, 5-fluorouracil and etoposide regimen in resected gastric cancer patients: a randomized phase III trial by the Gruppo Oncologico Italia Meridionale (GOIM 9602 Study). Ann Oncol. 2007;18(8):1354–8.

13. Bang YJ, et al. Adjuvant capecitabine and oxaliplatin for gastric cancer after D2 gastrectomy (CLASSIC): a phase 3 open-label, randomised controlled trial. Lancet. 2012;379(9813):315–21.

14. Noh SH, et al. O-0007 adjuvant Capecitabine and Oxaliplatin (XELOX) for gastric cancer after D2 gastrectomy: final results from the classic trial. Ann Oncol. 2013;24(suppl 4):iv14.

15. Diaz-Nieto R, Orti-Rodriguez R, Winslet M. Postsurgical chemotherapy versus surgery alone for resectable gastric cancer. Cochrane Database Syst Rev. 2013;9, CD008415.

16. Boku N, et al. Fluorouracil versus combination of irinotecan plus cisplatin versus S-1 in metastatic gastric cancer: a randomised phase 3 study. Lancet Oncol. 2009;10(11):1063–9.

17. Bleiberg H, et al. Adjuvant radiotherapy and chemotherapy in resectable gastric cancer. A randomized trial of the gastro-intestinal tract cancer cooperative group of the EORTC. Eur J Surg Oncol. 1989;15(6):535–43.

18. Macdonald JS, et al. Chemoradiotherapy after surgery compared with surgery alone for adenocarcinoma of the stomach or gastroesophageal junction. N Engl J Med. 2001;345(10):725–30.

19. Smalley SR, et al. Updated analysis of SWOG-directed intergroup study 0116: a phase III trial of adjuvant radiochemotherapy versus observation after curative gastric cancer resection. J Clin Oncol. 2012;30(19):2327–33.

20. Fuchs CS, et al. Postoperative adjuvant chemoradiation for gastric or gastroesophageal junction (GEJ) adenocarcinoma using epirubicin, cisplatin, and infusional (CI) 5-FU (ECF) before and after CI 5-FU and radiotherapy (CRT) compared with bolus 5-FU/LV before and after CRT: Intergroup trial CALGB 80101. ASCO Meet Abstr. 2011;29(15_suppl):4003.

21. Ajani JA, et al. Paclitaxel-based chemoradiotherapy in localized gastric carcinoma: degree of pathologic response and not clinical parameters dictated patient outcome. J Clin Oncol. 2005;23(6):1237–44.

22. Schwartz GK, et al. Randomized Phase II Trial Evaluating Two Paclitaxel and Cisplatin, ÄìContaining Chemoradiation Regimens As Adjuvant Therapy in Resected Gastric Cancer (RTOG-0114). J Clin Oncol. 2009;27(12):1956–62.

23. Lee J, et al. Phase III trial comparing capecitabine plus cisplatin versus capecitabine plus cisplatin with concurrent capecitabine radiotherapy in completely resected gastric cancer with D2 lymph node dissection: the ARTIST trial. J Clin Oncol. 2012;30(3):268–73.

24. Wagner AD, et al. Chemotherapy in advanced gastric cancer: a systematic review and meta-analysis based on aggregate data. J Clin Oncol. 2006;24(18):2903–9.

25. Shah MA, Kelsen DP. Gastric cancer: a primer on the epidemiology and biology of the disease and an overview of the medical management of advanced disease. J Natl Compr Canc Netw. 2010;8(4):437–47.

26. Vanhoefer U, et al. Final results of a randomized phase III trial of sequential high-dose methotrexate, fluorouracil, and doxorubicin versus etoposide, leucovorin, and fluorouracil versus infusional fluorouracil and cisplatin in advanced gastric cancer: a trial of the European Organization for Research and Treatment of Cancer Gastrointestinal Tract Cancer Cooperative Group. J Clin Oncol. 2000;18(14):2648–57.

27. Dank M, et al. Randomized phase III study comparing irinotecan combined with 5-fluorouracil and folinic acid to cisplatin combined with 5-fluorouracil in chemotherapy naive patients with advanced adenocarcinoma of the stomach or esophagogastric junction. Ann Oncol. 2008;19(8):1450–7.

28. Van Cutsem E, et al. Phase III study of docetaxel and cisplatin plus fluorouracil compared with cisplatin and fluorouracil as first-line therapy for advanced gastric cancer: a report of the V325 Study Group. J Clin Oncol. 2006;24(31):4991–7.

29. Ajani JA, et al. Quality of life with docetaxel plus cisplatin and fluorouracil compared with cisplatin and fluorouracil from a phase III trial for advanced gastric or gastroesophageal adenocarcinoma: the V-325 Study Group. J Clin Oncol. 2007;25(22):3210–6.

30. Shah MA, et al. Random assignment multicenter phase II study of modified docetaxel, cisplatin, fluorouracil (mDCF) versus DCF with growth factor support (GCSF) in metastatic gastroesophageal adenocarcinoma (GE). ASCO Meet Abstr. 2010;28(15_suppl):4014.

31. Mathe G, et al. Oxalato-platinum or 1-OHP, a third-generation platinum complex: an experimental and clinical appraisal and preliminary comparison with cisplatinum and carboplatinum. Biomed Pharmacother. 1989;43(4):237–50.

32. Rixe O, et al. Oxaliplatin, tetraplatin, cisplatin, and carboplatin: spectrum of activity in drug-resistant cell

lines and in the cell lines of the National Cancer Institute's Anticancer Drug Screen panel. Biochem Pharmacol. 1996;52(12):1855–65.

33. Cunningham D, et al. Capecitabine and oxaliplatin for advanced esophagogastric cancer. N Engl J Med. 2008; 358(1):36–46.

34. Shah MA, Schwartz GK. Treatment of metastatic esophagus and gastric cancer. Semin Oncol. 2004; 31(4):574–87.

35. Shah MA, et al. Multicenter phase II study of irinotecan, cisplatin, and bevacizumab in patients with metastatic gastric or gastroesophageal junction adenocarcinoma. J Clin Oncol. 2006;24(33):5201–6.

36. Shah MA, et al. Phase II study of modified docetaxel, cisplatin, and fluorouracil with bevacizumab in patients with metastatic gastroesophageal adenocarcinoma. J Clin Oncol. 2011;29(7):868–74.

37. Bang YJ, et al. Trastuzumab in combination with chemotherapy versus chemotherapy alone for treatment of HER2-positive advanced gastric or gastro-oesophageal junction cancer (ToGA): a phase 3, open-label, randomised controlled trial. Lancet. 2010;376(9742): 687–97.

38. Kang JH, et al. Salvage chemotherapy for pretreated gastric cancer: a randomized phase III trial comparing chemotherapy plus best supportive care with best supportive care alone. J Clin Oncol. 2012;30(13): 1513–8.

39. Spratlin JL, et al. Phase I pharmacologic and biologic study of ramucirumab (IMC-1121B), a fully human immunoglobulin G1 monoclonal antibody targeting the vascular endothelial growth factor receptor-2. J Clin Oncol. 2010;28(5):780–7.

40. Fuchs CS, et al. Ramucirumab monotherapy for previously treated advanced gastric or gastro-oesophageal junction adenocarcinoma (REGARD): an international, randomised, multicentre, placebo-controlled, phase 3 trial. Lancet. 2014 Jan 4;383(9911):31–9.

Laparoscopic Transhiatal Esophagectomy for Esophageal Cancer

10

Dido Franceschi, Elizabeth Paulus, and Danny Yakoub

Introduction

The incidence of esophageal cancer has increased over the last several decades, and the incidence of adenocarcinoma now surpasses that of squamous cell carcinoma [1]. Esophagectomy is the best curative option for the treatment of resectable esophageal cancer but is a complex operation with significant morbidity and mortality. While the overall morbidity and mortality in those who are surgically treated has declined, approaching 40–50 and 8–11 %, respectively, it is still significant [2, 3].

Over the past decade, minimally invasive esophagectomy (MIE) has been gaining favor as an attractive alternative to open resection with the potential to reduce surgical trauma, decrease morbidity, and shorten the length of hospital stay [4–8].

Electronic supplementary material Supplementary material is available in the online version of this chapter at 10.1007/978-3-319-09342-0_10. Videos can also be accessed at http://www.springerimages.com/videos/978-3-319-09341-3.

D. Franceschi, MD (✉)
Department of Surgery, University of Miami Hospital and Jackson Memorial Hospital,
1120 NW 14th Street, Clinical Research Building – 4th Floor, Miami, FL 33136, USA
e-mail: dfrances@med.miami.edu

E. Paulus, MD • D. Yakoub, MD, PhD
Division of Surgical Oncology,
University of Miami – Miller School of Medicine/Jackson Memorial Hospital, Miami, FL, USA

Laparoscopic techniques were first adapted into the field of esophageal disease in 1991 with laparoscopic fundoplication, performed by Dallemagne et al. [9]. With this, the shift toward minimally invasive esophageal surgery began. Traditional approaches via open transhiatal or transthoracic (Ivor Lewis) resections were first "hybridized" with minimally invasive techniques, where parts of the procedure were performed in a minimally invasive fashion and other parts via standard incisions. In 1993, Collard and colleagues [10] published their initial experience with thoracoscopic mobilization of the esophagus. The first esophagectomy performed completely via laparoscopy through a transhiatal approach was in 1995 by DePaula et al. [11]. In 1999, Watson et al. first described a completely minimally invasive Ivor Lewis technique [12].

However, unlike laparoscopic procedures for other malignancies such as the colon, stomach, and even liver, laparoscopic esophagectomies have not become commonplace in the management of esophageal cancer. The procedure is technically demanding requiring expertise in advanced laparoscopy and esophageal surgery. There is also the perceived lack of traditional benefits from laparoscopic approach such as decreased hospital stay, ICU stay, or morbidity. Some centers that initially embraced it abandoned the routine use of MIE [13].

Just like the open approach, there are several variations of minimally invasive esophagectomy. They include thoracoscopy combined with laparotomy, thoracoscopy combined with laparoscopy, hand-assisted thoracotomy, hand-assisted laparotomy or minilaparotomy, and laparoscopic transhiatal or hand-assisted laparoscopic transhiatal [14]. Most experience has been gained with a combined thoracoscopic and laparoscopic approach [4, 5].

Herein, we describe a completely laparoscopic approach with a cervical esophagogastric anastomosis for tumors located mainly in the gastro-esophageal junction.

Indications

Minimally invasive approaches to treatment of benign esophageal diseases have been met with widespread acceptance. This includes diseases such as achalasia, paraesophageal hernia, and other complex esophageal disorders [15–18]. This has not been the case with malignant disease of the esophagus. Currently, no criteria define when a minimally invasive procedure should be performed over an open procedure [19]. However, an increasing trend exists for many high-volume institutions to use minimally invasive esophagectomy (MIE) in treatment of Barrett's disease with high-grade dysplasia and in patients with small resectable lesions that have limited nodal involvement (N0-1). This includes T1 (invasion of the lamina propria or submucosa), T2 (invasion of the muscularis propria), and some instances of T3 lesions (invasion of the adventitia). Neoadjuvant chemoradiation is not a contraindication to a minimally invasive approach [7].

Contraindications

Currently, no standardized contraindications exist regarding the use of minimally invasive esophagectomy. However, T4 lesions (invasion of surrounding tissues) are generally not amenable to any form of surgical resection. Extensive nodal disease and metastatic disease are also advanced stages that may require an open surgical approach or even endoscopic stenting for palliation instead of an attempt at MIE. Furthermore,

any patient with a lesion that bridges the gastroesophageal (GE) junction may not be considered a candidate for this approach unless the gastric margin can be cleared and an esophagogastrectomy can be done either via open approach or minimally invasively. As with other laparoscopic procedures, patients with extensive adhesions and scar tissue over the abdomen or chest wall, particularly in areas where the thoracoscope or laparoscope would be placed, are a higher-risk group for treatment with MIE. Older patients and those with comorbid conditions are not candidates for surgery due to the high morbidity with either a MIE or standard procedure, but they may benefit more from nonsurgical therapy [20].

Surgical Technique (Video 10.1)

Positioning

The patient is positioned in a supine position, with the left arm tucked to the side. The patient is secured to the laparoscopic table and a footboard is used. The abdomen, chest, and neck are prepped under sterile condition.

Abdominal Dissection

Positioning of the ports is a modification of that described by Hochwald and Ben-David [4]; as for our approach, the ports are placed closer to the costal margin. Pneumoperitoneum is established either through a 5 mm Optiview trocar inserted under direct vision into the lateral aspect of the left subcostal region or alternatively with a traditional Hasson technique above the umbilicus. A 30° scope is inserted, and the abdomen is explored for the presence of metastases. Once the decision is made to proceed, the remaining ports can now be placed under laparoscopic visualization to avoid intra-abdominal injury. A 5-mm port is inserted at the subxiphoid area and replaced with a Nathanson liver retractor and secured to the right side of the table for liver retraction. Two 12-mm ports are placed, one on the right midclavicular line and the other on the left midclavicu-

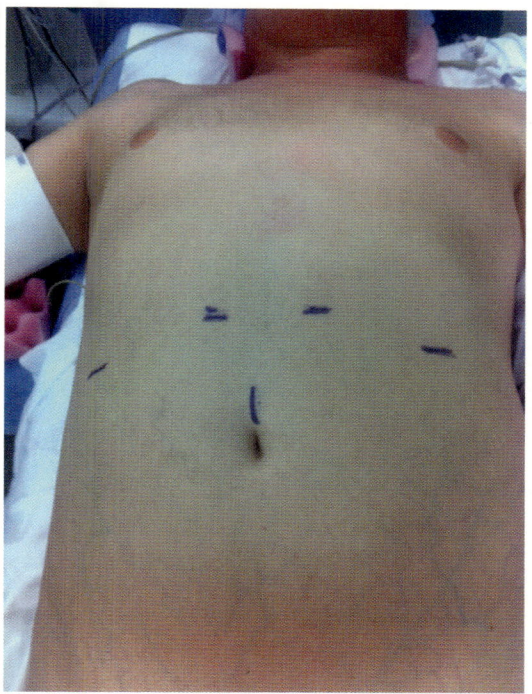

Fig. 10.1 Port placement for a laparoscopic transhiatal esophagectomy

lar line a few centimeters below the costal margin (Fig. 10.1). This varies depending on the patient's body habitus. The final 5-mm port is inserted at the right lateral subcostal region for additional retraction.

To start, the left lobe of the liver is retracted and the lesser omentum is incised and entered. The fascia covering the right crus of the diaphragm is incised sharply and an attempt is made to create a retrogastric tunnel exiting to the left and superior to the gastric cardia. Generally, the connective alveolar tissue in this area is loose and permits passage of a blunt grasper to the left of the gastroesophageal junction. The stomach is retracted inferiorly during this maneuver to enhance visualization. Occasionally, especially with bulky tumors of the GE junction, posterior visualization is not optimal and we prefer to complete the mobilization of the upper half of the greater curvature of the stomach prior to completing the retrogastric tunnel. When we are able to visualize the grasper as it exits the left side of the GE junction, above the left crus, we pass a

½-inch Penrose around the GE junction and secure it with an endo-loop.

Mobilization of the upper greater curvature is done by the surgeon on the right side of the patient. The stomach is retracted superiorly and to the right. The assistant surgeon provides countertraction of the omentum, and the lesser sac is entered at a point generally halfway up the greater curvature of the stomach. We utilize the Articulating Tissue Sealer (ENSEAL® G2, Ethicon, USA) to divide the gastrocolic omentum in a standard fashion. Care is taken to preserve the right gastroepiploic vessels. Dissection is carried out toward the gastrosplenic ligament, and the short gastric vessels are divided. The fundus is further released by dissection from the superior splenic pole and division of the pancreaticogastric attachments and the posterior vagus nerve. Dissection progresses until the left crus is identified. The fascia over it is incised sharply, and the posteroinferior mediastinum is entered. If successfully completed initially, the surgeon should be able to visualize the Penrose drain previously placed around the GE junction. If not previously placed, the Penrose can be secured at this time.

We now proceed to mobilize the lower half of the greater curvature of the stomach in a similar fashion. This is performed from the left side of the table. All adhesions of the gastric posterior wall to the pancreas are dissected until full mobilization of the stomach is achieved. A Kocher maneuver is performed to ensure optimal gastric mobilization to the thorax. Adhesions of the duodenum to the liver, gallbladder, or porta hepatis are divided.

Attention is now directed toward isolating the left gastric artery and vein. The stomach is retracted superiorly, and surrounding lymph nodes and fatty tissues are dissected to adequately visualize the celiac axis and origin of the common hepatic artery and splenic artery. Retropancreatic lymph nodes along the proximal splenic artery may be included in the dissection. Lymphatic and fatty tissue is cleared up to the crus which should have been previously dissected, guaranteeing the stomach is completely free except for the left gastric vessels. The left gastric artery and vein are divided and ligated

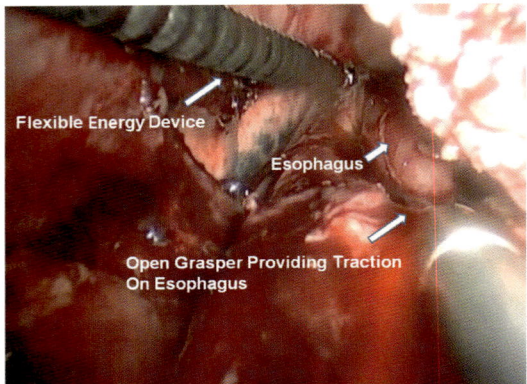

Fig. 10.2 The use of open grasper on esophagus to facilitate mediastinal dissection

with the ECHELON FLEX™ Powered ENDOPATH® Stapler (Ethicon, USA) utilizing a vascular load (1.5 mm staples).

The gastric conduit is created with a series of firings of the 6 cm ECHELON FLEX™ Powered ENDOPATH® Stapler (Ethicon, USA) along the lesser curvature of the stomach. Care is taken to pull the nasogastric tube back into the GE junction prior to stapler application. The stapler is applied from the right 12 mm port. Stapling is completed except for the final centimeter, leaving the esophagus attached to the conduit so it can be used to transfer the stomach into the posterior mediastinum.

Attention is returned to the hiatus where the distal esophagus is further mobilized circumferentially while utilizing retraction on the Penrose previously placed. Included in this step should be wide division of the phrenoesophageal ligament. After this, the posterior mediastinum can be entered to continue dissection with mediastinal lymph node dissection up to the level of the carina.

At this level, superior dissection continues close to the esophagus with mobilization of the proximal esophagus away from the trachea and prevertebral fascia. Traction of the Penrose located at the GE junction inferiorly and laterally aides with the dissection. The use of an open grasper on the esophagus (Fig. 10.2) to generate posterior or anterior traction close to the area of dissection is also useful. Generally, dissection

can be carried up to the thoracic inlet and distal cervical esophagus.

Cervical Component

A left cervical incision is performed along the anterior sternocleidomastoid muscle. We routinely incise the strap muscles transversely and expose the middle thyroid vein which is commonly divided and ligated with sutures. The jugular vein and carotid artery are retracted laterally as the thyroid is retracted superiorly and laterally. This exposes the cervical esophagus. Care is taken to identify the recurrent laryngeal nerve. The esophagus is circumferentially dissected and a Penrose is secured around it. Using mild traction of the proximal cervical esophagus, blunt dissection is used to free the cervical esophagus to the thoracic inlet. The degree of dissection will depend on the degree of success of our mediastinal dissection. Once the esophagus is completely free from adjacent tissues, the esophagus and gastric tube can be pulled through the cervicotomy. The nasogastric tube is pulled into the cervical esophagus, and after completing transection of the stomach, an end-to-end esophagogastric anastomosis is performed. Care is taken to bring the gastric tube oriented correctly, with the staple line toward the right mediastinum. Laparoscopic visualization as well as assistance with the transfer is performed through the abdominal ports.

For bulky tumors that may not be able to be successfully pulled through the mediastinum, we vary the technique by amputating the proximal esophagus and pulling the esophagus into the abdomen. A small upper midline incision is made, and the specimen is then removed abdominally after completing transection of the stomach. The gastric conduit is brought up to the posterior mediastinum by using a large Foley attached to the end of a thin laparoscopy bag that drapes over the conduit. The Foley is introduced into the neck and brought out the hiatus. By applying suction and traction to the Foley, the plastic adheres to the viscera and allows for gentle traction and correct orientation of the gastric tube as it is brought out the neck (Fig. 10.3).

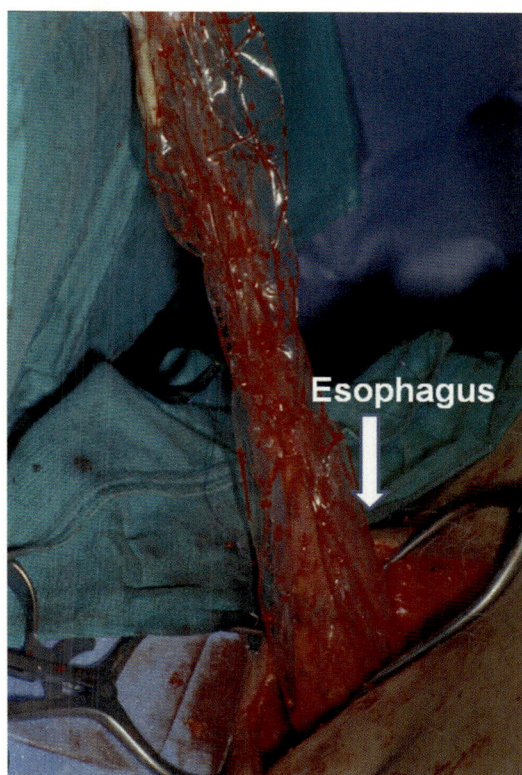

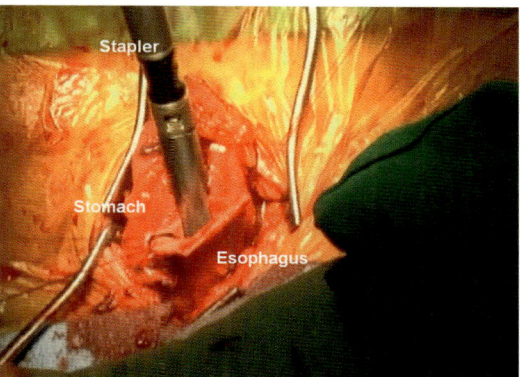

Fig. 10.4 Side-to-side anastomosis from the cervical esophagus to the gastric tube, utilizing a 6 cm stapler

Fig. 10.3 Gastric tube is placed in a plastic laparoscopy bag attached to a Foley previously passed from the neck through the mediastinum. Suction on the Foley collapses the plastic on the viscera and allows for gentle traction into the neck

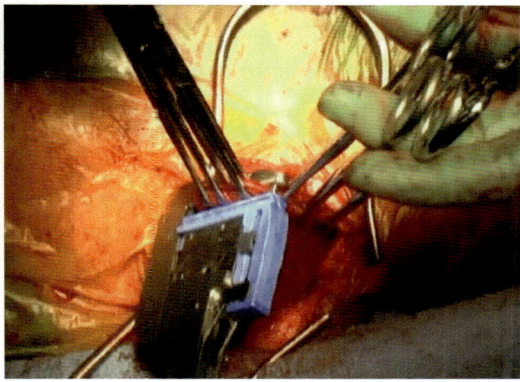

Fig. 10.5 Closure of anterior wall of anastomosis with a triangulation technique

For the esophagogastric anastomosis, we prefer a modification of the technique described by Collard et al. [21], utilizing a side-to-side anastomosis. The back wall is created with an application of the 6 mm ECHELON FLEX™ Powered ENDOPATH® Stapler (Ethicon, USA) (2.5 mm) (Fig. 10.4). The anterior layer is closed utilizing a triangulation technique with a PROXIMATE® Reloadable Staplers (TX) 30 mm (Ethicon, USA) (Fig. 10.5). The nasogastric tube is advanced to just proximal to the pylorus. A pyloromyotomy is not performed. A 19-round Jackson-Pratt drain is placed in each pleural cavity and brought out through the hiatus into the abdomen and out of the abdominal port sites. A jejunal feeding tube is placed, and all incisions are closed.

Outcomes

Complications and outcomes are significantly influenced by the volume of patients, because a large learning curve exists. High-volume centers tend to have more experience and, therefore, better outcomes than smaller-volume hospitals [22, 23]. Minimally invasive techniques for esophageal resection have been reported to have acceptably reduced procedure-related morbidity without compromising disease-free survival rates. Luketich et al. have the largest reported experience to date. Their initial series of 222 patients has now grown to more than 1,000 patients. In this series, mortality was 1.4 % versus 5.5 % for an open approach [5]. Furthermore, the survival curve at 19 months of follow-up was comparable in both groups. In another analysis of 41 elderly patients over the age of 75 years who underwent minimally invasive esophagectomy, no operative deaths occurred, with a survival of 81 % at 20 months of follow-up [24]. A recent meta-analysis of the available literature suggests that patients undergoing MIE had better operative and postoperative outcomes with no compromise in oncologic outcomes (as assessed by lymph node retrieval) [14]. Patients receiving MIE had significantly lower blood loss and shorter postoperative ICU and hospital stay. There was a 50 % decrease in total morbidity in the MIE group. Subgroup analysis of comorbidities demonstrated significantly lower incidence of respiratory complications after MIE; however, other postoperative outcomes such as anastomotic leak, anastomotic stricture, gastric conduit ischemia, chyle leak, vocal cord palsy, and 30-day mortality were comparable between the two techniques.

The only reported trial of minimally invasive esophagectomy versus open esophagectomy performed in the Netherlands [25] randomized 56 patients to open esophagectomy and 59 patients to MIE. 16 (29 %) patients in the open esophagectomy group had pulmonary infection in the first 2 weeks compared with five (9 %) in the minimally invasive group (relative risk (RR) 0.30, 95 % CI 0.12–0.76; $p=0.005$). 19 (34 %) patients in the open esophagectomy group had pulmonary infection in the hospital compared with seven (12 %) in the minimally invasive group (0.35, 0.16–0.8; $p=0.005$).

These findings suggest that minimally invasive esophagectomy can be safely performed in selected patients and even those considered high risk that might not otherwise be considered for an open surgery. Likewise, there seems to be good evidence of short-term benefits when compared to open procedures. A recent analysis also suggests that MIE is cost-effective compared to open esophagectomy in patients with resectable esophageal cancer [26].

The short-term results of several series of laparoscopic transhiatal esophagectomies (11, 27–30) are listed in Table 10.1. The number of surgical cases in these five studies ranged from 9 [27] to

Table 10.1 Short-term results for laparoscopic transhiatal esophagectomy

Parameter	Result
Mean operative time	160–390 min
Mean blood loss	220–400 cc
Conversion rate	0–16.6 %
Anastomotic leak	0–8.3 %
Mean number of retrieved lymph nodes	8–14
Mean hospital stay	6.4–12.1 days
Thirty-day mortality	0–13.6 %

22 [28, 30] with the percentage of cancer patients ranged from 17 [11] to 100 % [28]. Results compare favorably with the open procedure. Mean operative time reported varies widely between studies from 160 to 390 min. Anastomotic leak rate varies between 0 and 8.3 % with 30-day mortality ranging from 0 to 13.6 %. Surgical margin data were satisfactory when stated but were not commented on in detail, and long-term oncologic outcomes are not reported in any study.

Summary

Laparoscopic transhiatal esophagectomy was the first totally minimally invasive approach to esophagectomy that did not include a thoracotomy or laparotomy. This technique is similar to that of open blunt transhiatal esophagectomy except that the blunt mediastinal esophageal dissection is replaced by a laparoscopic transhiatal dissection of the mediastinal esophagus. The indications for a total laparoscopic transhiatal esophagectomy are similar to those of standard open transhiatal esophagectomy, and the procedure is particularly useful for patients who have lower- or middle-third tumors with significant proximal involvement or in conjunction with long-segment Barrett's esophagus. The anastomosis is performed in the neck and allows the surgeon to maximize the proximal margin. The main limitations of this technique include a limited view of the middle and upper third of the mediastinum; however, that can be improved by the use of long instruments and adequate port positioning.

Review of the literature suggests that the short-term outcomes are superior to the open approach; however, there is no data about the long-term survival. The procedure should be done in a high-volume center.

References

1. Eslik GD. Epidemiology of esophageal cancer. Gastroenterol Clin North Am. 2009;38:17–25.
2. Chang AC, Ji H, Birkmeyer NJ, Orringer MB, Birkmeyer JD. Outcomes after transhiatal and transthoracic esophagectomy for cancer. Ann Thorac Surg. 2008;85(2):424–9.
3. Connors RC, Reuben BC, Neumayer LA, et al. Comparing outcomes after transthoracic and transhiatal esophagectomy: a 5-year prospective cohort of 17,395 patients. J Am Coll Surg. 2007;205:735–40.
4. Hochwald SN, Ben-David K. Minimally invasive esophagectomy with cervical anastomosis. J Gastrointest Surg. 2012;16:1775–81.
5. Luketich JD, Pennathur A, Awais O, et al. Outcomes after minimally invasive esophagectomy: review of over 1000 patients. Ann Surg. 2012;256(1):95–103.
6. Hoppo T, Jobe BA, Hunter JG. Minimally invasive esophagectomy: the evolution and technique of minimally invasive surgery for esophageal cancer. World J Surg. 2011;35(7):1454–63.
7. Ben-David K, Rossidis G, Zlotecki RA, et al. Minimally invasive esophagectomy is safe and effective following neoadjuvant chemoradiation therapy. Ann Surg Oncol. 2011;18(12):3324–9.
8. Peyre CG, Peters JH. Minimally invasive surgery for esophageal cancer. Surg Oncol Clin N Am. 2013;22:15–25.
9. Dallemagne B, Weerts JM, Jehaes C, et al. Laparoscopic Nissen fundoplication: preliminary report. Surg Laparosc Endosc. 1991;1:138–43.
10. Collard JM, Lengele B, Otte JB, et al. En bloc and standard esophagectomies by thoracoscopy. Ann Thorac Surg. 1993;56(3):675–9.
11. DePaula AL, Hashiba K, Ferreira EA, et al. Laparoscopic transhiatal esophagectomy with esophagogastroplasty. Surg Laparosc Endosc. 1995;5:1–5.
12. Watson DI, Davies N, Jamieson GG. Totally endoscopic Ivor Lewis esophagectomy. Surg Endosc. 1999;13:293–7.
13. Smithers BM, Gotley DC, Martin I, et al. Comparison of the outcomes between open and minimally invasive esophagectomy. Ann Surg. 2007;245:232–40.
14. Nagpal K, Kamran A, Vats A, et al. Is minimally invasive surgery beneficial in the management of esophageal cancer? A meta-analysis. Surg Endosc. 2010;24:1621–9
15. Luketich JD, Fernando HC, Christie NA, et al. Outcomes after minimally invasive esophagomyotomy. Ann Thorac Surg. 2001;72:1909–13.
16. Pierre A, Luketich JD, Fernando HC, et al. Results of laparoscopic repair of giant paraesophageal hernia: 200 consecutive patients. Ann Thorac Surg. 2002;74:1909–15.
17. Krasna MJ, Jiao X. Thoracoscopic and laparoscopic staging for esophageal cancer. Semin Thorac Cardiovasc Surg. 2000;12:186–94.
18. Luketich JD, Schauer P, Landreneau R, et al. Minimally invasive surgical staging is superior to endoscopic ultrasound in detecting lymph node metastases in esophageal cancer. J Thorac Cardiovasc Surg. 1997;114:817–23.
19. Pennathur A, Zhang J, Chen H, Luketich JD. The 'Best Operation' for esophageal cancer. Ann Thorac Surg. 2010;89:2163–7.
20. Luketich JD, Alvelo-Rivera M, Buenaventura PO, et al. Minimally invasive esophagectomy: outcomes in 222 patients. Ann Surg. 2003;238:486–95.
21. Collard JM, Romagnoli R, Goncette L, et al. Terminalized semimechanical side-to-side suture technique for cervical esophagogastrostomy. Ann Thorac Surg. 1998;65:814–7.
22. Birkmeyer JD, Siewers A, Finlayson E, et al. Hospital volume and surgical mortality in the United States. N Engl J Med. 2002;346:1128–37.
23. Birkmeyer JD, Stukel TA, Siewers AE, et al. Surgeon volume and operative mortality in the United States. N Engl J Med. 2003;349(22):2117–27.
24. Perry Y, Fernando HC, Buenaventura PO, et al. Minimally invasive esophagectomy in the elderly. JSLS. 2002;6:299–304.
25. Biere SS, van Berge Henegouwen MI, Maas KW, et al. Minimally invasive versus open oesophagectomy for patients with oesophageal cancer: a multicentre, open-label, randomised controlled trial. Lancet. 2012;379(9829):1887–92.
26. Lee L, Sudarshan M, Li C, et al. Cost-effectiveness of minimally invasive versus open esophagectomy for esophageal cancer. Ann Surg Oncol. 2013;20:3732–9.
27. Swanstrom L, Hansen P. Laparoscopic total esophagectomy. Arch Surg. 1997;132:943–7.
28. Del Genio A, Rossetti G, Napolitano V, et al. Laparoscopic esophagectomy in the palliation treatment of advanced esophageal cancer after radiochemotherapy. Surg Endosc. 2004;18:1789–94.
29. Bonavina L, Incarbone R, Bona D, Peracchia A. Esophagectomy via laparoscopy and transmediastinal endodissection. J Laparoendosc Adv Surg Tech A. 2004;14:13–6.
30. Avital S, Zundel N, Szomstein S, Rosenthal R. Laparoscopic transhiatal esophagectomy for esophageal cancer. Am J Surg. 2005;190:69–74.

Laparoscopic and Thoracoscopic Esophagectomy with EEA Anastomosis

R. Taylor Ripley, David D. Odell, and James D. Luketich

Introduction

Minimally invasive esophagectomy (MIE) is now an accepted surgical approach for esophageal malignancy and the occasional benign conditions. Meta-analyses evaluating the results of MIE have shown improved perioperative outcomes and similar oncologic outcomes when compared to open esophagectomy with the advantages of minimally invasive surgery. MIE techniques are now a combination of laparoscopy and thoracoscopy for a totally minimally invasive esophagectomy. While this approach is technically demanding and associated with a significant learning curve, it is an excellent option for esophageal resection. In our experience, MIE is associated with a reduction in blood loss, decreased respiratory complications, lower

Electronic supplementary material Supplementary material is available in the online version of this chapter at 10.1007/978-3-319-09342-0_11. Videos can also be accessed at http://www.springerimages.com/videos/978-3-319-09341-3.

R.T. Ripley, MD (✉)
Division of Thoracic Surgery, Memorial Sloan-Kettering Cancer Center,
1275 York Avenue, New York, NY 10065, USA
e-mail: ripleyr@mskcc.org

D.D. Odell, MD, MMSc • J.D. Luketich, MD
Department of Cardiothoracic Surgery, University of Pittsburgh Medical Center, UPMC Presbyterian, Pittsburgh, PA, USA

mortality, improved pain control, and a decrease in hospital length of stay.

Currently, minimally invasive approaches for esophagectomy include laparoscopic transhiatal, laparoscopic-thoracoscopic 3-hole (McKeown), and laparoscopic-thoracoscopic Ivor Lewis esophagectomy. The choice between MIE approaches is often based on surgeon preference, but tumor location may influence the surgical approach. For example, a mid-esophageal squamous cell carcinoma is often best treated by a McKeown esophagectomy. The anticipated morbidity of the operation varies with the choice of surgical approach. The creation of a cervical anastomosis has a higher incidence of recurrent laryngeal nerve injury, anastomotic leak, stricture, and pharyngoesophageal swallowing dysfunction. In contrast, transthoracic approaches have a higher incidence of cardiopulmonary complications and potentially greater morbidity if an anastomotic leak occurs.

Our initial approach to MIE utilized a modified McKeown (3-hole) technique that proved to have equivalent oncologic outcome and morbidity to the open technique. Secondary to the morbidity of the cervical neck dissection, and the current predominance of adenocarcinoma with primarily lower third esophageal tumors, our preferred approach is now a laparoscopic-thoracoscopic (Ivor Lewis) esophagectomy and a

The authors have nothing to disclose.

two-field lymphadenectomy (celiac, left gastric, splenic, paraesophageal, and subcarinal lymph nodes). The minimally invasive Ivor Lewis is appropriate for most distal esophageal cancers, GE junction tumors with cardia extension, and short-to-moderate length Barrett's esophagus with high-grade dysplasia. In addition, when the length of the gastric conduit is compromised by either not enough stomach or a close margin, an intrathoracic anastomosis decreases the necessary length of the conduit. Total laparoscopic and thoracoscopic Ivor Lewis resections should not be performed for upper third or high mid-esophageal cancers. The following describes our current technique for laparoscopic-thoracoscopic Ivor Lewis minimally invasive esophagectomy.

Surgical Technique

Anesthetic Considerations

Anesthetic management during MIE poses specific challenges. All patients receive an arterial blood pressure monitoring line; a central venous catheter placement is not routine. A double-lumen endotracheal tube is placed initially in anticipation of the thoracoscopic phase. In patients with mid- or upper-thoracic tumors, a single-lumen endotracheal tube is initially placed for preoperative bronchoscopy to evaluate airway involvement.

Patients generally require volume loading during the laparoscopic phase secondary to the pneumoperitoneum and reverse Trendelenburg. The patient can develop significant hypercarbia and acidosis secondary to CO_2 insufflation. The surgeon must communicate with the anesthesiologists about vasopressors because they can directly impact the viability of the gastric conduit. Simple measures to correct these problems include lowering the insufflation pressure, decreasing the degree of the reverse Trendelenburg, and increasing volume. In addition to changing ventilator settings, hypercarbia can be corrected by reversing the pneumoperitoneum. Communication throughout the procedure between the surgeon and the anesthesiologist is imperative.

Endoscopic Evaluation

The operation begins with esophagogastroduodenoscopy (EGD). The location of the tumor is confirmed and the proximal and distal extents are assessed. The esophagus is examined for evidence of Barrett's changes proximal to the intended resection margin with four quadrant biopsies in areas of concern. Endoscopic examination of the stomach is necessary to assess suitability for use as a conduit. Insufflation should be a minimum to reduce small bowel distention which may significantly decrease domain and increase the difficulty of laparoscopy.

Laparoscopic Phase

Positioning and Laparoscopic Port Placement

The patient is supine with the arms at a 60° angle. A foot board is placed to allow steep reverse Trendelenburg during the hiatal dissection. The costal margin is identified and a line is drawn from the xiphoid to the umbilicus. This line is then divided into thirds. The first port placed using a direct Hassan cutdown approach in the right paramedian position roughly 2 cm lateral to the midline just cephalad to the junction of the lower and middle thirds of the described line. For patients with a protuberant abdomen or unusually long distance from the xiphoid to the umbilicus, the "thirds rule" may need to be modified by paying attention to the absolute distance from the xiphoid to the middle ports. If this distance is too great, adequate visualization in the crural area will be difficult. Five abdominal ports are used for gastric mobilization (10 mm right and 5 or 10 left paramedian, 5 mm right and left subcostal, and a second 5 mm right lateral subcostal port for liver retraction (Fig. 11.1)). After the Hassan cutdown, the remaining ports are placed under direct laparoscopic vision. A sixth port is placed in the right paraumbilical region to assist in placement of the feeding jejunostomy tube. All ports should be at least a hand's breadth apart to avoid interference between instruments. Additionally, skin and fascial incisions should be small to avoid

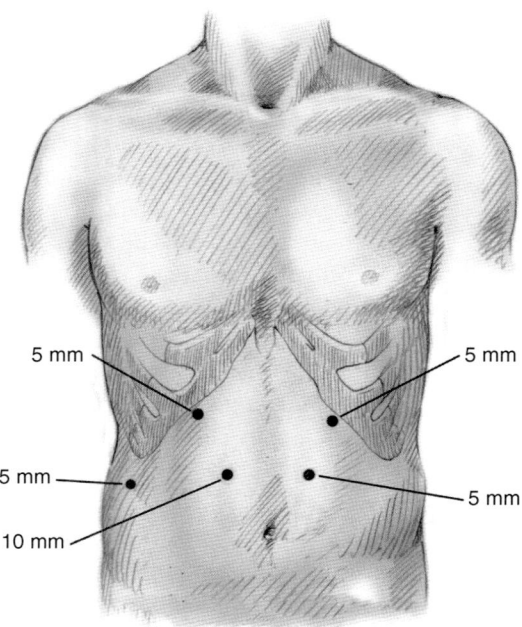

Fig. 11.1 Laparoscopic port placement. The 10 mm port in the right paramedian position is placed first via a direct cutdown technique. The left paramedian port may be converted from a 5 mm port (as shown) to a 10 mm port if a larger camera is desired (© Heart, Lung and Esophageal Surgery Institute University of Pittsburgh Medical Center)

subcutaneous emphysema. The liver retractor is brought in through the right lateral subcostal port and positioned to elevate the left lobe of the liver and expose the hiatus. This retractor is most effective if the port is as posterior and cephalad as possible in Morrison's pouch.

The camera is placed in the left paramedian port position for the majority of the laparoscopic phase. The surgeon works from the right side of the table using the right paramedian and subcostal ports. From the left, the assistant controls the camera and a second grasper for retraction (through the left subcostal port).

Gastric Mobilization

Inspection of the abdomen is performed to evaluate injuries occurring during port placement and to check for liver, omental, or other intraperitoneal metastasis. Biopsies of suspicious lesions are sent for frozen section evaluation. The gastrohepatic ligament is opened and the left gastric

vascular pedicle identified. A complete lymph node dissection is performed by dissection of the left gastric and celiac lymph nodes toward the specimen. This dissection is continued laterally along the splenic artery, the superior border of the pancreas, and superiorly toward the crura along the preaortic plane. If the nodes appear bulky or otherwise malignant, they are sent for frozen section evaluation. Once assured of the resectability of the tumor and nodal disease, the crural dissection and complete mobilization of the lower esophagus are performed. The right crus is dissected first; this dissection is continued anterior by transecting the phrenoesophageal ligaments to expose the anterior hiatus. The left crus is often exposed either by a combination of the anterior dissection along the medial crural border and by mobilizing the fundus of the stomach. This combined dissection exposes the retroesophageal window which ensures complete mobilization of the superior portion of the lesser curve completing 360° exposure of the gastroesophageal junction. During this dissection, the exposure is maximized by dividing the left gastric artery and vein with endovascular GIA stapler.

After identifying the gastrocolic omentum, the antrum of the stomach is retracted, and a window is created in the greater omentum, allowing access to the lesser sac. The remaining short gastric vessels are divided while ensuring the dissection is above the gastroepiploic arcade. The fundus is retracted to the right to dissect the remaining retro-gastric short gastric arteries while exposing the left gastric artery and vein. Care should be taken to ensure that all nodes are swept toward the specimen side and to avoid narrowing of the splenic or hepatic arteries. This dissection should complete the mobilization of the fundus and proximal stomach. Gastric mobilization is carried inferiorly to the pyloro-antral region. Meticulous attention must be paid during this phase of the dissection to avoid injury to the gastroepiploic arcade. Mistakenly transecting the arcade often renders the conduit unusable. Direct handling and instrumentation of the conduit portion of the stomach should be avoided. Adequate mobilization has been achieved when the pylorus reaches the caudate lobe. Depending on prior

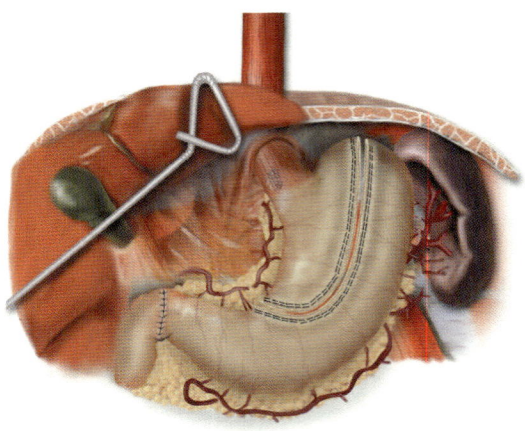

Fig. 11.2 Anatomy of the completed gastric conduit. The right gastroepiploic arcade forms the primary blood supply. The right gastric artery is also preserved and contributes some blood supply to the gastric antrum (© Jennifer Dallal, James D. Luketich, MD)

operations and adhesions, enough mobility may require a lysis of adhesions and a partial or a complete Kocher maneuver.

Creation of Gastric Tube

The gastric tube is created prior to the pyloroplasty and placement of the feeding jejunostomy tube to allow time for assessment of conduit viability prior to transition to the thoracoscopic phase. The gastric tube follows the arc of the greater curve of the stomach and is based on the right gastroepiploic artery (Fig. 11.2). Prior to creating the gastric conduit, the nasogastric tube, if previously placed, is pulled back to the midesophagus. An endovascular stapling technique allows for a controlled creation of the gastric tube conduit. The first staple load is a vascular (gold) load for the adipose tissue and vessels along the lesser curve above the level of the right gastric artery. No stomach is divided with this firing. The remainder of the firings divides the stomach with 45 mm purple loads (Endo GIA Reloads with Tristaple Technology, Covidien, Mansfield, MA). The course of the greater curvature is precisely followed by applying traction to the fundus and antrum by the assistants and by traction on the specimen side with the surgeon's left hand. This three-point traction provides a clear view of the location for gastric transection. Starting at the antrum, the staple line is then directed superiorly, toward the fundus, parallel to the line of the short gastric vessels along the greater curvature. A conduit width of 3–4 cm is preferred (Fig. 11.2). An unusually thick antrum may require that one chooses a greater staple height (e.g., the black Endo GIA loads) to get an adequate staple line integrity. The length of the conduit and margin of resected stomach should be assessed and modified if there is concern for extension of the tumor onto the gastric cardia. Sutures may be placed to reinforce the staple line if there is concern about its integrity though usually not necessary.

Pyloroplasty

The pylorus is identified and 2-0 Surgidac (Covidien, Mansfield, MA) stay sutures are placed on the superior and inferior aspects using the Endostitch device (US Surgical, Norwalk, CT) (Fig. 11.3). The anterior wall of the pylorus is transected with an ultrasonic shears. The pyloromyotomy is closed transversely in a Heineke-Mikulicz fashion using simple, interrupted 2.0 Surgidac sutures. An omental patch is placed over the pyloroplasty and sutured in place.

Feeding Jejunostomy Tube Placement

A 12 Fr jejunostomy catheter is placed in the left lower quadrant using a percutaneous technique. The transverse colon is retracted superiorly to expose the ligament of Treitz, and a position on the jejunum 30–40 cm downstream is identified. The antimesenteric border of the bowel is sutured to the abdominal wall with a 2-0 Surgidac suture. The 12 mm right paraumbilical port is used with the camera positioned in the right paramedian location. A Seldinger technique is used to introduce the catheter into the jejunum under direct laparoscopic vision. Air insufflation is used to verify luminal placement. The jejunum is tacked circumferentially to the abdominal wall. An additional suture is placed in the distal limb of the jejunum to prevent volvulus and obstruction.

Preparation for Thoracoscopic Phase

The gastric conduit is assessed for viability. Once viability of the conduit is assured, the most

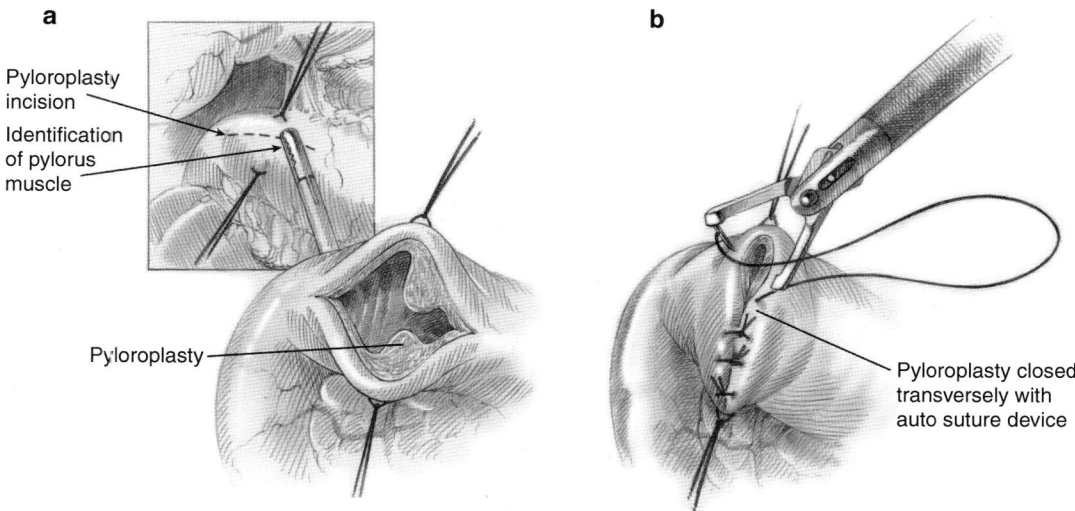

a

Pyloroplasty incision

Identification of pylorus muscle

Pyloroplasty

b

Pyloroplasty closed transversely with auto suture device

Fig. 11.3 Laparoscopic creation of a pyloroplasty (**a**) with vertical closure in a Heineke-Mikulicz fashion (**b**) (© Heart, Lung and Esophageal Surgery Institute University of Pittsburgh Medical Center)

superior portion of the gastric tube is stitched to the specimen (Fig. 11.4). Maintaining the alignment of the conduit to avoid twisting as the stomach is brought into the chest is imperative. The greater curvature along the short gastric vessels is sutured to the staple line of the proximal gastric remnant. If an omental flap has been created, the distal end is sutured to the conduit tip. If hemostasis of the staple line is needed, clips are applied. The specimen and gastric conduit are placed in the lower mediastinum while preserving the proper orientation. If the hiatal opening is large, the crura are reapproximated with a stitch to prevent delayed thoracic herniation of the distal conduit. This step requires considerable judgment by an experienced surgeon because a tight hiatus may compromise the venous drainage of the conduit. A nasogastric tube (if not previously placed) is placed in the esophagus prior to thoracic positioning.

Thoracoscopic Phase

Positioning and Port Placement

The patient is turned to the left lateral decubitus position, and location of the double-lumen endotracheal tube is reconfirmed. The surgeon stands on the right side and the assistant stands on the left side of the table. Five thoracoscopic ports are used (Fig. 11.5). A 10-mm camera port is placed in the 8th or 9th intercostal space slightly anterior to the midaxillary line. A 10-mm working port is placed in the 8th or 9th intercostal space posterior to the posterior axillary line. Another 10-mm port is placed in the anterior axillary line at the 4th intercostal space for a fan-shaped lung retractor aids in retracting the lung to expose the esophagus. A 5-mm port is placed just inferior to the tip of the scapula.

Thoracoscopic Dissection and Resection of the Esophagogastric Specimen

Retraction of the diaphragm is essential to the thoracoscopic phase of the dissection. A 48 in., 0 Surgidac suture is placed through the central tendon of the diaphragm using the Endostitch. The suture is brought out through the lateral chest wall at the level of the insertion of the diaphragm through a small stab incision, retracting the diaphragm inferiorly and exposing the distal esophagus. The inferior pulmonary ligament is divided to the inferior pulmonary vein to maximize retraction of the lung. The esophageal dissection is started on the avascular plane along the surface

Fig. 11.4 The gastric
conduit is sutured to the
distal portion of the
specimen. The lesser
curvature staple line faces
toward the right so as to
preserve orientation
(© Heart, Lung and
Esophageal Surgery Institute
University of Pittsburgh
Medical Center)

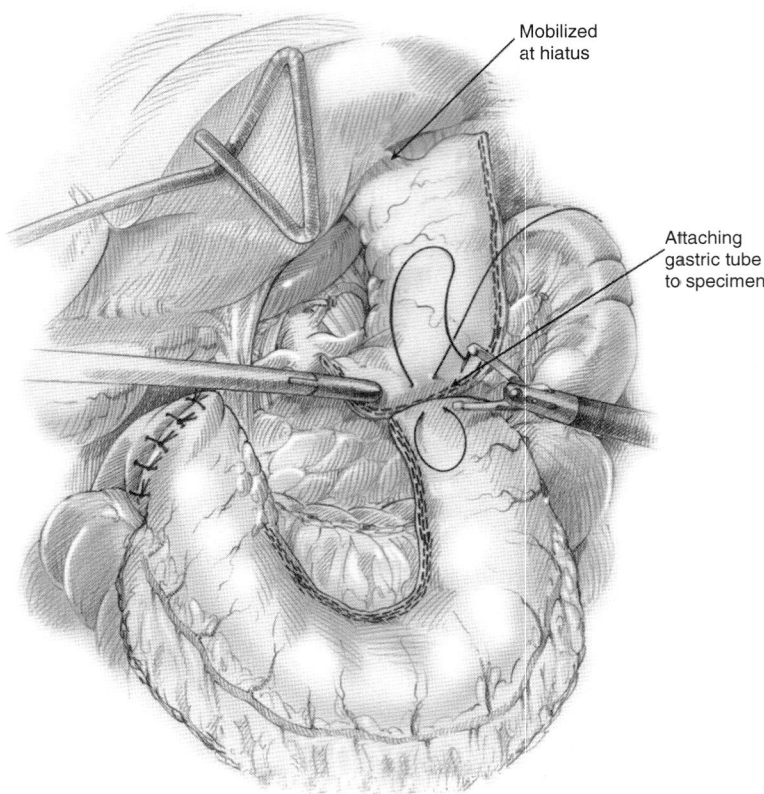

Mobilized
at hiatus

Attaching
gastric tube
to specimen

Fig. 11.5 Thoracoscopic
port placement

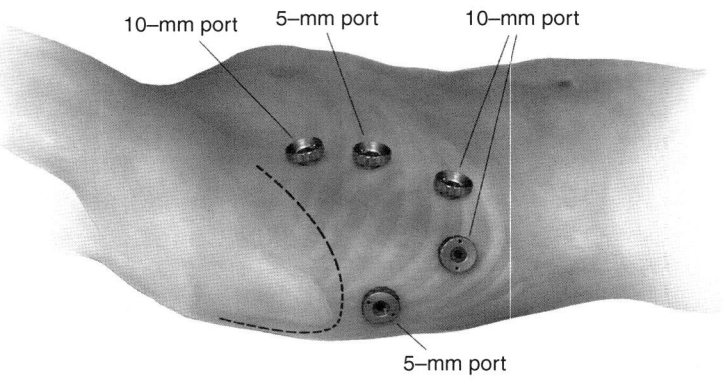

10–mm port   5–mm port   10–mm port

5–mm port

of the pericardium. This dissection is carried
superiorly to the subcarinal space ensuring that
the lymph nodes are dissected with the esophagus (Fig. 11.6). Care must be taken to identify the
membranous wall of the right mainstem bronchus because it is at risk of injury during this
phase of the dissection. Removing suction from
the right lung will prevent the membranous wall

from collapsing and can aid in visualization
while removing subcarinal lymph nodes. The
lung is retracted anteriorly and the pleura incised
along the anterior border of the esophagus to the
level of the azygous vein. The pleura above the
azygous vein is opened to facilitate the exposure
of the vein with division with the endo-GIA vascular (gold) load. Above the level of the azygous

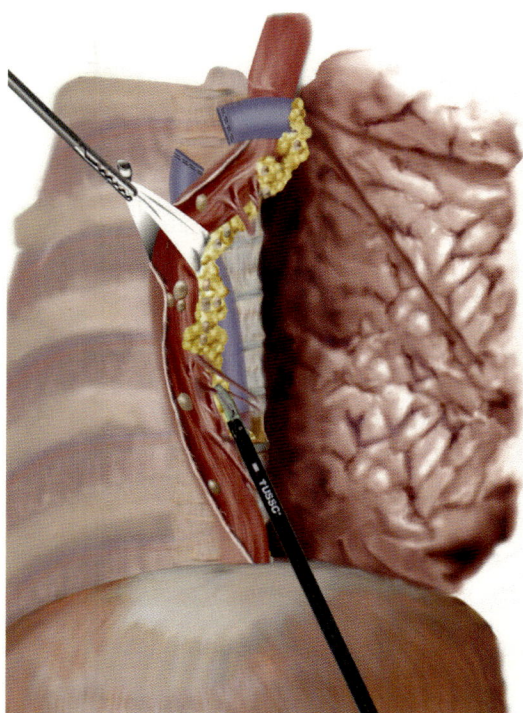

Fig. 11.6 Thoracoscopic mobilization of the esophagus. The pleura is incised longitudinally in line with the esophagus. The lung is anteriorly retracted to provide adequate exposure. All nodal tissue is excised en bloc with the esophageal tissue (© Jennifer Dallal, James D. Luketich, MD)

vein, the dissection no longer includes periesophageal tissue to avoid injury to the recurrent laryngeal nerve and the airway. The vagus is cut at this level to prevent traction injury to the recurrent laryngeal nerve. The extent of superior dissection and mobilization depends upon the location of the tumor and the intended site of resection. Next, the posterior mobilization is begun. The pleura is divided in the groove posterior to the esophagus near the diaphragm. This dissection is kept superficial to avoid injury to the thoracic duct and underlying thoracic aorta. Bridging lymphatics and aortoesophageal vessels are controlled with endoclips. Thoracic duct ligation should be considered if there is concern for trauma to the duct or tumor extension into the duct. This lateral dissection is carried along the length of the esophagus from the gastroesophageal junction to above the azygous vein. The contralateral pleura is the deep margin of the dissection. This dissection is

facilitated by lifting the specimen into the chest, cutting the suture between the conduit and the specimen, and tacking the proximal conduit to the diaphragm. As the specimen is rolled toward the apex, the remaining adhesions to the deep margin are transected. The left pleural space may be entered if needed to remove a bulky tumor.

Once mobilization of the esophagus has been completed, a 4–5 cm mini-thoracotomy without rib spreading is created between the surgeon's working port and the tip of the scapula. A wound protector (Applied Medical, Rancho Santa Margarita, CA) is placed to protect the skin and chest wall. The esophagus is sharply transected using laparoscopic scissors at or above the level of the azygous vein determined by the proximal extent of tumor. The nasogastric tube is pulled back into the proximal esophagus under direct vision during transection. The esophagogastrectomy specimen is then withdrawn through the wound protector, opened, grossly examined, and sent for frozen section evaluation of the margins.

Creation of Gastroesophageal Anastomosis (Video 11.1)

Next, the esophagogastric anastomosis is created. An EEA stapling device is utilized (Fig. 11.7). The anvil of the stapler is placed in the proximal end of the esophagus and sutured with two purse-string 2-0 Surgidac. All layers of the esophagus must be included to ensure a competent anastomosis. The ideal size is a 28 mm EEA stapler which will help to minimize stricture formation and to reduce postoperative dilation. If the proximal esophagus is not large enough to accommodate the 28 mm anvil, a Foley catheter with a 30 cc balloon can be used to gently dilate the esophageal lumen in an attempt to facilitate placement of the anvil. If dilatation fails, the 25 mm EEA may be necessary. The gastric conduit is pulled further into the chest and angled toward the mini-thoracotomy. The orientation of the gastric tube requires that the staple is facing the lateral chest wall. The tip of the gastric conduit is opened using ultrasonic shears to the right side of the staple line. The EEA stapler is placed through the wound protector and inserted into the conduit using the atraumatic graspers to pull the

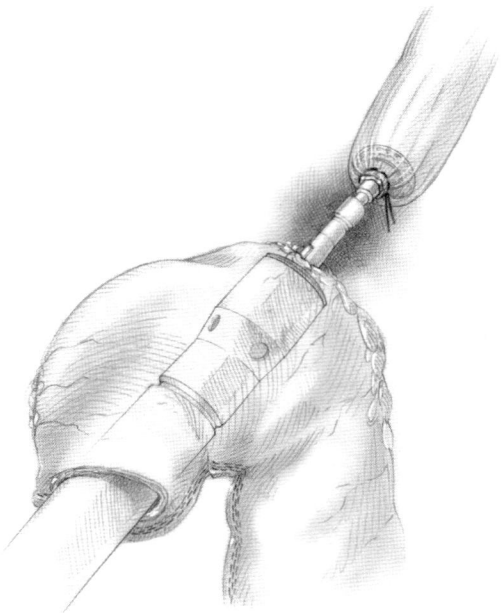

Fig. 11.7 Creation of the esophagogastric anastomosis using the EEA stapler. The anvil is sewn into the esophagus with 2 concentric sutures and the stapler introduced through a gastrotomy in the gastric conduit. Conduit orientation is maintained by keeping the lesser curvature staple line facing the camera while the stapler is docked (© Heart, Lung and Esophageal Surgery Institute University of Pittsburgh Medical Center)

conduit over the EEA stapler while gently pushing the stapler toward the mediastinum. The EEA is advanced to a position on the conduit appropriate for an anastomosis. While maintaining traction with the graspers on the gastrotomy edges, the EEA is shifted toward the proximal anastomosis to gently slide additional conduit into the mediastinum without lifting redundant conduit into the pleural space. Bringing excess stomach into the chest with the intent of minimizing tension on the anastomosis is a mistake. A redundant conduit above the diaphragm can lead to significant problems with conduit emptying. Once the appropriate length has determined, the stapler spike is brought out along the greater curve of the gastric conduit. The spike is carefully docked with the anvil. Prior to creating the anastomosis, the EEA spike is turned without moving the stapler to lift the esophagus until it is

on slight tension. Once the proximal esophagus is taught, the EEA is turned and advanced toward the esophagus to prevent additional tension on the esophagus. An estimate of the amount of conduit that will lie in the chest is performed at this point. The stapler is then fired and withdrawn. The tissue rings are inspected grossly to insure that they are complete and sent for permanent pathology.

After creating the anastomosis, the remaining gastric tip with the gastrotomy is resected with 2–3 loads of the endovascular GIA stapler (Fig. 11.8). The anastomosis and conduit resection need to be sufficiently separated to prevent ischemia of the intervening tissue. If an omental flap was created during the abdominal dissection, it is wrapped around the anastomosis by placing between the airway and the anastomosis and suturing into place. The chest is then thoroughly irrigated and inspected for hemostasis.

Drain Placement and Closure

Adequate drainage of the mediastinum surrounding the anastomosis is imperative to minimize complications in the event of an anastomotic leak. A 10 mm Jackson-Pratt drain is placed posteriorly along the anastomosis and a 28-French chest tube is placed in the pleural space. The nasogastric tube is advanced past the anastomosis under thoracoscopic visualization. The gastric conduit is sutured to the right crus and the diaphragm edge with a single 2-0 Endostitch to prevent delayed herniation. A long aspirating needle is used to instill a multilevel intercostal nerve block. The access incision is closed. The Jackson-Pratt drain is secured with multiple sutures to the skin to prevent dislodgement. Once all the incisions are closed, the patient is turned to the supine position and the oropharynx and nasopharynx are suctioned of all secretions. The patient is reintubated with a single-lumen endotracheal tube. If a tube exchange catheter is necessary, it should be used with caution because it may injure the right mainstem bronchus. A toilet bronchoscopy is performed while examining the right and left mainstem bronchi for injury.

Fig. 11.8 Closure of the gastrotomy is performed using a reticulating Endo GIA stapler. This portion of resected stomach represents the final gastric margin (© Heart, Lung and Esophageal Surgery Institute University of Pittsburgh Medical Center)

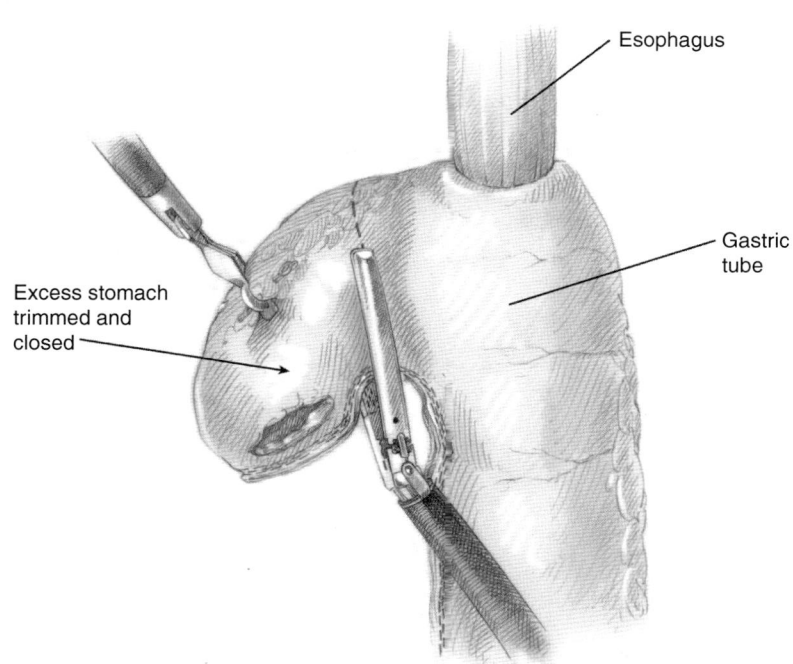

Esophagus

Gastric tube

Excess stomach trimmed and closed

Postoperative Care

Patients are transferred to the intensive care unit and usually transition to the ward on postoperative day 1. The typical hospital stay is 7 days in patients with an uncomplicated postoperative course. The nasogastric tube may be removed on postoperative day 2 if the patient is awake and alert and nasogastric drainage is minimal. Enteral nutrition, in the form of "trickle" (30 cc/h) jejunostomy tube feeds, is started typically on postoperative day 2. On day 3, tube feeds are advanced to goal nutritional intake and cycled over an 18 h period to facilitate ambulation during the daytime hours. A contrast esophagram is obtained on day 3–4 if the patient has adequate pulmonary toilet and a good cough. If there is no evidence of leak, oral intake is initiated as 1–2 oz of clear liquids per hour. This amount is advanced over 2 days to full liquids with no more than 3–4 oz/h while continuing cycled tube feeds. The chest tube on the operative side is removed once the volume of drainage is acceptable (typically 200 cc/24 h). The Jackson-Pratt drain is pulled back 3–5 cm on postoperative day 5 so as to prevent delayed fistulization to the anastomosis and resecured. The drain is removed at the first postoperative clinic visit in about 2 weeks.

Outcomes

Our group has refined the minimally invasive approach to esophageal resection over a period of several years in an effort to decrease the morbidity and mortality of open esophagectomy [1–5]. Our minimally invasive approach to esophageal resection was first described in 1998 [3], followed by the description of the initial experience in 77 patients undergoing minimally invasive esophagectomy (MIE) in 2000 [5]. We described the further experience with 222 patients in 2003 [2]. In 2011, we reported a large series of over 1,000 MIEs [4], and currently are approaching the 2,000 mark, with mortality rates in the range of 1 % [4]. In a recent prospective study of 17 centers experienced in minimally invasive esophageal surgery, minimally invasive esophagectomy was associated with a 2 % mortality rate and offered a safe and oncologically equivalent alternative to open esophagectomy [6].

References

1. Bizekis C, Kent MS, Luketich JD, et al. Initial experience with minimally invasive Ivor Lewis esophagectomy. Ann Thorac Surg. 2006;82:402–6; discussion 406–7.

2. Luketich JD, Alvelo-Rivera M, Buenaventura PO, et al. Minimally invasive esophagectomy: outcomes in 222 patients. Ann Surg. 2003;238:486–94; discussion 494–5.
3. Luketich JD, Nguyen NT, Weigel T, et al. Minimally invasive approach to esophagectomy. JSLS. 1998;2:243–7.
4. Luketich JD, Pennathur A, Awais O, et al. Outcomes after minimally invasive esophagectomy: review of over 1000 patients. Ann Surg. 2012;256:95–103.
5. Luketich JD, Schauer PR, Christie NA, et al. Minimally invasive esophagectomy. Ann Thorac Surg. 2000;70:906–11; discussion 911–2.
6. Pennathur A, Luketich JD, Landreneau RJ, et al. Long-term results of a phase II trial of neoadjuvant chemotherapy followed by esophagectomy for locally advanced esophageal neoplasm. Ann Thorac Surg. 2008;85:1930–6; discussion 1936–7.

Laparoscopic and Thoracoscopic Esophagectomy with Side-Side Thoracic Anastomosis

Kfir Ben-David and Isaac P. Motamarry

Over the past few decades, there has been a constant increase in the number of patients diagnosed with esophageal cancer in the United States. There were 17,990 newly diagnosed patients with esophageal cancer in 2013, and 15,210 patients died from this malignancy. Although squamous cell carcinoma is the most common malignancy of the esophagus worldwide, adenocarcinoma is considerably more prevalent in the United States. Regardless of histologic character, this malignancy has a reported overall 5-year survival rate of 13–18 % since most patients have advance disease at initial presentation [1].

Esophageal carcinomas are generally asymptomatic, with patients typically complaining of dysphagia or odynophagia. These symptoms are generally considered late manifestations of the disease process. The esophagus lacks a serosa, which gives way to dilation, and patients are usually not symptomatic until 60 % of the circumference is obstructed. Consequently, one of the

Electronic supplementary material Supplementary material is available in the online version of this chapter at 10.1007/978-3-319-09342-0_12. Videos can also be accessed at http://www.springerimages.com/videos/978-3-319-09341-3.

K. Ben-David, MD (✉)
Department of Surgery, University of Florida Health, Gainesville, FL, USA
e-mail: kfir.bendavid@surgery.ufl.edu

I.P. Motamarry, MD
Department of General Surgery,
University of Florida Shands, Gainesville, FL, USA

major difficulties for patients with esophageal cancer is accurate preoperative staging. Noninvasive staging modalities include computed tomography (CT) of the chest, abdomen, and pelvis and endoscopic ultrasound (EUS). EUS has become more sensitive with greater than 93 % accuracy in differentiating mucosal versus submucosal lesions. However, there are multiple limiting factors including the location, type of lesion, method and frequency of EUS probe, and the experience of the endosonographer [2]. EUS-guided fine-needle aspiration (FNA) for lymph node staging has been compared to PET/CT in recent studies, and PET/CT has consistently predicted nodal status as well as response to neoadjuvant therapy [3].

The initial workup includes: a barium swallow to assess anatomy and esophageal function, followed by an EGD for tissue biopsy. An EUS can also be used for biopsy but is more frequently used to assess depth of malignant penetration. CT and PET-CT are used to evaluate for metastatic disease, and a PET-CT is obtained post neoadjuvant chemoradiation to assess response to treatment at our institution. Neoadjuvant therapy is performed for T2–T4 and/or node-positive, M0 malignancy [4]. Following the completion of neoadjuvant therapy, patients are restaged with radiographic CT/PET imaging, and surgery is offered to medically fit patients who do not have metastatic disease.

Minimally invasive esophagectomy was first described by DePaula and was a primarily laparoscopic transhiatal approach with a cervical anastomosis [5]. Since then, multiple publications have surfaced regarding various techniques and outcomes shifting from open esophagectomy to a minimally invasive approach which has greatly decreased the overall morbidity and mortality of the operation [6]. In fact, Luketich has recently reported the largest MIE series with over 1,000 patients with a surgical mortality rate less than 2 % for the first 500 cases and 0.9 % for the latter 500 [7]. Similarly, our institution reported a mortality rate of 1 %, pneumonia 9 %, anastomotic leak 4 %, and median length of stay of 7.5 days, utilizing the three-field esophagectomy approach [8]. Consequently, there have been many controversies regarding the optimal minimally invasive surgical treatment of esophageal cancer. More specifically, a three-field esophagectomy is superior to a two-field with regards to lymphadenectomy, 5-year survival rate, perioperative morbidities and mortality [9]. Although many prefer an Ivor Lewis minimally invasive esophagectomy with circular anastomosis [7], we prefer the side-side thoracic anastomosis [10] since we have noticed a reduced anastomotic stricture formation. It also provides an excellent option for patient with previous neck dissections, foregut surgery, or gastroesophageal tumors extending into the proximal stomach.

Operative Description

The patient is intubated with a double-lumen endotracheal tube to achieve isolated left lung ventilation. An 18-gauge nasogastric tube is placed to help with gastric decompression. The abdominal cavity is entered with a 5-mm trocar under direct vision into the lateral aspect of the left subcostal region. The abdomen is evaluated for evidence of metastatic disease. If there is no evidence of metastatic disease, additional trocars are placed under direct visualization. These include a 5-mm camera port, 2 cm to the left and superior to the umbilicus to be controlled by the operative assistant. A 12-mm port is placed at the same level as the previous port just lateral to the rectus muscle on the right side. An additional

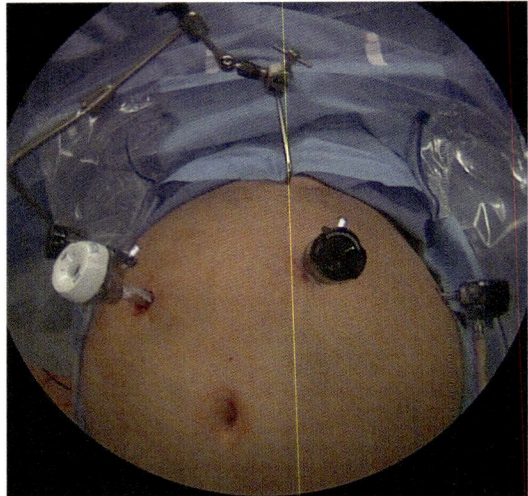

Fig. 12.1 Abdominal trocar placement

12 mm port is placed 6 cm superior and lateral to this port on the right side. These will serve as the surgeon's working ports. The patient is placed in steep reverse Trendelenburg position. A 5-mm incision is created inferior and to the left of the xiphoid process to allow for the placement of a liver retractor (Fig. 12.1). The surgeon stands on the patient's right side while the assistant is on the contralateral side.

Abdominal Dissection

The gastrohepatic ligament is divided. The dissection is continued to the right crus up toward the phrenoesophageal ligament and across the diaphragm to the left crus. A retrogastric tunnel is created by incising the tissue along the right crus of the diaphragm. Care is taken to visualize the left crus posteriorly and place a blunt grasper behind the gastroesophageal junction (GEJ) from right to left just inferior to the crura. The blunt grasper is visualized as it exits the loose connective alveolar tissue at the angle of His. A Penrose drain is placed around the gastroesophageal junction. The Penrose is secured around the GE junction with an endo-loop.

Following this portion, the operating surgeon grasps the anterior aspect of the stomach, and the lesser sac is entered about halfway up the greater curvature of the stomach. A tissue sealing device is utilized to divide the gastrocolic omentum and short gastric vessels. Great care is taken to preserve the right gastroepiploic vessels (Fig. 12.2). The stomach is mobilized all the way until the left crus and Penrose drain are visualized at the angle of His. Mobilization of the lower half of the greater curvature of the stomach is created between the right transverse colon and the right gastroepiploic vessels. The gastropancreatic folds are divided inferiorly and the stomach is mobilized away from the pancreas until the gastroduodenal artery is visualized. The surgeon on the right side of the table mobilizes the first and second portions of the duodenum along the superior aspect of the duodenum until the common bile duct is reached. Adhesions between the first portion of the duodenum to the liver, gallbladder, or porta hepatis are carefully divided. A formal Kocher maneuver is often not necessary for an intrathoracic esophagogastric anastomosis.

The right gastric artery along the superior aspect of the lesser curvature of the stomach is divided with a laparoscopic sealing device. The lesser curvature of the stomach is elevated. The surgeon skeletonizes the left gastric artery and vein at their base to assure an extensive lymphadenectomy is achieved. Subsequently, the left gastric artery and vein are stapled and divided with a vascular load. The lymphadenectomy dissection is continued along the common hepatic artery, splenic artery, and superior portion of the pancreas toward the left crus (Fig. 12.3).

The gastric conduit is created by a series of laparoscopic stapler firings along the lesser curvature of the stomach. The nasogastric tube is pulled back above the gastroesophageal junction. The first firing is done via the right upper abdominal 12 mm port. The stapler is introduced onto

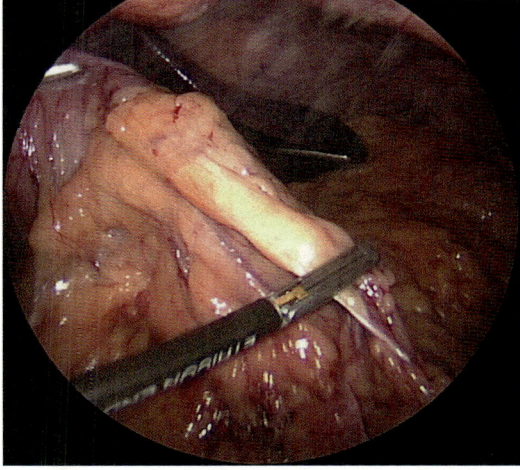

Fig. 12.2 Division of the gastrocolic omentum

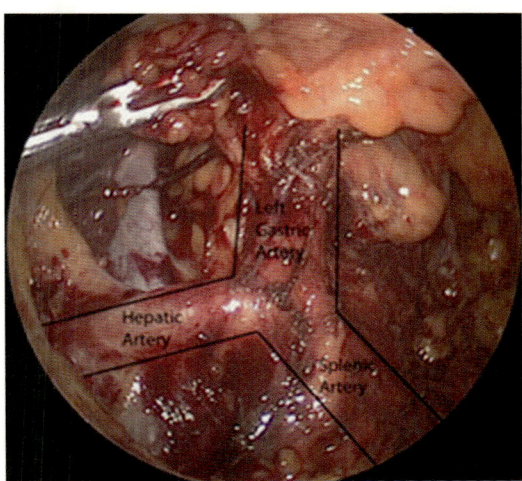
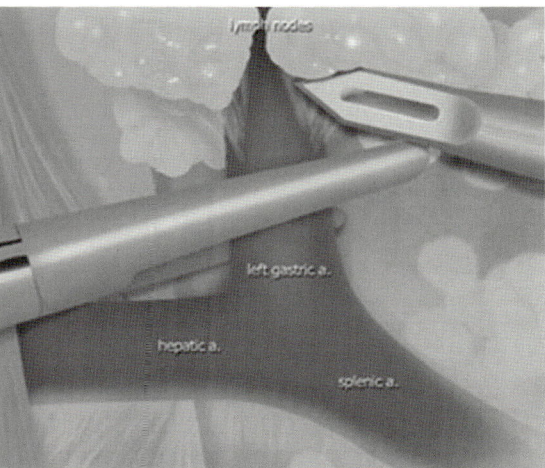

Fig. 12.3 Skeletonization and division of left gastric artery and vein (From Hochwald and Ben-David [16] with permission)

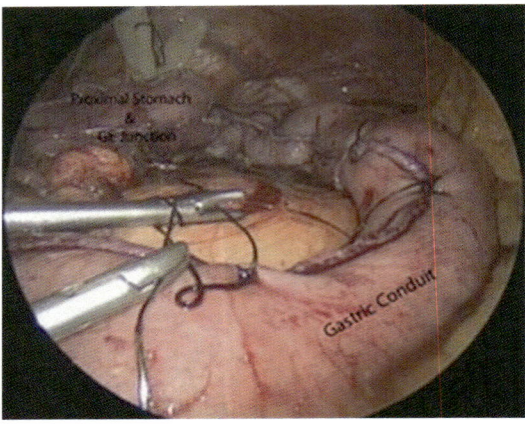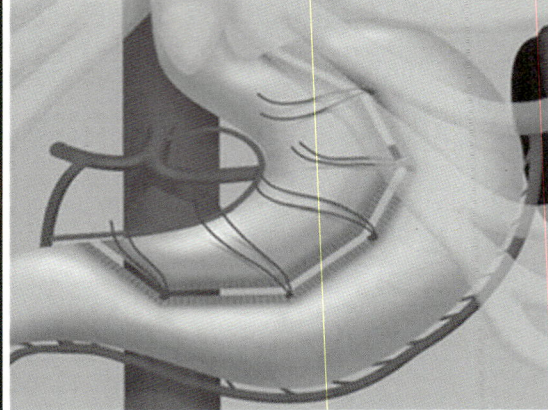

Fig. 12.4 Creation of the gastric conduit (From Hochwald and Ben-David [16] with permission)

the stomach 4 cm proximal to the pylorus along the lesser curvature of the stomach just proximal to the divided right gastric vessels. The stapler firings continue along the body and fundus of the stomach. The final division of the stomach is not done until after each staple line is reinforced with a single interrupted inverting suture of 2-0 silk. These sutures are placed at the junction of the staple lines and are used as handles for subsequent transfer of the stomach to the posterior mediastinum into the right chest (Fig. 12.4).

Following the final application of the stapler and division of the gastric conduit from the proximal stomach and GEJ, the esophagus is further mobilized. The Penrose drain is pulled laterally and medially enabling mobilization of the distal esophagus through the hiatus into the posterior mediastinum. The lower esophagus is widely dissected incorporating all lymphatic tissue. Subsequently, the gastric tube is sutured to the lesser curvature side of the upper divided stomach utilizing two interrupted 2-0 silk sutures.

The Penrose is placed through the hiatus into the posterior mediastinum while maintaining appropriate orientation of the gastric conduit to prevent organoaxial rotation of the gastric tube when it is being pulled into the right chest cavity. This is done by aligning the sutures placed along the lesser curvature of the stomach and straightening the gastric tube. A 16-French feeding tube is inserted into the proximal jejunum as we have

previously described [11]. The port site incisions and liver retractor incision are sutured closed and dressed appropriately after expelling the pneumoperitoneum.

Thoracic Dissection

The patient is placed in the left lateral decubitus position ensuring that all of their bony prominences are well padded. The right lung is deflated and a 5-mm trocar is placed under direct vision using a 5-mm 0° scope just inferior to the tip of the right scapula. This serves as the camera port for the duration of the case, and the scope is switched to a 5 mm 30° scope. The right chest cavity is insufflated with 8 mmHg of carbon dioxide (CO_2) pressure. This allows for further lung collapse during the thoracic portion of the procedure. A 5-mm port is placed in the seventh intercostal space along the posterior axillary line. A 12-mm trocar is placed in the tenth intercostal space just above the diaphragmatic insertion slightly anterior to the vertebral bodies. A 12-mm port is placed anteriorly in the seventh intercostal space and is utilized for the lung retractor (Fig. 12.5).

The lung is retracted anteriorly. The inferior pulmonary ligament is divided. The lower esophagus is widely dissected with an ENSEAL® tissue sealing device (Ethicon Endo-Surgery, Inc., Cincinnati, OH), and the Penrose drain is

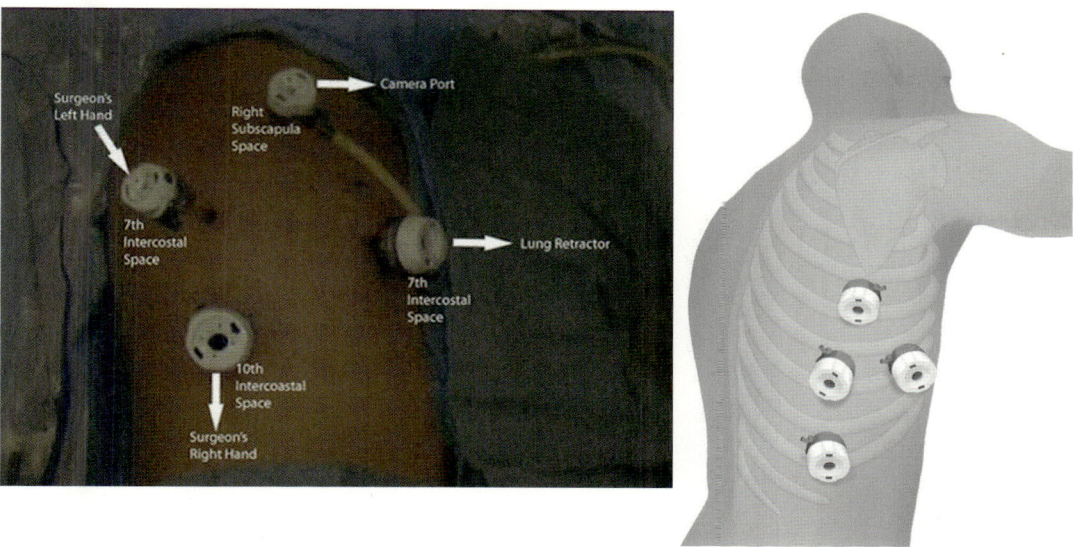

Fig. 12.5 Thoracic port placement (From Hochwald and Ben-David [16] with permission)

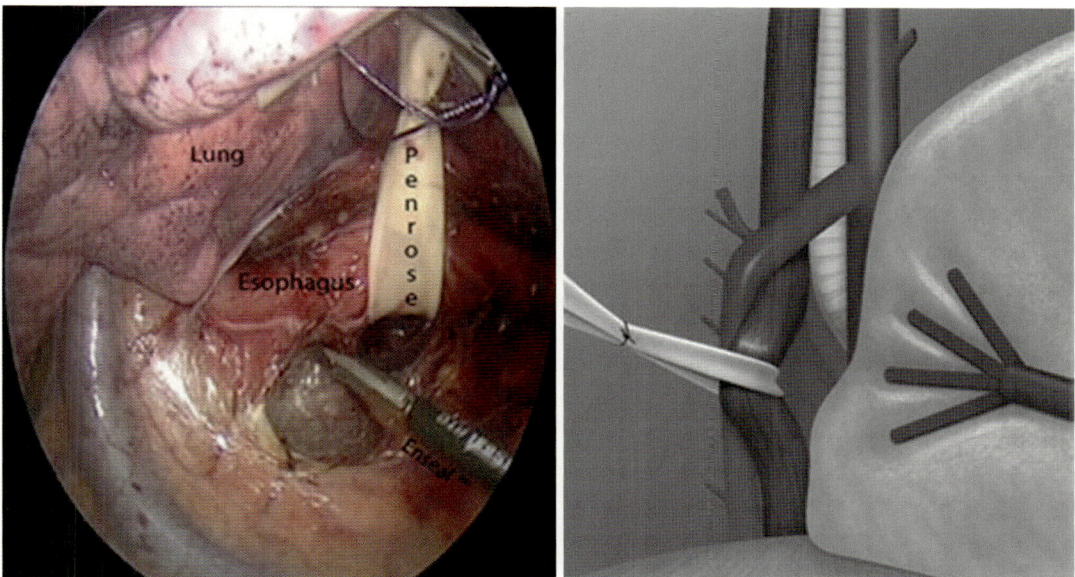

Fig. 12.6 Dissection of the distal esophagus (From Hochwald and Ben-David [16] with permission)

identified in the posterior mediastinum from our previous abdominal dissection. Care is taken not to enter into the left pleural space during this portion of the dissection. The esophagus is mobilized from its distal end to the level of the azygos vein. The Penrose is advanced along the esophagus during this dissection (Fig. 12.6). Periesophageal and subcarinal lymph nodes are included with the specimen. If the thoracic duct is identified, it is suture ligated or clipped. The azygous vein is divided with a 45- or 60-mm vascular load stapler (Fig. 12.7). The dissection continues with mobilization of the proximal esophagus away from the trachea. It is important to continue the esophageal mobilization just distal to the thoracic inlet.

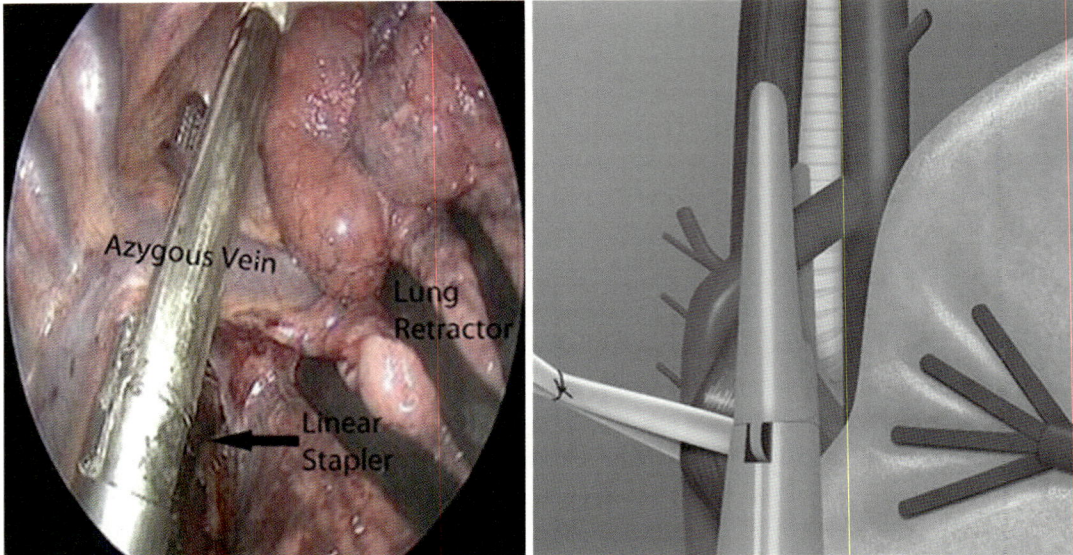

Fig. 12.7 Division of azygous vein (From Hochwald and Ben-David [16] with permission)

Thoracic Anastomosis (Video 12.1)

The gastroesophageal junction and gastric conduit are pulled into the chest cavity. The surgeon keeps the orientation of the gastric tube so that it does not twist. This is done by pulling on the sutures placed along the lesser curvature of the stomach and straightening the gastric tube as it is pulled through the posterior mediastinum. The proximal stomach specimen is separated from the gastric conduit by dividing the previously placed 2-0 silk sutures that were tethering them together. The posterior aspect of the gastric tube is placed alongside the anterior aspect of the esophagus with gentle tension superiorly. Cautery is utilized to make an opening in the medial aspect of the esophagus, 4–5 cm above the divided azygous vein. The tip of the nasogastric tube is pulled out from the esophagotomy (Fig. 12.8). Similarly, electrocautery is used to create a gastrotomy on the posterior aspect of the gastric conduit (Fig. 12.9). The anvil of a 6-cm staple load is introduced alongside the nasogastric tube into the esophagus, and the staple cartridge is placed in the stomach (Fig. 12.10). The stapler is closed, and care is taken to make sure the nasogastric tube is not caught in the staple

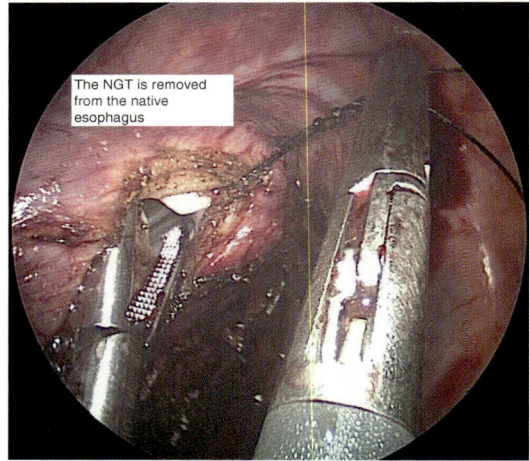

Fig. 12.8 Esophagotomy at the native esophagus

line. The stapler is fired and removed (Fig. 12.11). The nasogastric tube is then advanced through the anastomosis and the tip left in the lower aspect of the gastric conduit (Fig. 12.12). The common openings in the stomach and esophagus are aligned with the aid of 2-0 silk stay sutures (Fig. 12.13), and the esophagogastrostomy is sealed with the firings of the 6-cm linear stapler (Fig. 12.14). The specimen is transected with these same stapler firings. The omentum left on

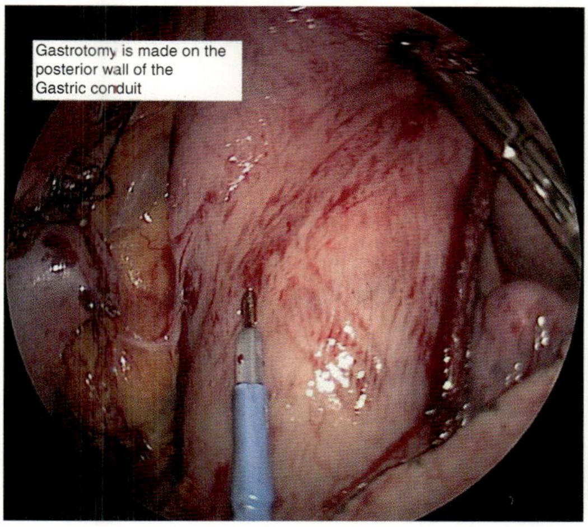

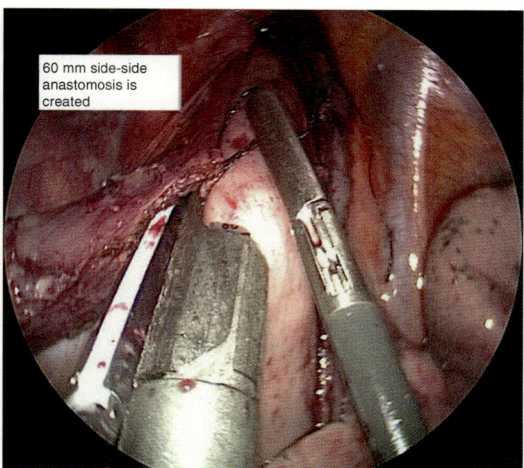

Fig. 12.9 Gastric conduit gastrotomy

Fig. 12.11 Side-to-side linear esophagogastrostomy anastomosis

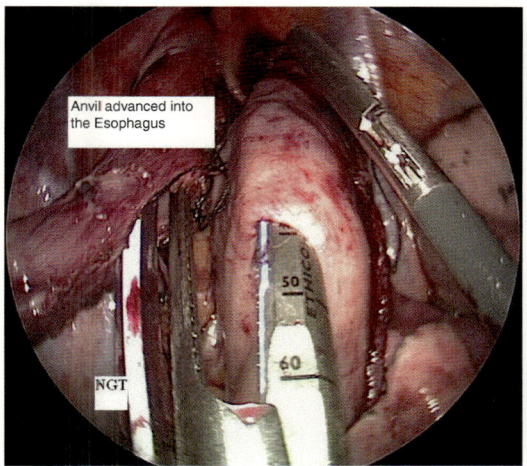

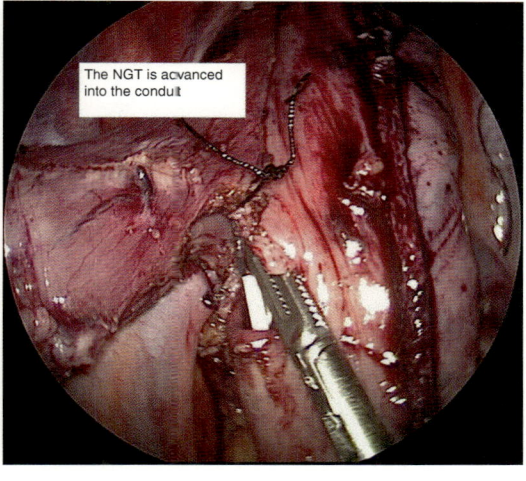

Fig. 12.10 The anvil of a 6-cm staple load is introduced alongside the nasogastric tube in the esophagus, and the staple cartridge is placed in the stomach

Fig. 12.12 Advancement of the nasogastric tube through the anastomosis into the gastric conduit

the gastric conduit is brought in a circumferential fashion around the anastomosis and sutured back to the gastric conduit as an additional buttressing layer (Fig. 12.15). A 24-French chest tube is placed through the inferior 12 mm port and positioned along the posterior mediastinum. The ports are removed and the incisions are closed with absorbable sutures.

Minimally invasive esophagectomy utilizing thoracoscopic and laparoscopic techniques with thoracic esophagogastric anastomosis has several

advantages. All components of the operation are done under direct vision with minimal blunt dissection. Appropriate lymphadenectomy can be easily accomplished as we have previously described [8, 10]. The intrathoracic anastomosis is performed utilizing a 6-cm stapler, without concern regarding the functional lumen size. Potential advantages of a long side-to-side stapled anastomosis include lower leak rates due to less tension and lower stenosis rates. In fact, a recent meta-analysis illustrated that anastomotic

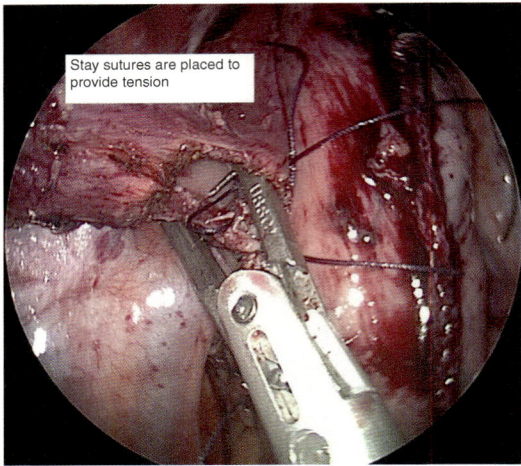

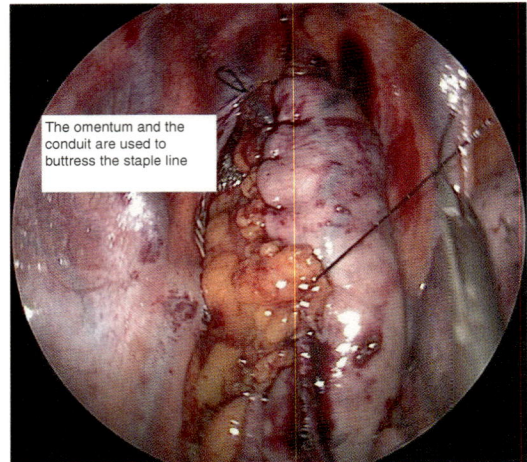

Fig. 12.13 Alignment of the esophagogastrostomy opening

Fig. 12.15 Buttressing the anastomosis with omental pedicle

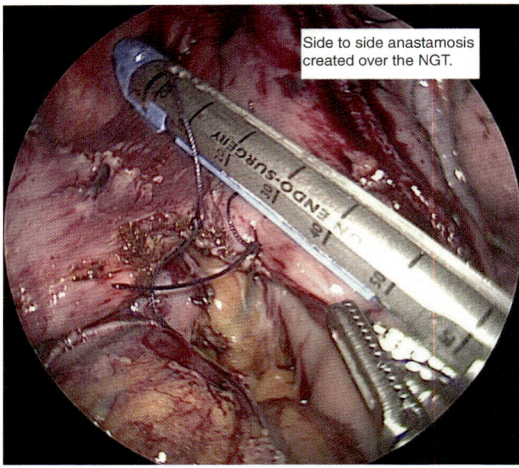

Fig. 12.14 Closure of the esophagogastrostomy opening with a linear stapler

hospital stay, decreasing morbidity and lower respiratory complications when compared with open esophagectomy [13, 14]. Despite these superior outcomes, patients undergoing a laparoscopic/thoracoscopic Ivor Lewis resection with a circular esophagogastric anastomosis have been shown to have a 26 % anastomotic stricture rate [15]. Hence, we have refined our technique for construction of a thoracic esophagogastrostomy using a 6-cm side-to-side linear stapled anastomosis. Although this method is applicable to the majority of patients undergoing minimally invasive resection of the esophagus for esophageal or GE junction cancer, it has become our procedure of choice for patients with previous neck dissections, foregut surgery, or gastroesophageal tumors extending into the proximal stomach.

leak was seen more commonly in the cervical group (13.64 %) than in the thoracic group (2.96 %) [12]. This group is also significantly less likely to experience vocal cord paresis/paralysis as noted by Luketich and colleagues [7]. In addition, although not common, anastomotic leaks can be managed with minimal intervention to the patient.

Minimally invasive esophagectomy is a safe alternative to the open technique. Patients undergoing these operations benefit from shorter

References

1. Worni M, Castleberry AW, Gloor B, et al. Trends and outcomes in the use of surgery and radiation for the treatment of locally advanced esophageal cancer: a propensity score adjusted analysis of the surveillance, epidemiology, and end results registry from 1998 to 2008. Dis Esophagus. 2014;27(7):662–9.
2. Thosani N, Singh H, Kapadia A, et al. Diagnostic accuracy of EUS in differentiating mucosal versus submucosal invasion of superficial esophageal cancers: a systematic review and meta-analysis. Gastrointest Endosc. 2012;75:242–53.

3. Cerfolio RJ, Bryant AS, Ohja B, et al. The accuracy of endoscopic ultrasonography with fine-needle aspiration, integrated positron emission tomography with computed tomography, and computed tomography in restaging patients with esophageal cancer after neoadjuvant chemoradiotherapy. J Thorac Cardiovasc Surg. 2005;129:1232–41.

4. Ben-David K, Rossidis G, Zlotecki RA, et al. Minimally invasive esophagectomy is safe and effective following neoadjuvant chemoradiation therapy. Ann Surg Oncol. 2011;18:3324–9.

5. DePaula AL, Hashiba K, Ferreira EA, et al. Laparoscopic transhiatal esophagectomy with esophagogastroplasty. Surg Laparosc Endosc. 1995;5:1–5.

6. Kim T, Hochwald SN, Sarosi GA, et al. Review of minimally invasive esophagectomy and current controversies. Gastroenterol Res Pract. 2012;2012:683213.

7. Luketich JD, Pennathur A, Awais O, et al. Outcomes after minimally invasive esophagectomy: review of over 1000 patients. Ann Surg. 2012;256:95–103.

8. Ben-David K, Sarosi GA, Cendan JC, et al. Decreasing morbidity and mortality in 100 consecutive minimally invasive esophagectomies. Surg Endosc. 2012;26: 162–7.

9. Ye T, Sun Y, Zhang Y, et al. Three-field or two-field resection for thoracic esophageal cancer: a meta-analysis. Ann Thorac Surg. 2013;96:1933–41.

10. Ben-David K, Sarosi GA, Cendan JC, et al. Technique of minimally invasive Ivor Lewis esophagogastrectomy with intrathoracic stapled side-to-side anastomosis. J Gastrointest Surg. 2010;14:1613–8.

11. Ben-David K, Kim T, Caban AM, et al. Pre-therapy laparoscopic feeding jejunostomy is safe and effective in patients undergoing minimally invasive esophagectomy for cancer. J Gastrointest Surg. 2013;17:1352–8.

12. Markar SR, Arya S, Karthikesalingam A, et al. Technical factors that affect anastomotic integrity following esophagectomy: systematic review and meta-analysis. Ann Surg Oncol. 2013;20:4274–81.

13. Biere SS, van Berge Henegouwen MI, Maas KW, et al. Minimally invasive versus open oesophagectomy for patients with oesophageal cancer: a multicentre, open-label, randomised controlled trial. Lancet. 2012;379:1887–92.

14. Biere SS, Maas KW, Bonavina L, et al. Traditional invasive vs. minimally invasive esophagectomy: a multicenter, randomized trial (TIME-trial). BMC Surg. 2011;11:2.

15. Nguyen NT, Hinojosa MW, Smith BR, et al. Minimally invasive esophagectomy: lessons learned from 104 operations. Ann Surg. 2008;248:1081–91.

16. Hochwald SN, Ben-David K. Minimally invasive esophagectomy with cervical esophagogastric anastomosis. J Gastrointest Surg. 2012;16(9):1775–81.

Moshim Kukar and Steven N. Hochwald

In this chapter, we will outline our technique for laparoscopic and thoracoscopic transhiatal esophagectomy with cervical anastomosis [1]. We utilize this technique routinely in patients with esophageal and Siewert's types 1 and 2 gastroesophageal junction cancer [2]. This technique has been shown to be safe in the setting of neoadjuvant chemoradiation since most patients in the western world present with locally advanced carcinoma and receive multimodality treatment [3]. This technique is best reserved for those patients who have no history of previous gastric surgery such as a Nissen fundoplication. In such patients, the amount of gastric conduit available to reach the neck may be limited and an intrathoracic esophagogastric anastomosis may be preferable as described in other portions of this book.

Preoperative Preparation

- The goals of surgery are to obtain a R0 resection and remove appropriate lymph nodes while minimizing morbidity. The extent of lymph node dissection has been previously reviewed elsewhere in this book and in previous publications [4].
- Review the details of endoscopy, extent of stomach involvement, and location of tumor in reference to the gastroesophageal (GE) junction. The surgeon should be prepared to perform an intraoperative endoscopy if needed.
- Patients are instructed to drink 6–8 oz of whole milk or cream 6 h prior to the start of the procedure. In those patients who are not able to tolerate this amount of liquid, the cream can be given through a gastrostomy or jejunostomy feeding tube. In our experience and others, it has been demonstrated to significantly reduce postoperative chyle leaks [5].

Anesthetic/Induction Phase

- Patient is intubated with double-lumen endotracheal tube. Under bronchoscopic guidance, the tube is confirmed in position so that patient can be maintained on single ventilation during thoracic dissection.
- Arterial line is placed.
- We do not routinely use central venous access/monitoring unless otherwise indicated.
- An 18 F nasogastric tube is placed carefully especially in patients with bulky lesions, and location is confirmed in the stomach. It is

Electronic supplementary material Supplementary material is available in the online version of this chapter at 10.1007/978-3-319-09342-0_13. Videos can also be accessed at http://www.springerimages.com/videos/978-3-319-09341-3.

M. Kukar, MD (✉) • S.N. Hochwald, MD, FACS
Department of Surgical Oncology,
Roswell Park Cancer Institute,
Elm & Carlton Streets, Buffalo, NY 14263, USA
e-mail: moshim.kukar@roswellpark.org

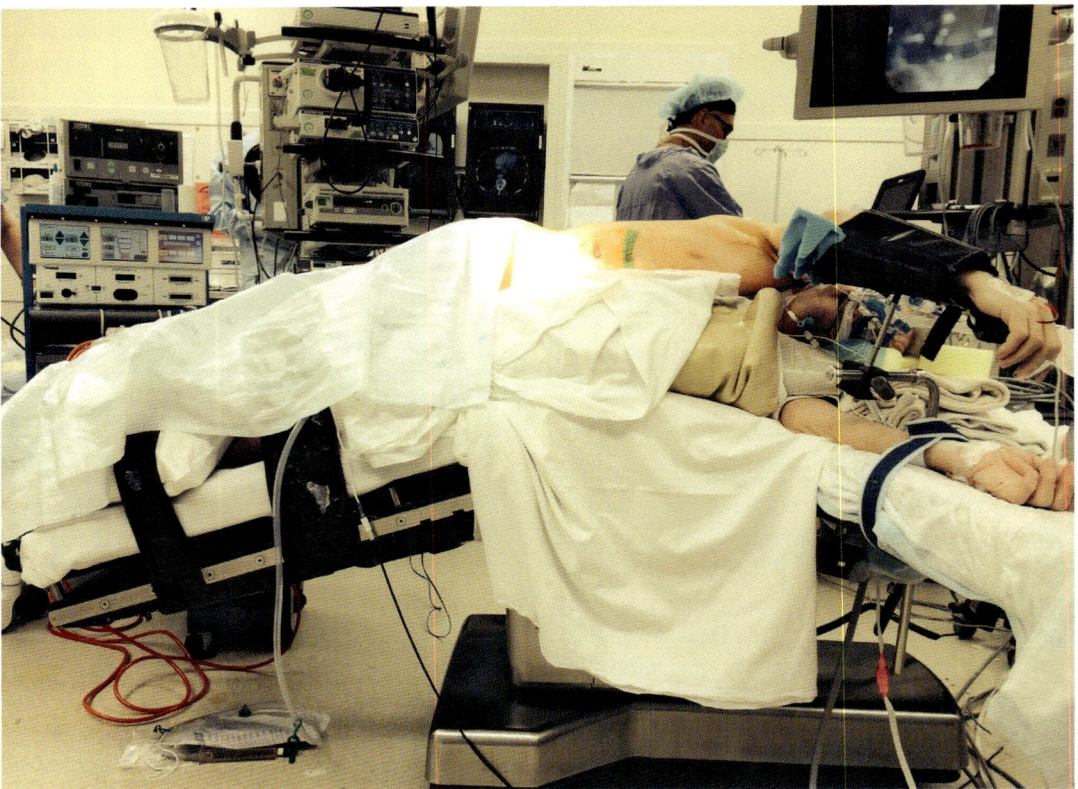

Fig. 13.1 Patient positioning

important that this tube is placed while the patient is in a supine position.
- Foley catheter is placed.

Patient Positioning (Fig. 13.1)

- A bean bag and an overlying gel pad are prepositioned on the operating table.
- The patient is positioned on the operating table so that the anterior superior iliac spine lies just inferior to the break of the table.
- Patient is positioned in left lateral decubitus position. The trough supporting the right arm is positioned so as to allow the right arm to fall forward. An axillary roll is placed and all areas are appropriately padded and secured.
- The table is raised and flexed so as to open the intercostal spaces and the subcostal spaces and rotate the hips down and away from the horizontal position.

- The bean bag is desufflated with patient in this position, making sure that the patient is not rotated.
- After positioning, repeat bronchoscopy is performed to confirm the location of endotracheal tube. The right lung is clamped and single-lung ventilation is begun.

Thoracoscopic Dissection (Video 13.1)

Port Placement (Fig. 13.2)

- Access: In most patients, two five and two twelve mm ports are necessary to perform the thoracic esophageal dissection. After desufflating the right lung, a 5 mm Optiview trocar with a 5 mm, 0° laparoscope is used to gain access and inserted under direct vision just inferior to the tip of the scapula. It is important

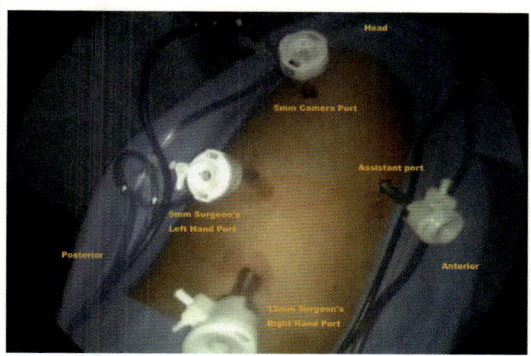

Fig. 13.2 Thoracoscopic port placement (From Hochwald and Ben-David [1] with permission)

that this port is placed about equidistant between the sternum and the vertebral bodies. This serves as the camera port. The chest is insufflated to a pressure of 8 mmHg. The camera is subsequently switched to a 5 mm, 30° scope after safe entry into the right pleural space is confirmed.

- A 5 mm port is then placed anteriorly in the seventh intercostal space. This port is utilized to retract the lung anteriorly during the initial dissection. If a 5 mm fan retractor is not available, a 12 mm port can be placed for a larger fan retractor. During the latter parts of the dissection, this port can be used by the assistant to help with the high thoracic dissection.
- A 12 mm port is inserted in the tenth intercostal space just above the diaphragmatic insertion in a straight line beneath the camera port.
- A 5 mm port is inserted in the seventh intercostal space midway between the inferior 12 mm and 5 mm camera ports. This along with the 12 mm port is used as the surgeon's working ports. It is critical that these two ports are not placed too posteriorly so that interference with the vertebral bodies is encountered.

Dissection

- 5 mm fan retractor is used to retract the lung anteriorly, exposing the esophagus. If a 5 mm fan is not available or adequate, this can be enlarged to a 12 mm port.

- Dissection is begun by dividing the inferior pulmonary ligament to the level of inferior pulmonary vein.
- The goal is to encircle the lower esophagus with a Penrose drain and to widely dissect the periesophageal tissue free from the posterior mediastinum. To accomplish this, the periesophageal tissue is widely opened anteriorly and posteriorly to the lower esophagus using the ENSEAL® tissue sealing device (Ethicon Endo-Surgery, Inc., Cincinnati, OH), carefully preserving the inferior pulmonary vein and avoiding entry into the pericardium and left pleural space.
- The esophagus is encircled carefully using a RealizeTM (Ethicon Endo-Surgery, Inc., Cincinnati, OH) dissector and a ¼-in. penrose is placed around the esophagus, and the ends are secured with an endoloop tie as shown in Fig. 13.3. It is critical to have a 2-0 silk tie sutured to one end of the penrose and a small loop fashioned in the suture that can be attached to the RealizeTM and subsequently pulled around the esophagus. The penrose is left slightly loose so as to allow its movement along the length of the esophagus.
- Both limbs of the penrose drain are grasped, and the esophagus is widely dissected from distal to proximal in the right chest. Periesophageal lymph nodes are left on the specimen. The vagus nerves are divided. The dissection is carried superiorly toward the azygous vein. The subcarinal lymph node packet is carefully dissected while preserving the membranous portions of the mainstem bronchi.
- During dissection of the lower esophagus from the inferior pulmonary ligament to the level of the azygous vein, it is critical to apply a generous amount of clips to the tissue between the aorta and the vertebral bodies and the esophagus. If the thoracic duct is visualized, it is ligated, otherwise, multiple clips are applied in this area to prevent injury to the thoracic duct or its branches.
- A window is made superior to the azygous vein and it is divided using a 45- or 60-mm vascular cartridge of the powered ECHELON

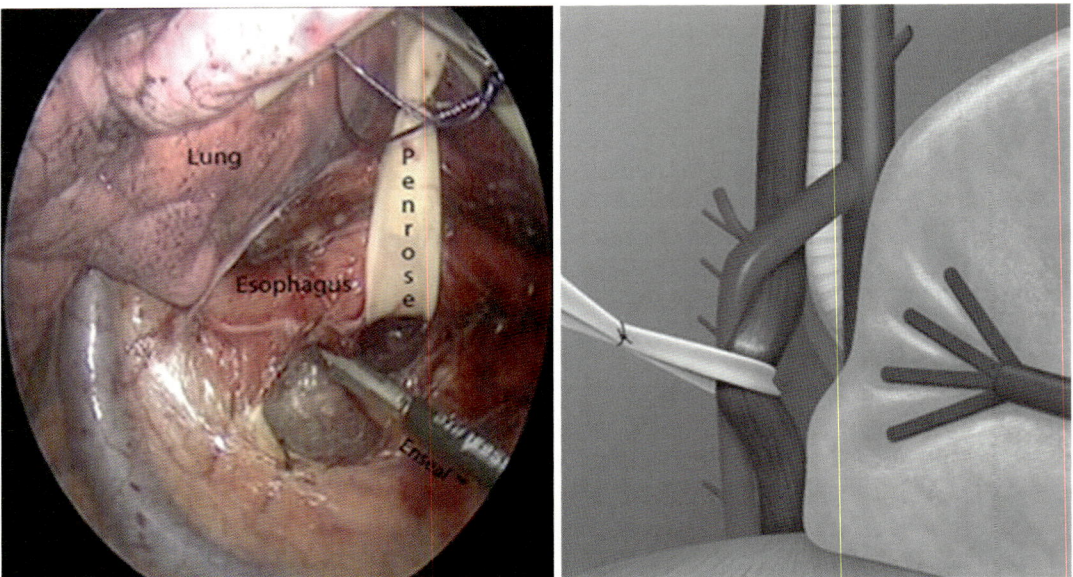

Fig. 13.3 Thoracoscopic mobilization of the esophagus (From Hochwald and Ben-David [1] with permission)

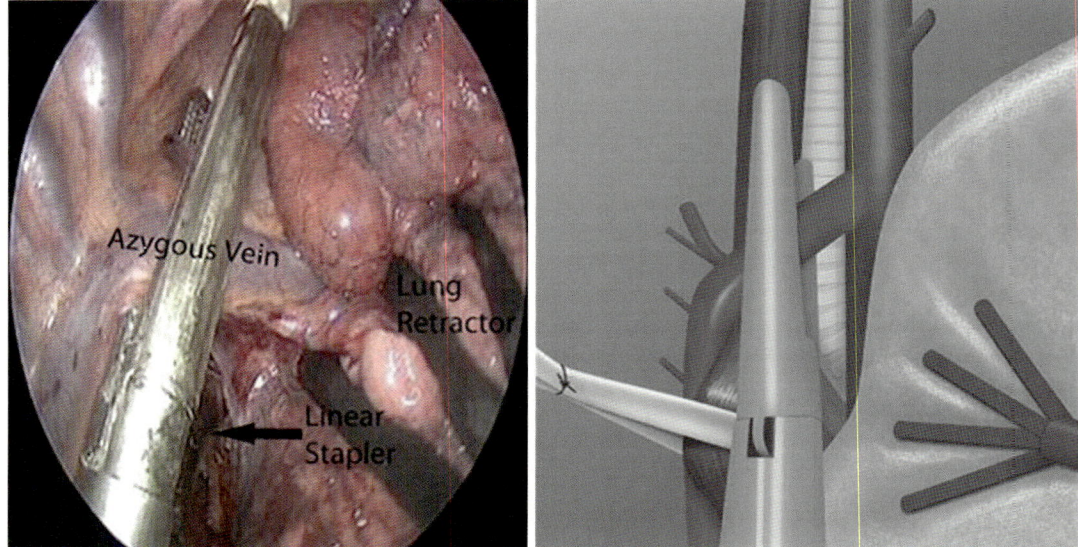

Fig. 13.4 Thoracoscopic division of azygous vein (From Hochwald and Ben-David [1] with permission)

FLEXTM ENDOPATH® stapler (Ethicon Endo-Surgery, Inc., Cincinnati, OH). Frequently the staple line on the azygous vein should be reinforced with titanium clips if there is any evidence of bleeding (Fig. 13.4).

• Dissection is carried superiorly to the azygous vein, and an attempt is made to stay close to the esophagus above the azygous vein to avoid injury to the recurrent laryngeal nerve (RLN).

• We make an attempt to complete the cervical esophageal mobilization through the thoracoscopic phase of the operation. Excellent visibility afforded by high-definition imaging and long instruments helps us accomplish this routinely. However, we try to minimize the use of energy devices on the tissue between the esophagus and the trachea to avoid injury to the RLN. The dissection is carried under the subclavian vessels up to the level of the clavicle.

- After the cervical esophagus is mobilized at a point superior to the thoracic inlet, we proceed with dissection toward the GE junction and care is taken to ensure that the esophagus is mobilized down to the diaphragm. However, it is important not to dissect into the abdominal cavity.
- After the esophageal mobilization is complete, the ¼-in. penrose is left in the superior apex of our dissection. The penrose should be above the subclavian vessels – in close proximity to the clavicle to ensure that the cervical esophageal dissection has been completed.
- Hemostasis is ensured and a 24 F Blake drain is left posteriorly in the thoracic cavity and brought out through the 12 mm port site, and a purse-string suture is used to secure it to the skin. This drain is connected to a pleuravac.
- The right lung is insufflated under direct vision and the port sites are closed with 4-0 Monocryl and Dermabond is applied.

Repositioning

- The chest tube is connected to −20 mmHg of wall suction.
- To recruit atelectatic right lung segments, the patient is put on dual lung ventilation with a PEEP set to 8 mmHg.
- The patient is placed supine and the left arm is tucked. A shoulder roll is inserted under the shoulder blades to optimize cervical exposure.
- The head is extended and tilted slightly to the right.
- The patient is placed supine on the operating table. Split-leg tables or stirrups are not used. A footboard is placed to facilitate steep reverse Trendelenburg position during the abdominal dissection.

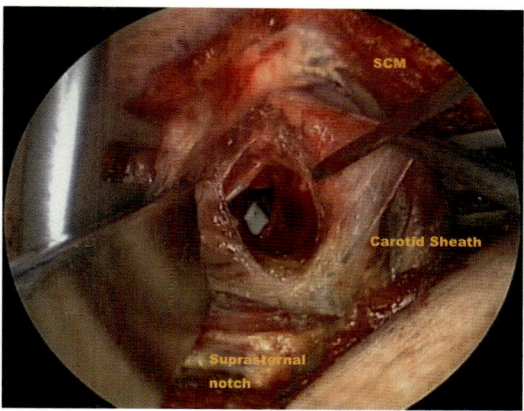

Fig. 13.5 Penrose easily identified after opening the prevertebral fascia

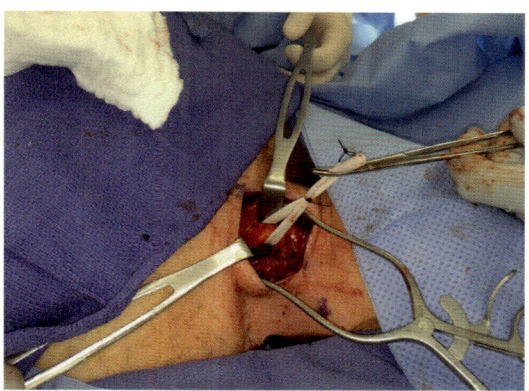

Fig. 13.6 Left cervical esophageal mobilization

Cervical Dissection (Video 13.2)

- A 6 cm skin incision is made along the anterior border of sternocleidomastoid starting from the suprasternal notch.
- The platysma is divided.
- Sternocleidomastoid muscle is identified and moved laterally, carefully ligating and dividing any crossing jugular vein branches.
- A self-retaining retractor is used to facilitate further dissection.
- The inferior belly of omohyoid is divided, exposing the prevertebral fascia.
- Keeping the jugular vein and carotid artery laterally, prevertebral fascia is opened and the penrose is identified (Fig. 13.5) and secured with a Kelly clamp (Fig. 13.6).

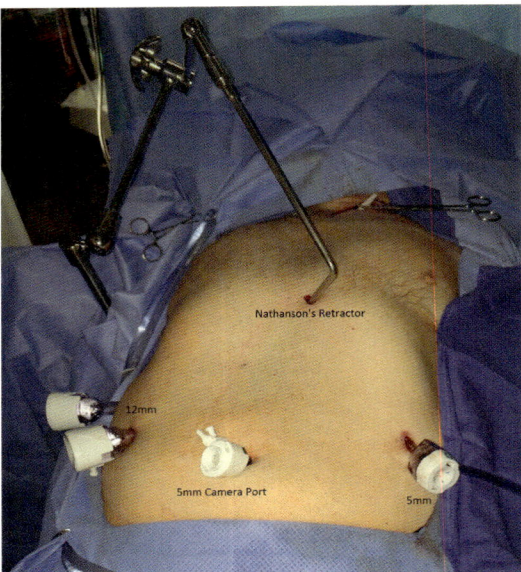

Fig. 13.7 Abdominal port placement

- Further dissection is done superiorly and inferiorly to ensure an adequate opening for easy retrieval of the specimen and the gastric conduit through this incision.
- Since most of the cervical dissection is completed thoracoscopically, blunt cervical dissection is minimized during this phase to avoid injury to the RLN, and this portion of the procedure takes only 5–10 min.

Abdominal Dissection (Video 13.3)

Port Placement (Fig. 13.7)

- 5 mm Optiview trocar with a 3-piece 5 mm, 0° laparoscope is inserted under direct vision in the left upper quadrant, just lateral to Palmer's point.
- A 5 mm trocar is inserted 22 cm below the xiphoid just to the left of the midline. This serves as the camera port and the camera is switched to a 5 mm, 30° scope.
- A 12 mm trocar is inserted at the same level of the camera port just to the right of the right rectus abdominis muscle.

- Another 12 mm trocar is inserted in the right upper quadrant 6 cm superior and lateral to the other 12 mm port.
- A 5 mm trocar is inserted just below and slightly to the left of the xiphoid process, the track is dilated with a hemostat clamp, and a Nathanson retractor is inserted to retract the left lobe of the liver anteriorly. The retractor is secured to the right side of the bed.

Dissection

- The patient is placed in steep reverse Trendelenburg position. The operating surgeon stands on the right side of the table and the assistant stands on the left side of the table.
- The abdomen is thoroughly inspected for any evidence of metastatic disease.
- Initial dissection is begun by opening the pars flaccida and the tissue along the right crus of the diaphragm. A retrogastric tunnel is made, carefully identifying the left crus, and a blunt grasper is passed from right to left and is visualized below the left crus by carefully grasping the gastric fundus and pulling inferiorly and to the right. Care is taken to avoid entry into the chest cavity and avoiding injury to the spleen. A penrose drain is encircled around the GE junction and secured with an endoloop tie.
- The lesser sac is entered halfway up along the greater curvature of the stomach, carefully preserving the right gastroepiploic arcade. After making an adequate window, the posterior wall of the stomach is grasped by the operating surgeon's left hand which allows the right gastroepiploic arcade to flip anteriorly. Care is taken to grasp the stomach to provide retraction. Minimal retraction of the omentum is performed.
- The dissection is continued along the greater curvature, dividing the short gastric vessels with the vessel sealing device until the left crus and the Penrose drains are visible. During this dissection, the left gastroepiploic vessels are ligated near their origin. In addition, the

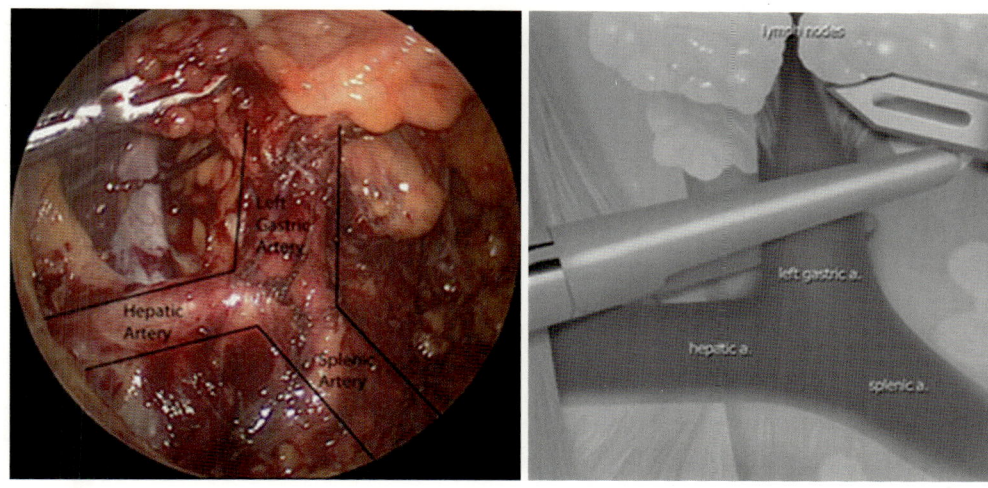

Fig. 13.8 Skeletonization of the celiac trunk and division of the left gastric artery (from Hochwald and Ben-David [1] with permission)

short gastric vessels are taken close to the spleen to assist in capturing splenic nodes.
- Further mobilization of the greater curvature toward the pylorus is performed by the assistant surgeon on the left side of the table. The transverse mesocolon is carefully mobilized off the right gastroepiploic arcade and the head of the pancreas.
- To facilitate this dissection, gastropancreatic folds are divided until the gastroduodenal artery is identified. Once the location of the gastroduodenal artery is known, even in obese patients, the location of the right gastroepiploic vessels can be determined.
- The operating surgeon performs a Kocher's maneuver to mobilize the duodenum so as to allow the pylorus to reach the GE junction with no tension. Most times, a full Kocher maneuver is not required. During this portion of the dissection, the assistant grasps the pylorus and retracts the stomach and duodenum to the patient's left.
- The right gastric artery is divided 4 cm proximal to the pylorus. Using a Maryland dissector, a window is made along the lesser curvature, and overlying tissue is divided with a sealing device.
- Nodal tissue along the left gastric vein and artery are dissected and swept up toward

the specimen. After skeletonizing the vessels, the pedicle is transected using a vascular staple load on the powered Endo GIA (Fig. 13.8). Sometimes the left gastric vein and artery are taken separately to facilitate a better nodal dissection. At this point, the stomach should be completely mobile.
- The gastric conduit is created using multiple 6 cm firings of 3.5 mm or 4.8 mm staple loads, depending on the thickness of the stomach. The operating surgeon's left-hand port is utilized to fire the first staple load, 4 cm proximal to the pylorus. Additional firings are done using the surgeon's right-hand port, following the curve of the stomach. We routinely use 5–6 staple loads (6 cm each), and care is taken to keep the width of the conduit around 5–6 cm. The stomach is not completely divided until sutures are used to reinforce the junction of the staple lines (Fig. 13.9).
- A 2-0 silk Endostitch is used to reinforce the intersecting staple lines, and the tails are left long to facilitate passage of the conduit through the mediastinum and out the cervical incision. After all the sutures are placed, an additional staple load is used to transect the upper fundus of the stomach.

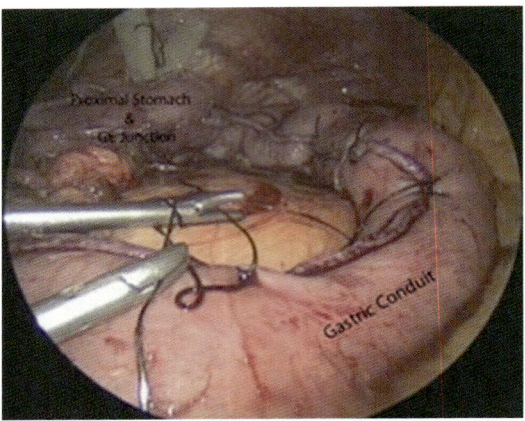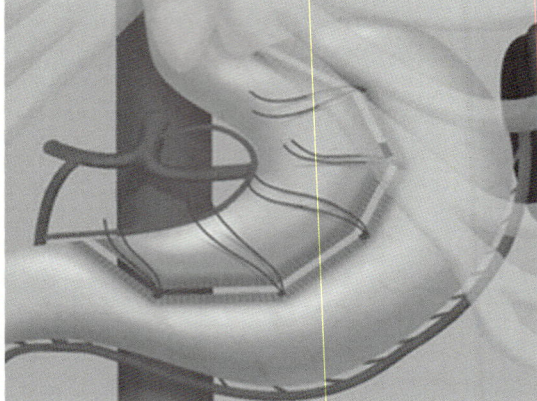

Fig. 13.9 Creation of gastric conduit (From Hochwald and Ben-David [1] with permission)

- Using the penrose as a handle, the GE junction is completely dissected free by widely dividing the phrenoesophageal membrane and connecting the abdominal with the thoracic dissection. The dissection is performed widely so that all the tissue between the left and right crura is left on the specimen. It is important to communicate with the anesthesia team as the patient may have some hemodynamic instability once the dissection is connected between the chest and abdomen.
- Two 2-0 silk Endostitches are used to anchor the tip of conduit to the most inferior and right part of the transected specimen side of the stomach so as to keep the correct orientation while pulling the gastric conduit through the mediastinum.
- Botulin toxin (100 units dissolved in 10 ml) is used to inject into the pylorus. A total of five to six ml is injected intramuscularly at 2–3 different areas in the anterior pyloric ring. We do not routinely perform a pyloroplasty.
- To facilitate the passage of the conduit to the posterior mediastinum, the operating surgeon grabs the silk tail ends of the sutures placed on the gastric conduit while the assistant pulls on the cervical esophagus. The specimen and gastric conduit are pulled out the cervical incision while the surgeon preserves the proper orientation at all times via visualization of the conduit both in the abdomen and the mediastinum.

Reconstruction (Video 13.4)

- The conduit is delivered out the neck incision, and the sutures holding it to the specimen are cut.
- The esophagus and the conduit are aligned so that a side-side anastomosis can be created between the posterior wall of the stomach and anteromedial aspect of the cervical esophagus. Judicious care is taken to ensure the correct orientation of the conduit at all times.
- An esophagotomy is made, and the NG tube is pulled out. A gastrostomy is made on the posterior wall of the stomach 4–5 cm proximal to the tip of the conduit.
- Using a 60, 3.5 mm load on the Endo GIA, a 6 cm side-to-side stapled anastomosis is created. After the stapler is closed, the NG tube is moved to ensure free mobility. The stapler is fired. The NG tube is advanced through the anastomosis and the tip left in the lower aspect of the gastric conduit (Fig. 13.10).
- The common channel is closed with a 60, 3.5 mm load of the TA stapler excising the tip of the conduit. After the stapler is fired, the TA stapler is left in place and serves as a handle to place two 3-0 silk sutures at the crotch of the staple line to decrease any tension.
- The TA staple line is suture inverted with a running 3-0 PDS suture. The anastomosis is carefully pushed back into the posterior-superior mediastinum. A 7 F Jackson-Pratt is placed along the anastomosis. The platysma is

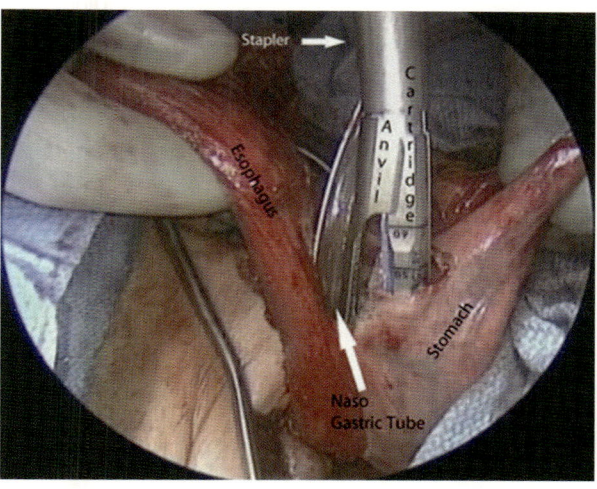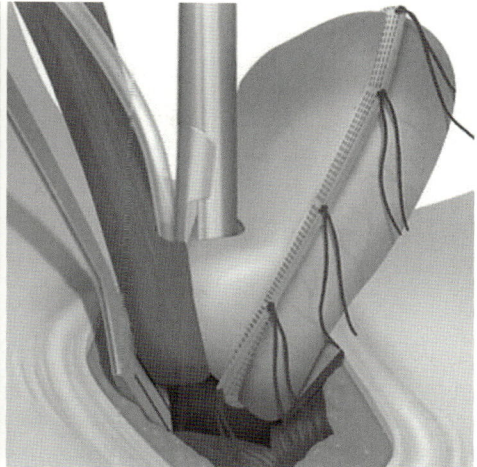

Fig. 13.10 Cervical linear-stapled esophagogastrostomy (From Hochwald and Ben-David [1] with permission)

approximated with interrupted 3-0 Vicryl sutures and skin closed with 4-0 Monocryl.
- The conduit is gently pulled down to ensure that redundant conduit is not left in the thoracic cavity. The gastric conduit is sutured to the left crus of the diaphragm with 2, 2-0 silk sutures to avoid herniation of intra-abdominal contents.
- A prefashioned 16 F T tube (back wall is cut and a portion is removed) is inserted in the proximal jejunum 15–20 cm from the ligament of Treitz. It is anchored to the abdominal wall with multiple transfacial sutures [6].
- The two 12 mm ports are closed with 0 Vicryl using a Carter Thompson device. All incisions are infiltrated with lidocaine and Marcaine and closed with 4-0 Monocryl and Dermabond applied.
- Table 13.1 details the pearls and pitfalls of each phase of dissection.

Postoperative Care

Results utilizing this anastomotic technique have been previously published [2]. Anastomotic leak rates are less than 5 % with a low stricture rate. For postoperative care, we follow an esophagectomy pathway at our institution.
- Patients are transferred to a monitored setting for overnight observation and transferred to the floor on postoperative day 1 with telemetry monitoring.

Table 13.1 Pearls and pitfalls

Preoperative
1. Patient's anterior superior iliac spine at the level of the break of the table
2. Right shoulder is slightly depressed and should fall forward
Thoracic dissection
1. Key anatomical structures to identify/preserve: Inferior pulmonary vein, thoracic duct, membranous portion of the trachea, recurrent laryngeal nerve
2. If thoracic duct is not visualized, multiple clips should be applied on the lymphatic tissue between the aorta and esophagus
3. Mobilize the esophagus past the level of thoracic inlet
4. Minimize the use of energy device during esophageal mobilization on the tracheal side to avoid thermal injury to the recurrent laryngeal nerve
Cervical dissection
1. Minimize blunt dissection
2. Ensure adequate opening so that the specimen and conduit can be delivered easily
Abdominal dissection
1. Holding the posterior wall of the stomach during mobilization of greater curvature prevents injury to right gastroepiploic vessels
2. Adequate mobilization of the first and second portions of the duodenum to allow the pylorus to reach the gastroesophageal junction
3. Pull the NG tube back into the esophagus during the creation of conduit
4. Conduit width should be approximately 5–6 cm, and a minimum of 5–6 staple load fires (6 cm loads) are needed for a conduit to reach the neck
5. Care is maintained to keep the right orientation while delivering the conduit into the mediastinum and during the anastomosis

- Day 2, they are started on trickle tube feeds and the Foley catheter is discontinued.
- Day 3, NG tube is removed if the chest x-ray shows a decompressed conduit.
- Day 4, they are given a trial of colored clears and the neck JP is removed.
- Day 5, they are advanced to full liquids and the right chest Blake drain is removed.
- Day 6–7, patients are advanced to goal tube feeds when they have full return of bowel function and usually discharged home on postoperative day 7 with tube feeds for 16 h and also maintaining a full liquid diet.

References

1. Hochwald SN, Ben-David K. Minimally invasive esophagectomy with cervical esophagogastric anastomosis. J Gastrointest Surg. 2012;16(9):1775–81.

2. Ben-David K, Sarosi GA, Cendan JC, Howard D, Rossidis G, Hochwald SN. Decreasing morbidity and mortality in 100 consecutive minimally invasive esophagectomies. Surg Endosc. 2012;26(1): 162–7.

3. Ben-David K, Rossidis G, Zlotecki RA, Grobmyer SR, Cendan JC, Sarosi GA, Hochwald SN. Minimally invasive esophagectomy is safe and effective following neoadjuvant chemoradiation therapy. Ann Surg Oncol. 2011;18(12):3324–9.

4. Kukar M, Hochwald SN. Operative and multimodal aspects of esophago-gastric junction (EGJ) cancer care: western viewpoints. Textbook of complex general surgical oncology (in press).

5. Shen Y, Feng M, Khan MA, Wang H, Tan L, Wang Q. A simple method minimizes chylothorax after minimally invasive esophagectomy. J Am Coll Surg. 2014;218(1):108–12.

6. Ben-David K, Kim T, Caban AM, Rossidis G, Rodriguez SS, Hochwald SN. Pre-therapy laparoscopic feeding jejunostomy is safe and effective in patients undergoing minimally invasive esophagectomy for cancer. J Gastrointest Surg. 2013;17(8): 1352–8.

Laparoscopic and Thoracoscopic Esophagectomy with Colonic Interposition

14

Christopher Armstrong, Monica T. Young, and Ninh T. Nguyen

Introduction

Surgical management of cancer of the thoracic esophagus and proximal stomach is complex. Various surgical approaches have been utilized for resection of these lesions [1]. The choice of approach is highly dependent on the location and extent of the tumor. Patients with a gastric cardia cancer without involvement of the esophagus but with significant involvement of the gastric body may be candidates for total gastrectomy with Roux-en-Y esophageal-jejunal reconstruction. Patients with isolated gastric cardia cancer may be candidates for an Ivor Lewis esophagogastrectomy, transhiatal esophagectomy, or a three-hole McKeown esophagectomy. In most cases, the stomach is the preferred conduit for reconstruction due to its robust blood supply and the technical advantages of a gastric pull-up with a single intra-thoracic or cervical anastomosis [2]. Occasionally, patients with proximal gastric or distal esophageal cancers will have extensive involvement of the stomach or a previous gastric resection rendering the stomach unusable as a conduit. In these situations, the colon or small bowel can be used as an alternative option. Advantages of colonic interposition include lack of acid reflux, preservation of the gastric reservoir (if the stomach is preserved), long length, and that it is outside the radiation field for those patients receiving neoadjuvant chemoradiotherapy [3]. These advantages are tempered by increased technical complexity, construction of three anastomoses, and a higher potential for anastomotic leak [4].

Although esophageal resection has been traditionally managed with open surgery, minimally invasive techniques have continued to evolve and now are increasingly utilized among specialized centers [2, 5, 6]. Colonic interposition adds further technical complexity to esophageal resection and is typically undertaken using an open approach. Currently only one case report authored by Nguyen et al. describes the surgical steps of a minimally invasive Ivor Lewis esophagectomy with colonic interposition [7]. In this chapter, we describe our technique of a laparoscopic and

Electronic supplementary material Supplementary material is available in the online version of this chapter at 10.1007/978-3-319-09342-0_14. Videos can also be accessed at http://www.springerimages.com/videos/978-3-319-09341-3.

C. Armstrong, MD, FRCSC
Department of General Surgery, Rockyview General Hospital and South Health Campus,
University of Calgary, 4448 Front St, SE,
Calgary, AB T3M 1M4, Canada
e-mail: csarmstrong1@me.com

M.T. Young, MD
Department of General Surgery,
University of California Irvine Medical Center,
Orange, CA, USA

N.T. Nguyen, MD (✉)
Department of Surgery,
University of California Irvine Medical Center,
Orange, CA, USA
e-mail: ninhn@uci.edu

S.N. Hochwald, M. Kukar (eds.), *Minimally Invasive Foregut Surgery for Malignancy: Principles and Practice*,
DOI 10.1007/978-3-319-09342-0_14, © Springer International Publishing Switzerland 2015

thoracoscopic esophagogastrectomy with colonic interposition.

Technique

Patient Selection/Evaluation

In all cases, preoperative assessment is a crucial component of the surgical process. Complete knowledge of the proximal and distal extent of the tumor is vitally important to planning the correct operative approach and reconstructive strategy. Patients undergo an extensive endoscopic evaluation of the proximal stomach and distal esophagus with biopsies to accurately determine the proximal and distal extent of the tumor. Patients also undergo a comprehensive staging workup which typically includes a CT-PET to exclude metastatic disease. If the colon is to be used for reconstruction, it is important that the patient also undergoes a colonoscopy to exclude the possibility of a synchronous colonic neoplasm. It is our practice that patients undergo CT angiography to more accurately assess the colonic blood supply. Patients are given a bowel preparation preoperatively. The points of proximal and distal transection of the colonic interponat are shown in Fig. 14.1.

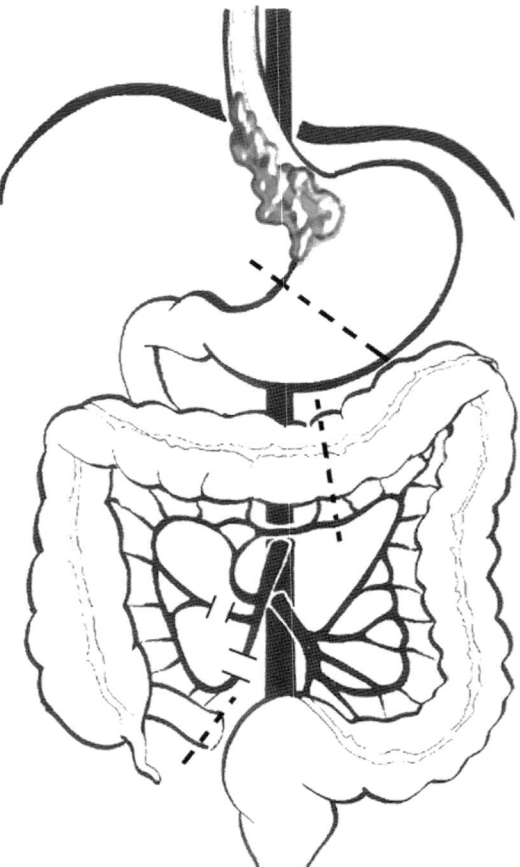

Fig. 14.1 Surgical plan for resection and reconstruction using the right colon to restore esophageal continuity (From Nguyen et al. [7] with permission)

Abdominal Phase

The patient is positioned supine for the initial abdominal phase of the surgery. We employ a standard port placement for most procedures involving the stomach or requiring dissection of the diaphragmatic hiatus (Fig. 14.2). This involves establishing pneumoperitoneum using a Veress needle placed in the left abdomen lateral to the umbilicus at the edge of the rectus abdominis. A 12-mm trocar is placed at this site. We then insert a 5-mm port in the right subcostal region beneath the inferior edge of the liver at the midaxillary line. This port is used for a fixed liver retractor. Another 5-mm port is placed in the right subcostal region at the midclavicular line and a 12-mm port is inserted slightly cephalad

and to the right of the umbilicus. These serve as the surgeon's main operating ports. A final 5-mm trocar is placed in the left upper quadrant and is utilized by the assistant. An initial staging laparoscopy is performed to exclude occult metastatic disease. We frequently do an intraoperative upper endoscopy as well to ensure accurate assessment of the proximal and distal extent of the tumor.

After staging laparoscopy excludes the presence of occult metastatic disease, the hepatogastric ligament is divided and the left gastric vessels are exposed. We perform a celiac lymphadenectomy en bloc and then proceed to divide the left gastric artery at the level of the celiac trunk with a single firing of a linear stapler. The stomach is further mobilized by dividing the gastrocolic

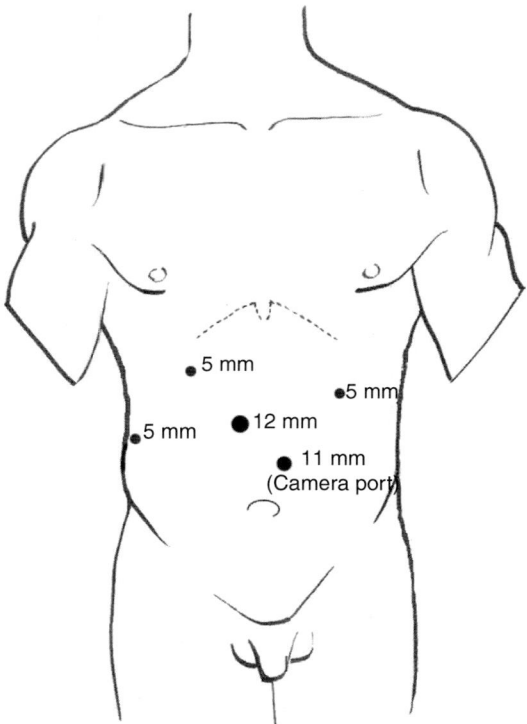

Fig. 14.2 Laparoscopic port placement

ligament and short gastric vessels. We routinely perform a partial omentectomy during this phase of the procedure.

After the gastric fundus has been fully dissected, the distal esophagus is mobilized into the mediastinum by opening the phrenoesophageal ligament. We routinely try to obtain at least 6 cm of mediastinal dissection transabdominally. Unlike a gastric pull-up, there is no need to preserve the right gastroepiploic vessels; therefore, these can be divided. The stomach is then transected using a linear cutting stapler. In this situation, it is our preference to leave a small remnant stomach rather than dividing distal to the pylorus as there is a lower risk of anastomotic disruption with a gastrocolic anastomosis compared to a duodenocolic anastomosis. In all cases, we routinely send a frozen section to ensure that a microscopically negative distal margin has been achieved.

At this point, the right colon is mobilized along the white line of Toldt toward the hepatic flexure. We routinely take down both flexures and the transverse colon to minimize tension on the esophagocolonic anastomosis in the chest. Since the blood supply for the colonic interponat is based on the middle colic vessels, it is critical to identify them early and ensure that they are carefully preserved. The ileocolic and right colic vessels are divided at the takeoff of the right colic with a linear stapler. The right colonic mesentery can usually be divided with bipolar cautery. The distal aspect of the colon is divided proximal to the splenic flexure. The proximal aspect of the divided terminal ileum is anastomosed to the colonic splenic flexure. Our preference is to construct a stapled side-to-side anastomosis using a 60-mm linear stapler. The remaining enterotomy is closed with a two-layer running suture using the Endo Stitch™ (Covidien, CT). The mesenteric defect should also be closed to avoid potential internal herniation postoperatively. The second anastomosis constructed is the gastrocolic anastomosis. The distal aspect of the colonic interponat is anastomosed to the prepyloric gastric remnant in a side-to-side fashion using a 60-mm linear stapler. Again it is our preference to close the remaining enterotomy using two-layer running suture.

Once these two anastomoses have been completed, we proceed with dividing the upper stomach or distal esophagus in the mediastinum. The cecal pole is sutured to the stomach or esophageal stump in preparation for a colonic pull-up into the thorax (Fig. 14.3). We routinely place a Penrose drain around the distal esophagus in the mediastinum to aid in identification and retrieval of esophagus once in the chest. Our preference during esophagectomy is to remove the tumor during the thoracic phase of the procedure via a small thoracotomy incision; however, in some instances, a large tumor may be extracted from the abdomen if required. We routinely use a plastic wound protector to protect the wound from direct contact with the tumor. The 12-mm trocar incision close to the midline is best suited for tumor extraction and can be enlarged as needed to permit tumor extraction. Our protocol during any esophagectomy is to place a needle catheter jejunostomy in the proximal jejunum to expedite

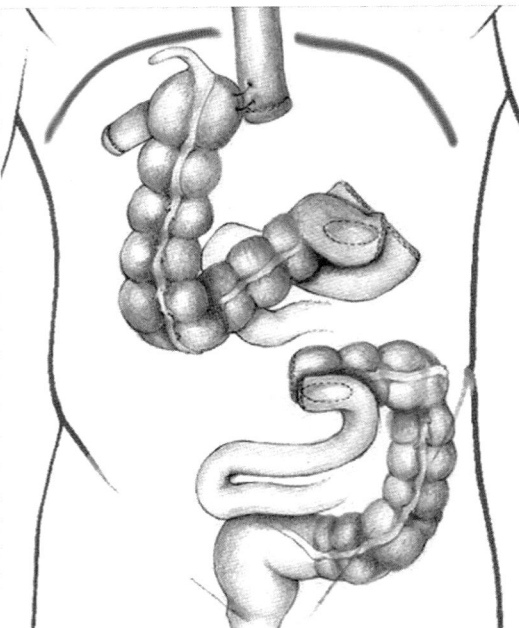

Fig. 14.3 Gastrocolic anastomosis has been performed and the cecum has been anchored to the distal esophagus for pull-up into the chest (From Nguyen et al. [7] with permission)

enteral feeding postoperatively while the patient is kept nil per os.

Thoracic Phase

The patient is then repositioned in left lateral decubitus position under single lung ventilation. Three trocars and a mini-thoracotomy incision (2–3 cm) are placed in the right chest. A plastic wound protector is used in the mini-thoracotomy incision to protect the chest wall from any direct contact with tumor cells. Dissection is initiated by mobilizing the inferior pulmonary ligament. The mediastinal pleura overlying the distal esophagus is incised using bipolar electrocautery, and the Penrose drain encircling the distal esophagus is retrieved. We have found that the Penrose drain greatly assists with esophageal retraction during intrathoracic esophageal mobilization. The esophagus is mobilized up to the level of the azygous vein. We routinely reevaluate the proximal extent of the tumor endoscopically at this

point. If the esophagus requires additional proximal mobilization, the azygous vein can be divided with a 60-mm linear stapler. The esophagus is then divided proximally using ultrasonic shears. The remaining distal esophagus and attached colonic interponat can then be pulled into the right chest and separated. The surgical specimen is removed from the chest through the mini-thoracotomy incision.

When we initially reported our technique of minimally invasive Ivor Lewis esophagectomy with colonic interposition, we used a circular stapled technique (Video 14.1). A 25-mm anvil was inserted into the esophageal stump and secured in place with a purse-string suture. The ileocecal valve was then dilated to permit passage of the 25-mm circular stapler. The stapler was inserted transthoracically through the 2.5-cm trocar site and positioned through the terminal ileum into the sidewall of the cecum. The esophagocolic anastomosis is then created by firing the circular stapler (Fig. 14.4). The anastomosis was reinforced with a second layer of Lembert sutures. The remaining enterotomy at the terminal ileum was closed using a linear stapler and similarly oversewn with a second layer of Lembert sutures. During our experience with minimally invasive esophagectomy with gastric pull-up, we subsequently changed our practice to construct an entirely hand-sewn thoracoscopically performed esophagogastric anastomosis. The esophagocolic anastomosis can also be constructed thoracoscopically using the Endo Stitch™. Our preferred technique is a double-layer closure with interrupted Surgidac™ sutures (Covidien, CT). We routinely position a nasogastric tube distal to the proximal anastomosis. We place an apically oriented 28-French chest tube as well as a basally oriented 10-French Blake drain (Johnson & Johnson Gateway, Livingston, UK) for postoperative drainage.

Postoperative Care

Following esophageal resection, our patients are routinely sent to the intensive care unit for the initial 24–48 h postoperative period.

Fig. 14.4 A circular stapled or hand-sewn esophagocolonic anastomosis is created in the chest. The three anastomosis are now completed: (1) ileocolic anastomosis, (2) gastrocolic anastomosis, and (3) esophagocolic anastomosis (From Nguyen et al. [7] with permission)

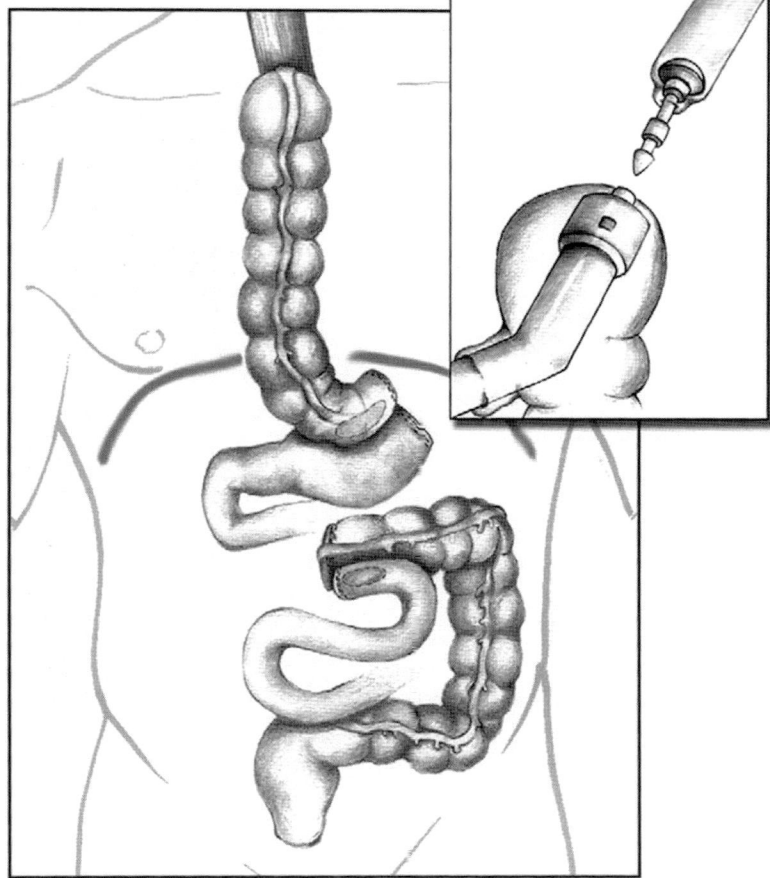

Patients are given patient-controlled analgesia with an opioid infusion. Enteral feeds are commenced via jejunostomy tube at 48 h and advanced toward goal caloric intake as the patient tolerates. The nasogastric tube is left to gravity drainage and suctioned twice a day by the surgical team during inpatient rounds. We routinely perform a water-soluble contrast study on postoperative day 5 to assess for anastomotic leakage (Fig. 14.5). Patients are typically discharged from the hospital by postoperative day 7 provided there is no clinical evidence of leak. Patients receive enteral feeds postoperatively and are allowed to start clear fluids by the second week after surgery. They are gradually advanced toward a soft diet over 3–4 weeks.

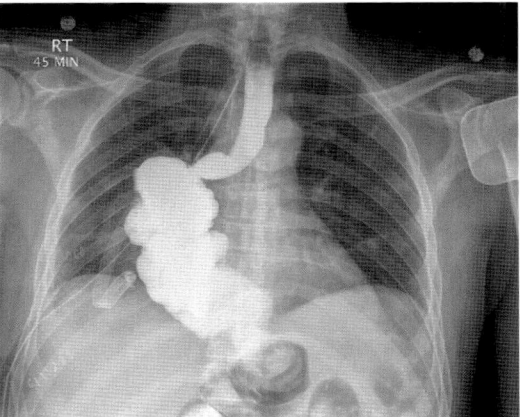

Fig. 14.5 Postoperative water-soluble contrast study demonstrating an intact proximal esophagocolonic and distal gastro-colonic anastomoses without evidence of anastomotic leak (From Nguyen et al. [7] with permission)

Table 14.1 Selected series demonstrating morbidity and mortality associated with esophagectomy with colonic interposition

Authors	Publication year	Patients (#)	Mortality (%)	Graft necrosis (%)	Anastomotic leakage (%)	Anastomotic strictures (%)
Wilkins [9]	1980	100	9	7	14	a
Isolauri et al. [8]	1987	248	16	3	4	a
DeMeester et al. [10]	1988	92	5	7.6	4.3	4.3
Cerfolio et al. [11]	1995	32	9.4	9.4	3.3	24
Mansour et al. [12]	1997	129	5.9	3.0	14.8	2.3
Thomas et al. [13]	1997	60	8.3	5.0	10.0	13.5
Kolh et al. [14]	2000	38	2.5	0	0	a
Hagen et al. [15]	2001	72	5.6	5.6	12.5	a
Popovici [16]	2003	347	4.6	1.2	6.9	6.3
Davis et al. [4]	2003	42	16.7	2.4	14.3	a
Knezevic' et al. [17]	2007	294	4.2	2.4	9.2	a
Motoyama et al. [18]	2007	34	0	0	9	6
Klink et al. [19]	2010	43	14	9	30	19
Hamai et al. [20]	2012	40	0	5	17.5	a

Adapted from Yasuda and Shiozaki [23] with permission
[a]Data not given

Discussion

There is only one published case report to date describing the technique of laparoscopic esophagectomy with colonic interposition [7]. In this paper, the patient had a large esophagogastric cancer involving the gastric body. He underwent laparoscopic/thoracoscopic esophagectomy with interposition of a proximal colonic segment based on the middle colic vessels. Total operative time was 4 h for the laparoscopic portion and 2 h for the thoracoscopic portion. Lymphadenectomy yielded 18 nodes, and microscopically negative proximal and distal margins were achieved at the time of resection. The patient tolerated the procedure well and did not have any evidence of radiologic leakage postoperatively.

Isolauri and colleagues have published the largest series of open esophagectomy with reconstruction by colonic interposition [8]. In that series of 248 patients, they describe an overall mortality of 16 %. Graft necrosis occurred in 3 %

of patients and they reported an anastomotic leak rate of 4 %. The major source of morbidity postoperatively in their series was pulmonary complications, which occurred in 8 % of patients. Other published series of open colonic interposition are shown in Table 14.1. These series demonstrate a large variation in overall mortality between 5 and 16 %. Anastomotic leak was noted to occur in 0–14.8 % of patients. The major source of postoperative morbidity in most published series of open esophagectomy with colonic interposition was pulmonary complications. A minimally invasive approach to esophageal resection appears to lessen the risk of postoperative pulmonary complications in high-volume centers. This may be associated with a reduction in overall mortality [21]. The recently published TIME trial that compared minimally invasive esophagectomy with traditional open esophagectomy demonstrated a major reduction in pulmonary complications between the open (29 %) and minimally invasive groups (9 %) [22]. Patients who underwent minimally invasive esophagectomy also had a shorter length of hospital stay and improved quality of life postoperatively compared to those patients undergoing traditional open esophagectomy. It is likely that the advantages observed during laparoscopic esophagectomy with gastric pull-up are transferrable to minimally invasive colonic interposition, although more published series of this technique are needed.

Conclusion

There are certain scenarios where it is not feasible to use the stomach as a conduit for esophageal reconstruction. Colonic interposition is a well-established alternative method of reconstruction following esophagectomy yet adds further complexity to an already high-risk surgical procedure. Minimally invasive techniques for esophageal resection are being increasingly utilized and appear to be advantageous in reducing pulmonary complications after esophagectomy. Although laparoscopic esophagectomy with colonic interposition is technically feasible [7], it is best undertaken at high-volume centers by surgeons with experience in both laparoscopic esophageal and colonic surgeries.

References

1. Kim T, et al. Review of minimally invasive esophagectomy and current controversies. Gastroenterol Res Pract. 2012;2012:683213.
2. Nguyen NT, et al. Minimally invasive esophagectomy: lessons learned from 104 operations. Ann Surg. 2008;248:1081–91.
3. DeMeester SR. Colon interposition following esophagectomy. Dis Esophagus. 2001;14:169–72.
4. Davis PA, Law S, Wong J. Colonic interposition after esophagectomy for cancer. Arch Surg. 2003;138:303–8.
5. Luketich JD, et al. Outcomes after minimally invasive esophagectomy: review of over 1000 patients. Ann Surg. 2012;256:95–103.
6. Lazzarino AI, et al. Open versus minimally invasive esophagectomy: trends of utilization and associated outcomes in England. Ann Surg. 2010;252:292–8.
7. Nguyen TN, et al. Laparoscopic and thoracoscopic Ivor Lewis esophagectomy with colonic interposition. Ann Thorac Surg. 2007;84:2120–4.
8. Isolauri J, Markkula H, Autio V. Colon interposition in the treatment of carcinoma of the esophagus and gastric cardia. Ann Thorac Surg. 1987;43:420–4.
9. Wilkins Jr EW. Long-segment colon substitution for the esophagus Ann Surg. 1980;192:722.
10. DeMeester TR, et al. Indications, surgical technique, and long-term functional results of colon interposition or bypass. Ann Surg. 1988;208:460–74.
11. Cerfolio RJ, Allen MS, Deschamps C, Trastek VF, Pairolero PC. Esophageal replacement by colon interposition. Ann Thorac Surg. 1995;59:1382–4.
12. Mansour KA. Bryan FC, Carlson GW. Bowel interposition for esophageal replacement: twenty-five – year experience. Ann Thorac Surg. 1997;64:752–6.
13. Thomas P, Fuentes P, Giudicelli R, Reboud E. Colon interposition for esophageal replacement: current indications and long-term function. Ann Thorac Surg. 1997;64:757–64.
14. Kolh P, et al. Early stage results after oesophageal resection for malignancy—colon interposition vs. gastric pull-up. Eur J Cardiothorac Surg. 2000;18:293–300.
15. Hagen JA, DeMeester SR, Peters JH, Chandrasoma P, DeMeester TR. Curative resection for esophageal adenocarcinoma: analysis of 100 en bloc esophagectomies. Ann Surg. 2001;234:520–30; discussion 530–1.
16. Popovici Z A new philosophy in esophageal reconstruction with colon. Thirty-years experience. Dis Esophagus. 2003;16:323–7.
17. Knežević JD, et al. Colon interposition in the treatment of esophageal caustic strictures: 40 years of experience Dis Esophagus. 2007;20:530–4.
18. Motoyama S, et al. Surgical outcome of colon interposition by the posterior mediastinal route for thoracic esophageal cancer. Ann Thorac Surg. 2007;83:1273–8.
19. Klink CD Binnebösel M, Schneider M, Ophoff K. Operative outcome of colon interposition in the treatment of esophageal cancer: a 20-year experience. Surgery. 2010. doi:10.1016/j.surg.2009.10.045.
20. Hamai Y. Hihara J, Emi M, Aoki Y, Okada M. Esophageal reconstruction using the terminal ileum and right colon in esophageal cancer surgery. Surg Today. 2012;42:342–50.
21. Biere SS Cuesta MA, van der Peet DL. Minimally invasive versus open esophagectomy for cancer: a systematic review and meta-analysis. Minerva Chir. 2009;64:121–33.
22. Biere SS, et al. Minimally invasive versus open oesophagectomy for patients with oesophageal cancer: a multicentre, open-label, randomised controlled trial. Lancet. 2012;379:1887–92.
23. Yasuda T, Shiozaki H. Esophageal reconstruction with colon tissue. Surg Today. 2011;41(6):745–53.

Thoracolaparoscopic Esophagectomy in the Prone Position for Carcinoma of the Esophagus

15

C. Palanivelu, Palanivelu Praveen Raj, Palanisami Senthilnathan, and R. Parthasarathi

In open surgery for intrathoracic esophageal tumors/carcinoma, transhiatal esophagectomy was used for tumors in the lower third [1] of the esophagus and a transthoracoscopic McKeown three-hole/three-field approach with cervical anastomosis was used for tumors in the middle and upper thirds of the esophagus [2]. Initially, we followed the same principles when using a laparoscopic approach [3]. Our standard approach for thoracoscopic esophagectomies is with the patient in the prone position [4].

Electronic supplementary material Supplementary material is available in the online version of this chapter at 10.1007/978-3-319-09342-0_15. Videos can also be accessed at http://www.springerimages.com/videos/978-3-319-09341-3.

C. Palanivelu, MS, MCh, FRCS, FACS (✉)
Division of Oesophagastric Surgery,
GEM Hospital and Research Centre,
Pankaja Mills Road, Ramanathapuram,
Coimbatore, Tamil Nadu 64105, India
e-mail: info@geminstitute.in

P.P. Raj, MS, DNB(GI), DNB(SGI), FALS, FMAS
P. Senthilnathan, MS, DNBGen, MRCSEd,
DNB GISurg, FACS
Department of Surgical Gastroenterology,
GEM Hospital and Research Centre,
Coimbatore, Tamil Nadu, India

R. Parthasarathi, MS, FMAS
Division of Advanced Minimally Invasive
and GI Surgery, GEM Hospital and Research Centre,
Coimbatore, Tamil Nadu, India

The use of thoracoscopic esophagectomy in the prone position for esophageal cancer was first reported by Cushieri et al. [5] in 1992. Subsequently, no other group reported using this approach. Many esophageal surgeons have been interested in performing minimally invasive esophagectomy for cancer. All of the cases reported in the literature reported using video-assisted thoracoscopic (VATS) esophagectomy with the patient in the lateral decubitus position [6–8]. 10 years after the original publication, our report of 130 cases using the approach with the patient in the prone position created great enthusiasm among many surgeons across the world, including those in Japan, Korea, and Europe [4]. The author's video using this approach received best technique awards in various congresses such as the American College of Surgeons (ACS) in 2005 [9], the 16th European Congress at Stockholm [10], and the 10th World Congress of the International Society for Diseases of the Esophagus [11]. The author performed a live thoracolaparoscopic esophagectomy on a patient in the prone position for esophageal cancer during the Hong Kong Asia Pacific Congress (ELSA) in 2005, which created great enthusiasm among the Asian group.

Two-field lymphadenectomy was used for surgeries up to the infracarinal group of lymph nodes. Decisions regarding the type of operation were based primarily on the location of the tumor with the goal of low morbidity; radical

S.N. Hochwald, M. Kukar (eds.), *Minimally Invasive Foregut Surgery for Malignancy: Principles and Practice*,
DOI 10.1007/978-3-319-09342-0_15, © Springer International Publishing Switzerland 2015

lymphadenectomy was not the surgical goal in the early 1990s.

Thoracoscopic en bloc esophagectomy [4] with the patient in the prone position and three-field radical lymphadenectomy (TLE–3H–3F) became our standard of practice. We found no significant change in the incidence of morbidity and mortality by adopting the three-hole trans-thoracic esophagectomy and cervical dissection approach in comparison with laparoscopic tran-shiatal esophagectomy [12].

More and more two-hole esophagectomies (TLE–2H) [13–15] with intrathoracic anastomosis are being performed, limiting the three-hole esoph-agectomy (TLE–3H) approach to removal of upper esophageal growths/cancer. Total mediastinal, extended two-field lymphadenectomy (TLE–2H–TM) for adenocarcinoma and thoracoscopic modi-fied three-field lymphadenectomy including the right cervicothoracic packet of lymph nodes (TLE–2H–3F) along the right recurrent laryngeal group are becoming the standard approaches [16–19]. Esophagogastrectomy for cancer of the cardia with shorter gastric tube thoracolaparoscopic esopha-gectomy with two-field lymphadenectomy (TLE–2H–2F) is also performed.

Advantages of the Prone Approach

Anatomical

1. Effects of gravity
   - Liver falls caudally
   - Heart falls anteriorly
   - Mediastinum widens
2. No lung ventilation is needed

In a lateral approach, the esophagus lies in the most dependent portion of the chest, where it is often obscured by overlying lung.

Surgeon

- Positioning is comfortable for the surgeon
- Blood does not accumulate near the dissection field

- Learning curve is shorter
- Pneumothorax partially collapses the lung
- Lung falls anteriorly
- Wide exposure is obtained without lung retraction

Physiological

- Single-lumen endotracheal tube
- Double-lung ventilation
- Improved ventilation/perfusion ratio
- Incidence of postoperative pulmonary compli-cations is lower
- Improved postoperative oxygenation

Anesthesia Effects

The TLE–3 F operative procedure can be divided into three steps (1) the thoracoscopic phase: en bloc esophagectomy and radical lymphadenec-tomy, (2) the abdominal phase: radical lymph-adenectomy and gastric tube formation, and (3) the cervical phase: specimen extraction, gastric pull up, and cervicogastric anastomosis. Ivor Lewis esophagogastrectomy (TLE–2F) is per-formed in two phases (1) the laparoscopic phase: gastric mobilization and lymph node dissection, gastric tube formation, and extraction of speci-men and (2) the thoracoscopic phase: esopha-gectomy, radical lymphadenectomy, and anastomosis. Rarely there is a second laparo-scopic phase wherein the specimen extraction is performed through a Pfanneiel incision after adjusting the patient's position to supine before extubation.

General anesthesia with a single-lumen endo-tracheal tube and the patient in a semiprone posi-tion is our standard practice, with a specially made mechanical support (Figs. 15.1 and 15.2). The semiprone position [11] allows for a lateral thoracotomy to be performed during an emer-gency without changing the patient's position. The operative field of the right chest is prepared and draped anteroposteriorly from midline to midline.

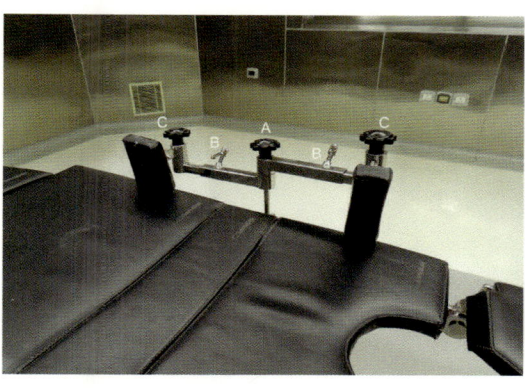

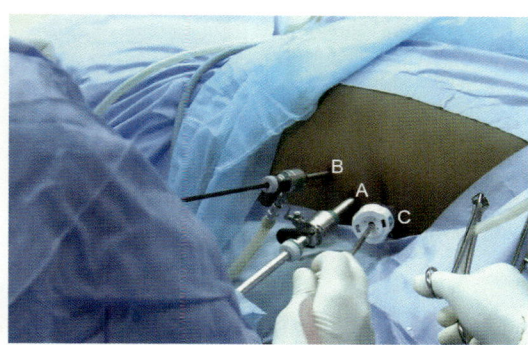

Fig. 15.1 Operating table side support is fixed to the table side rails. (*A*) Center knob to adjust the arm. (*B*) Side knob to pull out the inner rod and adjust the length. (*C*) Outer knob to turn the pad in either direction

Fig. 15.3 Thoracoscopic ports. (*A*) Camera 10-mm port. (*B*) Left-hand working 5-mm port. (*C*) Right-hand working 5-mm port

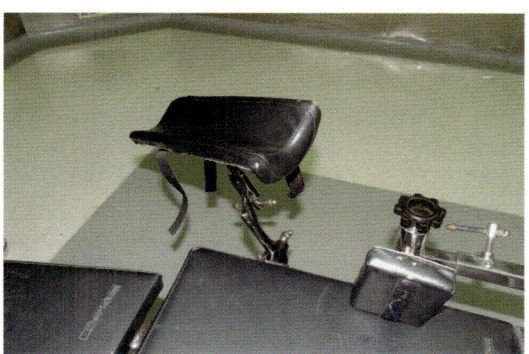

Fig. 15.2 Right forearm support

Thoracolaparoscopic Esophagectomy and Three-Field Lymphadenectomy in the Prone Position (Video 15.1)

TLE–3F: Thoracoscopic Phase

A right pneumothorax is created either by using a closed Veress needle technique or by using Visiport. Four trocars are placed into the right thoracic cavity (Fig. 15.2). The first trocar (10 mm) for the camera is placed in the fifth intercostal space corresponding to the level of the arch of the azygos vein. The second trocar (5 mm)

for the work performed with the right hand is placed in the third intercostal space. The third trocar (10 mm) is placed in the seventh intercostal space. The fourth trocar (5 mm) is placed in the ninth intercostal space. The 10-mm trocar in the seventh space is useful for applying clips, vascular clamps, and taking sutures into the thorax; the camera is sometimes used in this trocar during mobilization of the lower esophagus (Fig. 15.3). Initially, the right pneumothorax at 10 mmHg partially collapses the right lung, which lies in the anterior compartment, and then the pressure is reduced to 6–8 mmHg. In addition to the pneumothorax, gravity also aids in keeping the collapsed lung in an anterior position. Two-lung ventilation is continued throughout the procedure.

The surgeon and camera operator stand at the patient's right side, and the video monitor is positioned directly opposite, on the patient's left side (Fig. 15.4). The surgeon, using a hook, incises the mediastinal pleura overlying the anterior aspect of the esophagus, and the inferior pulmonary ligament is released up to the right pulmonary vein. Anterior dissection is begun by mobilizing the esophagus away from the hilum and the pericardium [20]. Because of gravity, the heart tends to fall down anteriorly; thus, the space in front of the esophagus is widened. The mobilization extends to the level of the azygos vein, which is skeletonized and divided with double

Fig. 15.4 Team setup for
thoracoscopy. The patient is
in the prone position, the
surgeon, camera surgeon,
and assisting surgeon stand
on the right side of the
patient and the monitor is on
the left side of the patient

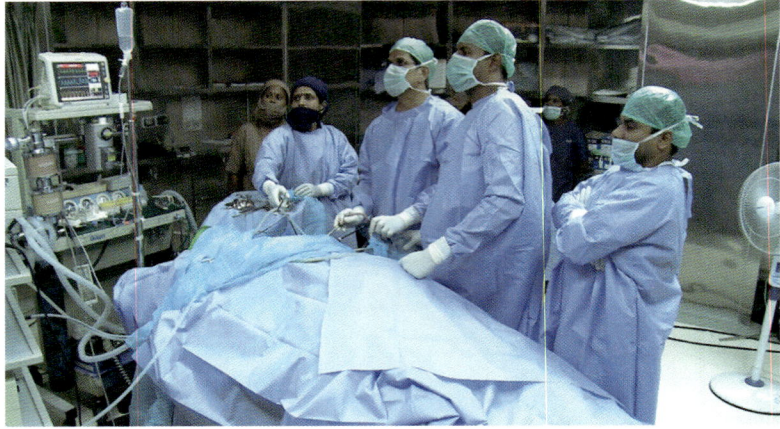

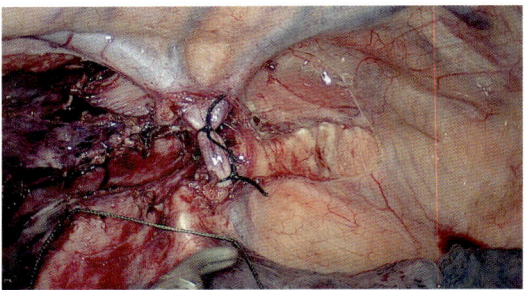

Fig. 15.5 After pleural incision and dissection of the azygos vein, the azygos arch is ligated doubly with silk

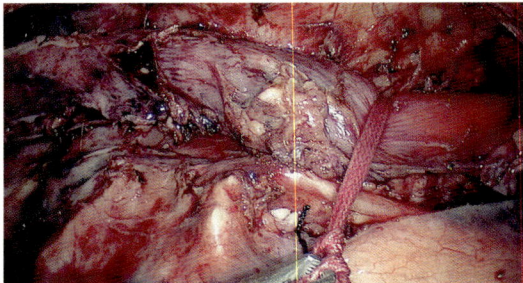

Fig. 15.7 Umbilical tape is tied around the esophagus
loosely for free sliding and retraction

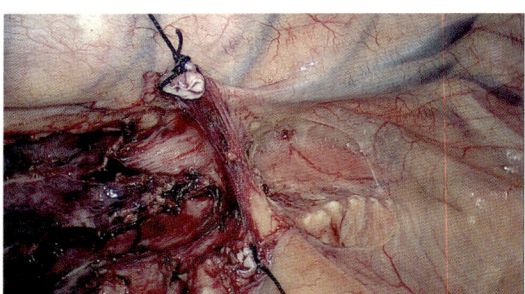

Fig. 15.6 The azygos arch is divided and the vertebral
side is retracted for exposure

ligatures on both sides (Fig. 15.5). The posterior
end of the thread is kept long and brought out
through the posterior chest wall. Retraction of the
thread dorsally separates the divided ends, providing a wider view. At the level of the aortic
arch (Fig. 15.6), the azygos vein is the only structure that lies between the esophagus and the

surgeon. Many surgeons prefer an endovascular
(Endo GIA) stapler to divide the arch of the azygos vein. The parietal pleura posterior to the
esophagus is incised from the level of the azygos
arch vein to the crus. Blunt dissection is used to
identify any potential thoracic duct branches and
perforator vessels from the aorta. The thoracic
duct is identified between the esophagus and
aorta, and is not routinely divided. In case of
tumor infiltration, the thoracic duct is clipped
caudally at the hiatus and at the thoracic inlet at
its insertion with the subclavian vein cranially
and is transected. The esophagus is encircled
with an umbilical tape, and traction by the assistant through the fourth port provides excellent
exposure (Figs. 15.7 and 15.8). The surgeon is
able to use both hands, simplifying the en bloc
mobilization and lymphadenectomy. Initially, we
used three ports, and have now changed to using
four ports; the fourth port is used for traction. The

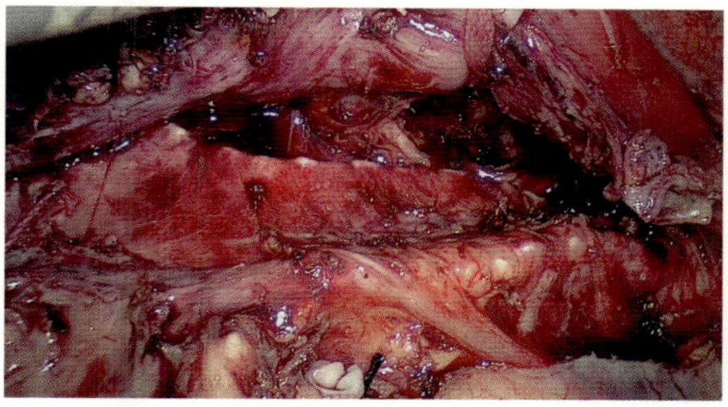

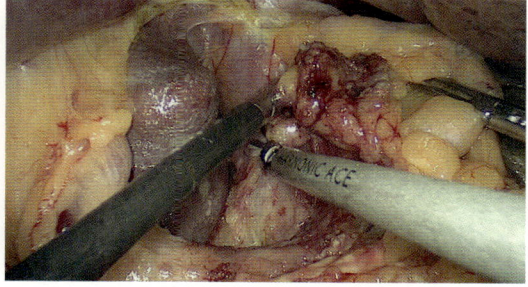

Fig. 15.8 Dissection of the esophagus from the trachea

Fig. 15.10 Clearance of lymph node stations 7, 8, and 9

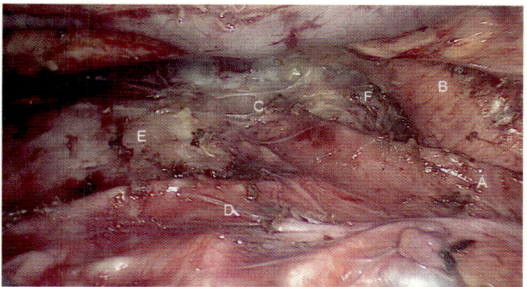

Fig. 15.9 Thoracoscopic view after complete mobilization. (*A*) Trachea. (*B*) Arch of aorta. (*C*) Left bronchus. (*D*) Right bronchus. (*E*) Pericardium. (*F*) Aortopulmonary window

operative time is shorter using the two-handed technique. The groups of lymph nodes are dissected sequentially, the subcarinal, aortobronchial, paratracheal, right recurrent laryngeal, and then left recurrent laryngeal groups (Fig. 15.9) are removed in that order [20]. The thoracoscopic approach enables removal of the cervicothoracic packet of lymph nodes along the right recurrent laryngeal nerve using a strictly "no touch" technique [16, 18].

If tumor is present in the lower esophagus, the dissection starts from the upper chest; for upper growths, the dissection may start from the lower mediastinum. The entire periesophageal tissue and the lymph nodes are removed. If the mediastinal pleura is infiltrated, it is also excised to obtain an R0 resection. In cases of advanced tumors, where we anticipate excision of both pleura, the dissection begins from the cranial end. The esophagus may be divided by stapling and retracted laterally, which exposes the entire mediastinum. Thorough irrigation and suction of the pleural cavity is performed. A single 28-F chest tube is placed through the seventh intercostal space and the lung is re-expanded.

Abdominal/Laparoscopic Phase

The patient is positioned supine and five ports are placed. The left lobe of the liver is retracted with instruments through the subxiphoid (epigastric) trocar. A 10-mm port for the camera is placed in the epigastrium. Two working ports, a 12-mm port in the right midclavicular line and a 5-mm port in the left midclavicular line are placed. One 5-mm port at the left anterior axillary line for gastric traction.

The lesser omentum is incised and the stomach retracted to the left and anteriorly with a grasper. The retroperitoneal lymphadenectomy (D2) is begun by incising the peritoneum at the upper border of the pancreas. The retroperitoneal lymphatic and areolar tissues are swept superiorly by skeletonizing the common hepatic artery, dissecting cranially along the lateral celiac group (Fig. 15.10). The left gastric vein is divided first at its insertion with the portal vein, followed by the left gastric artery, and then the celiac axis is completely cleared. The left gastric artery is clipped with Hem-o-lok and divided. The dissection is continued along the splenic artery up to the splenic hilum. This retroperitoneal dissection extends up to the dissected esophageal hiatus superiorly, the hilum of the spleen laterally, and the common hepatic artery and inferior vena cava medially. Finally, the lesser curvature and left

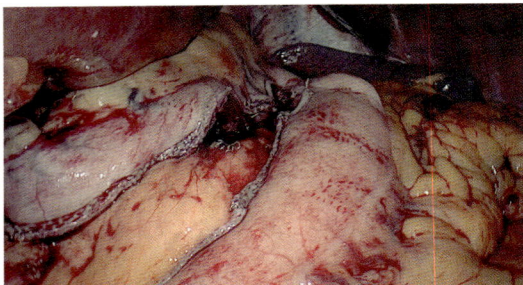

Fig. 15.11 Intracorporeal formation of the gastric tube using an Endo GIA stapler

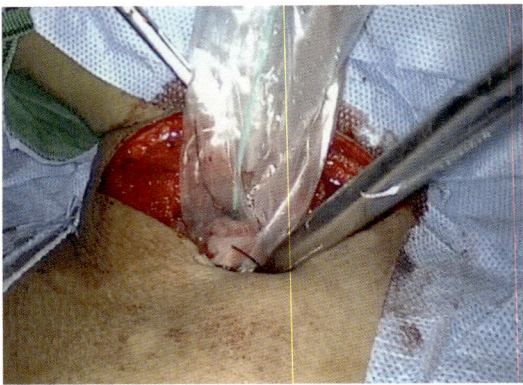

Fig. 15.12 Divided esophagus, Ryle's tube with a covering plastic sleeve is being pushed into the posterior mediastinum

gastric nodes are included with the specimen as the gastric tube is prepared.

The right gastroepiploic artery and the arterial arcade along the greater curve is carefully assessed early to ensure its suitability as a vascular supply to the gastric conduit. The greater omentum is divided at a safe distance from the gastroepiploic arcade, and the dissection is continued upward and to the left to divide the gastrocolic and gastrosplenic ligaments by dividing the short gastric vessels, keeping the dissection closer to the origin of the left gastroepiploic artery from the splenic origin. On the right side, the dissection continues up to the second part of the duodenum. The right gastroepiploic vein is carefully protected from injury.

Gastric Tube Formation

A 5-cm-wide gastric conduit is created by means of multiple firings of an Endo GIA 6-cm cartridge (Echelon–Ethicon) through the right midclavicle port. The stomach is stretched when stapling starts on the lesser curvature, 5 cm away from the pylorus, and progressing toward the fundus of the stomach. A golden cartridge is used to staple the antrum and blue cartridges are used for dividing the body of the stomach (Fig. 15.11).

A pyloroplasty or pyloromyotomy is performed by incising the pylorus longitudinally and the closure is performed transversely with interrupted sutures using 3-0 PDS suture. The placement of the feeding jejunostomy is at the discretion of the surgeon. Our preference is to place a nasojejunal feeding tube. Only in selected cases in which the patient develops a leak do we perform a feeding jejunostomy. The incidence of developing a leak is very low [13] and feeding jejunostomy is not without morbidity.

Cervical Phase

Specimen Extraction and Gastric Pull Up

The cervical esophagus is dissected through a left collar incision and divided. The distal end of the esophagus in the neck is over sewn and attached to a long Ryles tube. A long plastic sleeve is used as a protective sheath and attached to the esophagus with a separate stitch (Fig. 15.12). The pneumoperitoneum is reestablished and the esophagus is pulled down until the protective sheath reaches the peritoneal cavity. The stitch is released and the lower end of the plastic sheath opened (Fig. 15.13). The Ryles tube in the neck is used to pull the esophagus into the plastic sheath by the assistant; the surgeon working on the anterior wall of the gastric tube pushes the tube carefully, using a hand-over-hand technique and avoiding twisting or spiraling (Fig. 15.14).

Esophagogastric Anastomosis

A small vertical gastrotomy is performed with electrocautery. The posterior wall of the esophagus and the anterior wall of the stomach are then

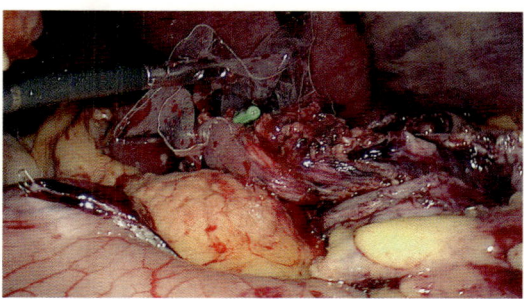

Fig. 15.13 Plastic sleeve in position (from neck wound connecting the peritoneal cavity) lying in the posterior mediastinum. (*A*) Nasogastric tube attached to the divided end of the cervical esophagus

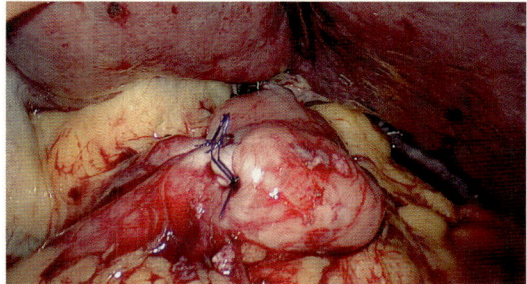

Fig. 15.14 Position of the stomach tube. The pyloroplasty wound is visible

aligned. A 3-cm long, 3.5-mm Endo GIA stapler is used to perform the posterior anastomosis. The anterior anastomosis is performed transversely using two staplers according to the modified Collard [19] or Orringer technique [21] and a wide stoma is obtained. The anterior wall may also be approximated with single-layer hand-sewn continuous suturing using a 3-0 monofilament absorbable suture, beginning at each corner and tied in the middle. After completion of the anastomosis, any redundant stomach is retracted into the abdomen. A nasogastric tube is passed carefully until it reaches the antrum of the stomach and its tip is kept above the pylorus. The gastric tube is then secured to the diaphragmatic hiatus anteriorly and laterally using long 2-0 nonabsorbable sutures to prevent intrathoracic herniation of the abdominal viscera. A nasojejunal tube is placed across the pylorus into the jejunum.

Two-Hole Esophagogastrectomy and Modified Three-Field Lymphadenectomy in the Prone Position

The abdominal dissection is performed first in the same way as in the three-hole approach. A gastric tube is formed, leaving adequate proximal stomach with the specimen. The mediastinal dissection is performed beyond the upper limit of the growth. For smaller growths confined to the cardia, the esophagus is divided transhiatally and extracted through a Pfannenstiel incision. For larger growths or if there is greater involvement of the esophagus, then the division is performed in the right pleural cavity during the thoracoscopic phase.

The patient is moved into a semiprone position. A mediastinal lymphadenectomy is performed similar to that described in the three-hole approach. The esophagus is divided high in the upper mediastinum, keeping an adequate distance from the upper limit of the growth, and is pushed into the peritoneal cavity to be removed after completing the thoracic phase. Stapling or a hand-sewn anastomosis is performed. Complete mediastinal lymphadenectomy for adenocarcinoma and a modified three-field or extended two-field lymphadenectomy by the thoracic approach is our preference [22].

Postoperative Care

Generally, the patient is extubated on the operating table and their recovery is good. Because of the absence of a thoracotomy, the patients have less pain and their breathing is comfortable. On the first day after the surgery, nothing is administered by mouth and the nasogastric tube is kept open for decompression of the gastric tube. On the second postoperative day, gastrografin contrast is administered and gastric emptying is assessed. Patients are administered enteral feeding through a nasojejunal tube, beginning with clear fluids. Between the third and fifth day, the nasogastric tube is removed and patients are allowed to take oral liquids followed by semi-solid followed soft diet by the end of first week. If dilation of the gastric tube or delayed emptying occurs, then the postoperative care changes.

If there is any doubt about the integrity of the anastomosis or delayed emptying of the gastric conduit longer than 5 days, endoscopy is performed with the patient under sedation. If there is an area of ischemic mucosa or a leak, then contrast-enhanced computed tomography (CECT) is performed, looking for collection. Small areas of mucosal ischemia can heal without additional intervention. In this group, placement of a feeding jejunostomy is performed for enteral feeding. Obvious anastomotic leaks are treated with an endoscopic stent. If drainage fails and the CT scan result shows collection, another thoracoscopy is performed for complete drainage.

Results

More than 765 patients with esophageal cancer were treated by minimally invasive esophagectomy between 1997 and 2013 at GEM Digestive Cancer Institute, Coimbatore, India. Transhiatal esophagectomy was performed in 165 patients and thoracolaparoscopic esophagectomy in 610 patients in the prone position. Of these, 132 patients received neoadjuvant chemotherapy and/or radiotherapy for locally advanced disease as determined by staging thoracoscopy. In all except 12 patients, esophagectomy was completed successfully. In 504 patients, TLE–3F with cervical anastomosis was performed and, in 106 patients, two-hole thoracolaparoscopic esophagectomy with intrathoracic anastomosis was performed.

The anastomotic leak rate was 3 % and the mortality was 1.1 %. The mean intensive care unit (ICU) stay was 2 days and the mean hospital stay was 7.2 days. Vocal cord palsy was identified in 1.5 % of the patients, most recovered in a few days, only one case lasted for 30 days. The median number of lymph nodes identified was 21. No tracheal or bronchial injury was noted. Two cases had azygos arch venous injury that was managed by a thoracoscopic method.

Demographic characteristics

Number of patients	610		
Age range	22–87 years		
Sex (men, women)	67 %, 33 %		
Period	1997–2002	2002–2007	2007–2012
Number of patients	45	180	385
Type of pathology (squamous cell carcinoma/ adenocarcinoma)	45/0	124/56	236/149
Tumor location	26 upper; 244 middle; 340 lower + cardia		

Preoperative comorbidity

	Number of patients
Hypertension	47 (8 %)
Diabetes	62 (10 %)
Cardiovascular disease	12 (2 %)
Pulmonary disease	27 (4 %)
Neoadjuvant therapy, chemotherapy and/or radiation therapy	135 (22 %)

Surgery

Type of surgery	Number of patients
Ivor Lewis	106 (17 %)
Two field (2F)	60
Modified three field (3F; 2F+cervicothoracic group)	46
Modified McKeown+neck anastomosis	504 (83 %)

Perioperative factors

Operative time	310 minutes
Blood loss	200–600 ml
ICU days	1.5 days
Anastomotic leakages	3 %
Gastric tip necrosis	1.35 %
Vocal cord paralysis/paresis	1.5 %
Pulmonary complications	2.4 %
Cardiovascular complications	3.75 %
Chylothorax	1 %
Overall morbidity	24 %
Hospital mortality	1.1 %

Pathology

Median tumor size	3.9 cm
T status	T0 8.7 %; T1 6.8 %; T2 25.2 %; T3 55.3 %; T4 3.9 %
N status	N0 42.7 %; N1 35.9 %; N2 8.7 %; N3 12.6 %
Margins positive	Proximal: 6 cases
	Distal: 0 cases
RO/R1	86 %/14 %

Number of lymph nodes harvested

Mean	24.4
Median	21
Hospital stay	7.2 days

Other complications

Pulmonary embolism	2 %
Reoperations (thoracoscopic revision)	1.15 %
Revision anastomosis	2 %
Drainage of abscess	3 %
Gastric tube pull out	2 %

Rethoracoscopy for Anastomotic Leak

After TLE with stapled anastomosis, two patients had leaks and rethoracoscopies were performed. In the first patient, the leak was diagnosed on the ninth postoperative day, just a day before their scheduled discharge. Endoscopy revealed the anastomotic leak and collection adjoining the leak. CT scanning results revealed the collection. Rethoracoscopy was performed and a pneumothorax was created using Visiport. The collection was drained, the pleural cavity thoroughly irrigated, and an intercostal drainage tube was placed next to the leak. A percutaneous feeding jejunostomy was performed. The fistula healed conservatively in 22 days. In the second patient, the fistula was a large opening and a stent was placed. After 2 weeks, the closure of the fistula was confirmed and the patient was moved to oral feeding. The stent was removed after 8 weeks. After an Ivor Lewis procedure, two patients experienced anastomotic leaks identified on the fourth and seventh postoperative days. Rethoracoscopies were performed and the anastomoses were revised. Both of these patients recovered well without further leaks. In one patient after TLE–3F, endoscopy revealed necrosis of the proximal part of the gastric tube approximately 3 cm from the tip. Rethoracoscopy was performed, the gastric tube was taken back, and a feeding gastrostomy and a cervicostomy were performed. After 2 months, coloplasty reconstruction was performed through the substernal route.

Discussion

Thoracoscopic view with the patient in the prone position is unfamiliar to most surgeons, but easily adaptable because of the excellent ergonomics. Using a single-lumen endotracheal tube and positioning the patient in a semiprone lateral approach position is easier and takes less time than using a double balloon and the prone position. The difficulty of an open conversion (posterior thoracotomy) in the case of massive hemorrhage is the only concern in an emergency with the patient in the prone position [20]. With the patient in the semiprone position, a lateral thoracotomy can be performed in an emergency without changing the position. However, we never had such an experience.

Thoracoscopic esophagectomy with the patient in the prone position has several advantages, including a wide working space, tendency of the blood to collect outside the operative field because of gravity, no need for skilled assistance, excellent ergonomic position for the surgeon, and reduction in lung injury because of the lack of lung handling [23, 24], and the two-lung anesthesia with continuous perfusion also significantly reduces postoperative pulmonary complications. The potential advantages of a prone thoracoscopic mobilization may also include shortened operative times, less surgeon fatigue, and shortening of the learning curve [25].

Use of a double-balloon endotracheal tube is not only time consuming, but also presents difficulties in exchanging the tube for a single-lumen endotracheal tube at the completion of the thoracic mobilization and repositioning the patient to a supine position for the abdominal phase. Dissection in front of the trachea and bronchus in the presence of a double-balloon endotracheal tube may precipitate traumatic injury and delayed leakage. Any untoward incidence, such as injury to the membranous bronchus or trachea, may be readily repaired as we do in open surgery [20].

Summary

Thoracoscopic esophagectomy with the patient in the prone position is a safe operation, and radical en bloc esophagectomy and lymphadenectomy may be performed perfectly in a shorter operative time, with less fatigue, reduced blood loss, and with a shortened learning curve for the surgeon. There are anatomic and physiologic advantages in addition to the ergonomic convenience for the surgeon. The thoracolaparoscopic esophagectomy with the patient in the prone position is likely to be the standard approach for this operation in the future; the two-hole or three-hole approach depends on the choice of the surgeon and the location of the tumor. The prone or semiprone approach is an excellent technique for extended radical lymphadenectomy and its aim should be to improve the survival rate. Modified thoracoscopic extended two-field and modified three-field lymphadenectomy and intrathoracic anastomosis are currently undergoing clinical trials and the early results are encouraging. A minimally invasive approach may be used with low morbidity and mortality.

References

1. Orringer MB, Sloan H. Esophagectomy without thoracotomy. J Thorac Cardiovasc Surg. 1978;76: 643–54.
2. McKeown KC. Total three-stage oesophaectomy for cancer of the oesophagus. Br J Surg. 1976;63:259.
3. Dantoc MM, Cox MR, Eslick GD. Does minimally invasive esophagectomy (MIE) provide for comparable oncologic outcomes to open techniques? A systematic review. J Gastrointest Surg. 2012;16(3):486–94.
4. Palanivelu C, Senthilnathan P, Parthasarathy R. Minimally invasive esophagectomy: thoracic mobilisation of the esophagus and mediastinal lymphadenectomy in prone position – experience of 130 cases. J Am Coll Surg. 2006;203(1):7–16.
5. Cushier A, Shimi S, Banting S. Endoscopic oesophagectomy through a right thoracoscopic approach. J R Coll Surg Edinb. 1992;37:7–11.
6. McAnena OJ, Rogers J, Williams NS. Right thoracoscopically assisted oesophagectomy for cancer. Br J Surg. 1994;81:236–8.
7. Gossot D, Cattan P, Fritsch S, Halimi B, Sarfati E, Celerier M. Can the morbidity of esophagectomy be reduced by the thoracoscopic approach? Surg Endosc. 1995;9:1113–5.
8. Robertson GS, Lloyd DM, Wicks AC, Veitch PS. No obvious advantages for thoracoscopic two-stage oesophagectomy. Br J Surg. 1996;83:675–8.
9. PraveenRaj P, Palanivelu C, Parthasarathy R. Video presentation international Award session annual conference of American College of Surgeons, New Orleans; 2007.
10. Palanivelu C, Parthasarthy R, Senthilnathan P. Award session; EAES best video session: 16th annual conference of European Society of Endo Surgeons, Stockholm; 2008.
11. Palanivelu C, Best abstract technique session: 10th world congress of International Society for Diseases of Esophagus, Kagoshima; 2010.
12. Hulsher JB, Tijseen JG, Overtop H, et al. Transthoracic verses transhiatal esophagectomy for carcinoma of the esophagus: a meta analysis. Ann Thorac Surg. 2001;72:306–13.
13. Pennathur A, Awais O, Luketich JD. Technique of minimally invasive Ivor Lewis esophagectomy. Ann Thorac Surg. 2010;89(6):S2159–62.
14. Watson DI, Davies N, Jamieson GG. Totally endoscopic Ivor Lewis esophagectomy. Surg Endosc. 1999;13(3):293–7.
15. Nguyen NT, Follette DM, Lemoine PH, et al. Minimally invasive Ivor Lewis esophagectomy. Ann Thorac Surg. 2001;72(2):593–6.
16. Lam KY, Ma LT, Wong J. Measurement of extend of spread of esophageal carcinoma by serial sectioning. J Clin Pathol. 1996;49:124–9.
17. Alkorki N, Skinner D. Should en bloc esophagectomy be the standard of care for esophageal carcinoma? Ann Surg. 2001;234:581–7.
18. Hegan JA, Peters PM, DeMeester TR. Superiority of extended enbloc esophagogastrectomy for carcinoma of the lower esophagus and cardia. J Thorac Cardiovasc Surg. 1993;106:850–8.
19. Collard JM, Romagnoli R, Goncette L, et al. Terminalised semi mechanical side to side technique for cervical esophagogastrostomy. Ann Thorac Surg. 1998;65(3):814–7.

20. Ozawa S, Ito E, Kazuno A, Chino O, Makuuchi H. Thoracosopic esophagectomy while in a prone position for esophageal cancer: a preceding anterior approach method. Surg Endosc. 2013;27:40–7.
21. Orringer MB, Marshall B, Iannettoni MD. Eliminating the cervical esophagogastric leak with a side to side stapled anastomosis. J Thorac Cardiovasc Surg. 2000;119(2):277–88.
22. Nishihira T, Hirayama K, Mori S. A prospective randomised trial of extended cervical and superior mediastinal lymphadenectomy for esophageal ca of the thoracic esophagus. Am J Surg. 1998;175:47–51.
23. Iwasaki H, Kobayashi K, Uchiyama A, Miyasaka Y, Masatsugu T, Koike K, Miyazaki K. Lymphadenectomy along the left recurrent laryngeal nerve by a minimally invasive esophagectomy in the prone position for thoracic esophageal cancer. Surg Endosc. 2010;24: 2965–73.
24. Akaishi T, Kaneda I, Higuchi N, Kuriya Y, Kuramoto J, Toyoda T, Wakabayashi A. Thoracoscopic en bloc total esophagectomy with radical mediastinal lymphadenectomy. J Thorac Cardiovasc Surg. 1996;112: 1533–40. discussion 1540–1.
25. Fabian T, Martin J, Katigbak M, McKelvey AA, Federico JA. Thoracoscopic esophageal mobilization during minimally invasive esophagectomy: a head-to-head comparison of prone versus decubitus positions. Surg Endosc. 2008;22:2485–91.

Thoracoscopic Enucleation of Esophageal Benign Tumors

Yusuke Kimura, Akira Sasaki, Toru Obuchi,
Takeshi Iwaya, Yuji Akiyama, Masafumi Konosu,
Fumitaka Endo, Koki Otsuka, Hiroyuki Nitta,
Keisuke Koeda, and Go Wakabayashi

Introduction

Benign esophageal tumors are rare, with a prevalence of 0.005–5.1 %, based on autopsy results, and account for <1–10 % of all esophageal neoplasms [1, 2]. Leiomyomas constitute 70–80 % of these benign esophageal neoplasms [1–3]. Other benign esophageal tumors, such as granular cell tumors or schwannomas, are extremely rare. Esophageal leiomyomas are usually detected in patients between 20 and 50 years of age, with a twofold male predominance, and most commonly occur in the lower third of the esophagus. At least 50 % of patients with esophageal leiomyomas are asymptomatic; in symptomatic individuals, dysphagia is the most commonly reported symptom, followed by chest tightness and pain. These tumors are usually discovered, incidentally, during esophagography or endoscopic examination of the upper gastrointestinal tract for unrelated reasons [4]. The treatment strategy for esophageal benign tumors, such as leiomyomas, involves continued monitoring of smaller tumors and surgical resection of larger or symptomatic tumors. Conventional, open thoracotomy for enucleation of this tumor type has been gradually replaced by less invasive thoracoscopic or laparoscopic approaches [1, 2, 5–7]. In the present report, we describe our experience with patients undergoing surgical enucleation of esophageal leiomyomas via thoracoscopic or laparoscopic approaches.

Management and Treatment

Surgical Indications

Surgical indications for thoracoscopic or laparoscopic enucleation of esophageal leiomyomas include the presence of dysphagia, foreign body sensations during swallowing, pathological confirmation that excludes malignancy, tumors greater than 3 cm in diameter, and tumors that show evidence of growth. Such patients underwent detailed assessment, including esophagography, endoscopy, endoscopic ultrasound (EUS), and computed tomography (CT) evaluations. Preoperative EUS-guided fine-needle aspiration (EUS-FNA) was performed only in cases where the morphologic appearance did not suggest that malignancy could be excluded with high probability.

Electronic supplementary material Supplementary material is available in the online version of this chapter at 10.1007/978-3-319-09342-0_16. Videos can also be accessed at http://www.springerimages.com/videos/978-3-319-09341-3.

Y. Kimura, MD, PhD (✉) • A. Sasaki, MD, PhD
T. Obuchi, MD, PhD • T. Iwaya, MD, PhD
Y. Akiyama, MD, PhD • M. Konosu, MD
F. Endo, MD, PhD • K. Otsuka, MD, PhD
H. Nitta, MD, PhD • K. Koeda, MD, PhD
G. Wakabayashi, MD, PhD
Department of Surgery,
Iwate Medical University School of Medicine,
19-1 Uchimaru, Morioka,
Iwate Prefecture 020-8505, Japan
e-mail: ykimura@iwate-med.ac.jp

It remains controversial whether esophageal submucosal tumors (SMT) should be preoperatively biopsied. The National Comprehensive Cancer Network (NCCN) guidelines do not suggest preoperative biopsy of esophageal SMTs because the biopsy may result in hemorrhaging and an increased risk of tumor dissemination [8]. Furthermore, surgeons who have performed enucleations have subjectively stated that biopsies increase the difficulty associated with identifying the dissection plane. Although we have also operated on patients who have undergone EUS-FNAB, we have not observed these complications. Esophageal gastrointestinal stromal tumor (GIST) resections are essentially limited to either simple enucleation or esophagectomy, but the specific procedure to be performed is controversial [9]. We believe that complete resection remains the standard surgical treatment for localized esophageal GISTs as the procedure reduces the risk of tumor rupture and the consequent risks of tumor relapse. In addition, complete resection also avoids the possibility of microscopic residual tumors; enucleation methods should not be indicated for esophageal GISTs.

Surgical Procedures (Video 16.1)

Thoracoscopic Approach

For tumors of the upper and middle thirds of the esophagus, we normally select a thoracoscopic approach utilizing a balloon-mounted endoscope. In our experience, thoracoscopic enucleations have been performed under general anesthesia, administered using a double-lumen endothoracheal tube for single-lung ventilation, with the patient in the left lateral decubitus position. We adopt four ports approach: the observation port lies at the midaxillary line in the eighth intercostal space (A), the main working ports are located at the posterior axillary line in the fifth (B) and the seventh (C) intercostal space, and the secondary working port is lying at the anterior axillary line in the fourth intercostal space (D) (Fig. 16.1). Thereafter, a flexible, 10-mm diameter endoscope is used for the entire procedure. First, the right lung is retracted to expose the

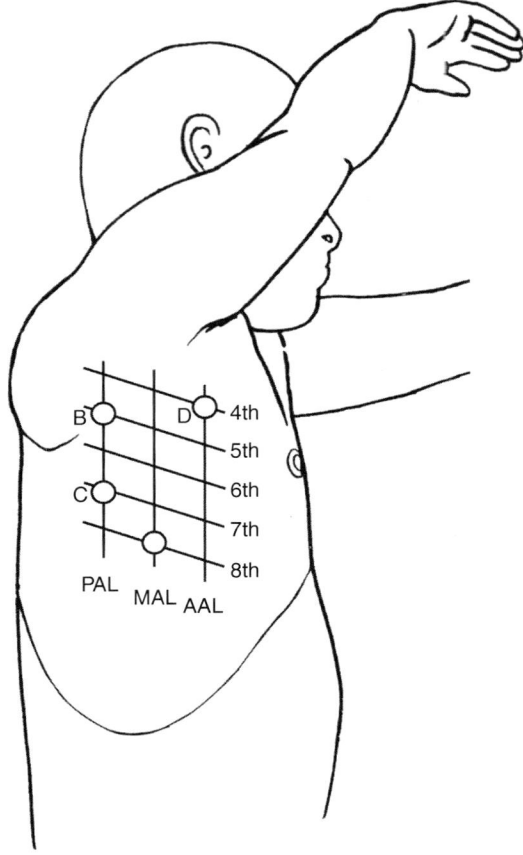

Fig. 16.1 Arrangement of ports in thoracoscopic approach. *AAL* anterior axillary line, *MAL* midaxillary line, *PAL* posterior axillary line

esophagus, which facilitates to confirm the tumor location by intraoperative endoscopy. An upper-GI balloon endoscope is simultaneously inserted in to the esophagus so that the tumor could be shifted toward adventitial layer by balloon pressure in the esophageal lumen (Fig. 16.2). The mediastinal pleura over the tumor is then longitudinally incised, and the tumor is pushed away from the esophageal wall using a balloon-mounted esophagoscope. The use of this type of esophagoscope improves the operative speed and safety. If necessary, the esophagus is circumferentially mobilized in order to expose the tumor, and a Penrose drain is placed around the esophagus. At this stage of the procedure, the esophagus can be rotated to some degree to allow visualization of the tumor. The mediastinal pleura over the esophageal tumor was divided to expose the tumor and the adjacent esophagus. An esophageal myotomy was performed using a

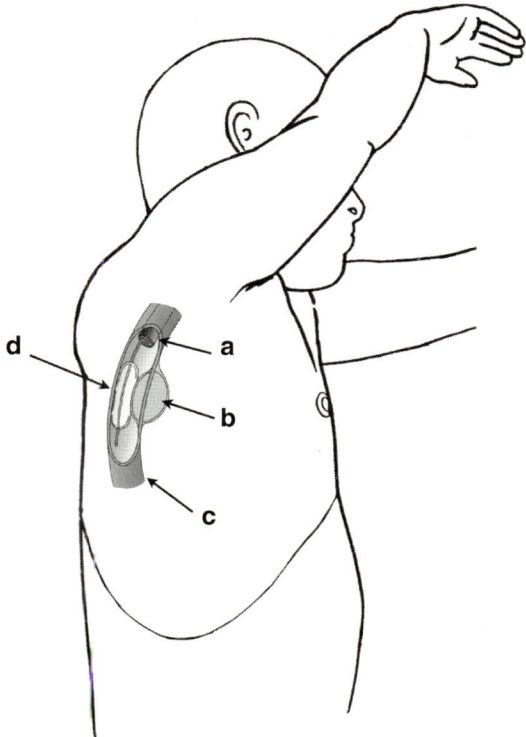

Fig. 16.2 The esophageal tumor is pushed away from the esophageal wall using a balloon-mounted esophagoscope. (*a*) esophagoscope, (*b*) esophageal leiomyoma, (*c*) esophagus, and (*d*) balloon

combination of laparoscopic coagulating shears (LCS) and Endo Peanut ™(Covidien company) avoiding injury to the mucosa. In order to avoid wound-healing delay, LCS is not used as much as possible.

After that blunt dissection was performed separating the tumor from the mucosa, followed by applying traction suture to the tumor to aid in tumor elevation as well as in the dissection which was done mostly by blunt dissection (Fig. 16.3a). After tumor enucleation, the specimen was placed in a retrieval bag introduced through anterior 10-mm trocar and was delivered through this trocar wound. The dissected area is thoroughly examined by endoluminal endoscopic inspection after air insufflation of the esophagus. Finally, the esophageal muscle layer is carefully closed using interrupted sutures to prevent the development of a pseudodiverticulum; a chest tube is also routinely inserted via a thoracoscopic approach (Fig. 16.3b). An alternative method for thoracoscopic resection of an esophageal leiomyoma is demonstrated in Video 16.2.

Laparoscopic Transhiatal Approach

A laparoscopic transhiatal approach is routinely used for tumors of the lower third of the esophagus. With the patient in a supine position, a pneumoperitoneum is established after the placement of a 12-mm trocar into the subumbilical area, using an open technique; CO_2 insufflation, to a

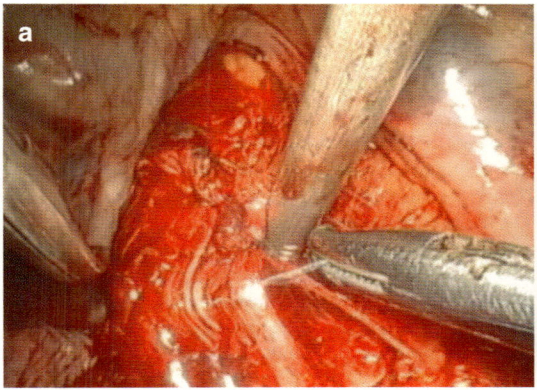
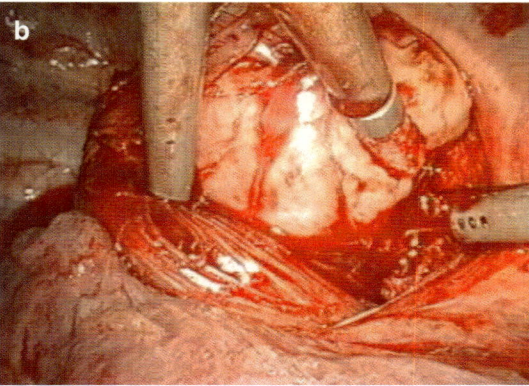

Fig. 16.3 Thoracoscopic enucleation for an esophageal leiomyoma. (**a**) The tumor was removed gently with particular attention for not damaging mucosa. (**b**) The esophageal muscle layer was carefully closed using interrupted sutures to prevent the development of pseudodiverticulum

pressure of 10 mmHg, is then maintained. Five trocars are inserted into the upper abdomen, and the phrenoesophageal ligament and the short gastric vessels are divided using a Harmonic scalpel (Johnson & Johnson Medical, Cincinnati, OH, USA). After dissection of the abdominal esophagus, a Penrose drain is placed around the esophagus to aid in esophageal retraction; dissection of the abdominal esophagus is very similar to a fundoplication dissection. After the esophageal SMT is identified, it is enucleated via a laparoscopic transhiatal approach, and a Dor or Toupet fundoplication was performed to restore the integrity of the anti-reflux mechanism.

Clinical and Technical Points

The first successful resection and enucleation of a benign esophageal tumor was reported by Sauerbrach in 1932 [10]. Traditionally, tumors of the upper and middle thirds of the esophagus have been approached by a right thoracotomy and tumors of the lower third have been approached by a left thoracotomy. Surgical enucleations of esophageal leiomyomas by video-assisted thoracoscopic surgery have also been reported and have contributed to the growing interest in the use of this approach in recent years [5, 11, 12]. There are some clinical and technical points that should also be considered during thoracoscopic/laparoscopic enucleations of esophageal leiomyomas. First, the myotomy must be performed in the correct direction and at the right level, and appropriate traction must be applied on the tumor to facilitate its subsequent enucleation. Second, a balloon-mounted esophagoscope allows the localization of small tumors and permits the confirmation of mucosal integrity and ensures safety. Third, an anti-reflux operation needs to be performed to restore the integrity of the anti-reflux mechanism, following dissection and mobilization of the esophagogastric junction and as a means of covering the myotomized esophageal mucosa. Finally, the difficulty of the cases, and thus, patient selection should be carefully considered. Conversion to an open procedure should be considered in cases in which technical problems or limitations are noted.

Conclusion

A thoracoscopic/laparoscopic approach offers potential advantages, compared with traditional thoracotomies. These advantages include its minimally invasive nature as well as the lower respiratory morbidity, reduced postoperative wound pain, and shorter hospital stay. In conclusion, thoracoscopic and laparoscopic transhiatal enucleations for esophageal leiomyomas are safe and feasible procedures. The optimal approach should be tailored for each patient, based on the location and size of the tumor.

References

1. Jiang G, Zhao H, Yang F, Li J, Li Y, Liu Y, Liu J, Wang J. Thoracoscopic enucleation of esophageal leiomyoma: a retrospective study on 40 cases. Dis Esophagus. 2009;22:279–83.
2. Kent M, D'Amato T, Nordman C, Schuchert M, Landreneau R, Alvelo-Rivera M, Luketich J. Minimally invasive resection of benign esophageal tumors. J Thorac Cardiovasc Surg. 2007;134:176–81.
3. Seremetis MG, Lyons WS, deGuzman VC, Peabody Jr JW. Leiomyomata of the esophagus. An analysis of 838 cases. Cancer. 1976;38:2166–77.
4. Zaninotto G, Portale G, Costantini M, Rizzetto C, Salvador R, Rampado S, Pennelli G, Ancona E. Minimally invasive enucleation of esophageal leiomyoma. Surg Endosc. 2006;20:1904–8.
5. Everitt NJ, Glinatsis M, McMahon MJ. Thoracoscopic enucleation of leiomyoma of the oesophagus. Br J Surg. 1992;79:643.
6. von Rahden BH, Stein HJ, Feussner H, Siewert JR. Enucleation of submucosal tumors of the esophagus: minimally invasive versus open approach. Surg Endosc. 2004;18:924–30.
7. Samphire J, Nafteux P, Luketich J. Minimally invasive techniques for resection of benign esophageal tumors. Semin Thorac Cardiovasc Surg. 2003;15:35–43.
8. Jiang P, Jiao Z, Han B, Zhang X, Sun X, Su J, Wang C, Gao B. Clinical characteristics and surgical treatment of oesophageal gastrointestinal stromal tumours. Eur J Cardiothorac Surg. 2010;38:223–7.
9. Demetri GD, Benjamin RS, Blanke CD, Blay JY, Casali P, Choi H, Corless CL, Debiec-Rychter M, DeMatteo RP, Ettinger DS, Fisher GA, Fletcher CD, Gronchi A, Hohenberger P, Hughes M, Joensuu H, Judson I, Le Cesne A, Maki RG, Morse M, Pappo AS,

Pisters PW, Raut CP, Reichardt P, Tyler DS, Van den Abbeele AD, von Mehren M, Wayne JD, Zalcberg J, NCCN Task Force. NCCN Task Force report: management of patients with gastrointestinal stromal tumor (GIST) – update of the NCCN clinical practice guidelines. J Natl Compr Canc Netw. 2007;5 suppl 2:S1–29.

10. Sauerbrach F. Presentations in the field of thoracic surgery. Arch Klin Chir. 1932;173:457.

11. Bardini R, Segalin A, Ruoi A, Pavanello M, Peracchia A. Videothoracoscopic enucleation of esophageal leiomyoma. Ann Thorac Surg. 1992;54: 576–7.

12. Obuchi T, Sasaki A, Nitta H, Koeda K, Ikeda K, Wakabayashi G. Minimally invasive surgical enucleation for esophageal leiomyoma: report of seven cases. Dis Esophagus. 2010;23:E1–4.

Minimally Invasive Feeding Tube and Esophageal Stent Placement

Erin Schumer and Robert C.G. Martin II

Introduction

Nutritional support for esophageal adenocarcinoma and squamous cell carcinoma present a difficult challenge as approximately 60–80 % of esophageal cancer patients present malnourished, which remains one of the highest rates among those diagnosed with cancer [1]. Poor nutrition has been shown to negatively affect survival and operative outcomes [2]. In addition to the well-recognized cachexia resulting from the tumor itself, esophageal cancers exacerbate this problem through dysphagia and obstruction. One current standard therapy for stage 2 and 3 esophageal adenocarcinomas includes neoadjuvant chemotherapy and/or radiation for those planning to undergo surgical resection. This regimen can include cisplatin and fluorouracil-based chemotherapy, which has side effects of nausea, vomiting, and diarrhea in addition to radiation-induced affects, further compounding

Electronic supplementary material Supplementary material is available in the online version of this chapter at 10.1007/978-3-319-09342-0_17. Videos can also be accessed at http://www.springerimages.com/videos/978-3-319-09341-3.

E. Schumer, MS, MD
Department of General Surgery, University of Louisville, 550 S. Jackson St., Louisville, KY 40202, USA
e-mail: emschu05@louisville.edu

R.C.G. Martin II, MD, PhD, FACS (✉)
Division of Surgical Oncology,
University of Louisville, Louisville, KY, USA
e-mail: Robert.Martin@louisville.edu

malnutrition [3]. In multiple reviews, patients have been shown to have difficulty tolerating these therapies and report decreased quality of life scores as well as worsening of their nutritional status [4]. This data has led to the development of multiple strategies to improve both the nutritional status and quality of life for patients with esophageal cancer.

Evaluation

A multidisciplinary team should be used to evaluate the patient presenting with esophageal cancer. All patients undergo a complete staging workup including imaging studies and an endoscopic ultrasound. Those patients deemed resectable based upon the staging workup and performance status undergo neoadjuvant chemotherapy and radiation. As part of the evaluation, the patient's nutritional status is assessed using a focused history and physical, the subjective global assessment (SGA), and serum protein markers such as prealbumin and albumin [5]. The SGA includes history of the patient's weight loss, GI symptoms, functional status, dietary intake, as well as examination focused on the presence of edema, ascites, muscle wasting, and loss of subcutaneous fat. In deciding the use of esophageal stenting or laparoscopic or percutaneous jejunostomy tube, a number of clinical factors are taken into account, including patients' education level, primary caregivers' educational level, dietary education/understanding, compliance estimation,

S.N. Hochwald, M. Kukar (eds.), *Minimally Invasive Foregut Surgery for Malignancy: Principles and Practice*,
DOI 10.1007/978-3-319-09342-0_17, © Springer International Publishing Switzerland 2015

Table 17.1 Outline of steps for placement of endoluminal esophageal stent

Step	Action
1	Insert endoscope
2	Dilate to 16 m with balloon dilator, if necessary
3	Place hemoclip 2 cm at planned distal end of stent
4	Insert wire and remove endoscope
5	Under fluoroscopic guidance, place stent over wire and advance distal end to hemoclip
6	Reintroduce endoscope and confirm placement

Mm millimeter, *Cm* centimeter

ability to calculate calories during neoadjuvant therapy, and the type of neoadjuvant therapy planned.

Esophageal Stent

Stent placements occur in either endoscopy or in combination with staging laparoscopy and infusaport placement in the operating suite by either the attending surgeon or gastroenterologist using intravenous conscious sedation (Video 17.1 and Table 17.1). A diagnostic endoscope (Olympus America Inc., Center Valley, PA, GIFQ180) is used with only the need to perform balloon dilation occurring if the diagnostic scope cannot traverse the stricture. Using a Controlled Radial Expansion Wireguided Balloon Dilator (Boston Scientific Inc, Microvasive, Natick, MA), the stricture is dilated to a maximum of 16 mm prior to stent placement. Care should be taken not to dilate >16 mm, since this will only lead to greater migration of the stent. After the stricture is dilated, a hemoclip is placed 2 cm at the planned distal extent of the stent, since all current stents are distal release (Video 17.2). A guidewire (Jagwire High Performance Guidewire, 0.89 mm, Boston Scientific, Natick, MA) is placed across the lesion and advanced into the distal stomach. A wire exchange is performed with removal of the endoscope keeping the guidewire in place. Using fluoroscopic guidance, either a fully covered metal stent (WallFlex, Boston Scientific), EndoMaxx, or Cook or a retrievable silicone-

covered stent (Polyflex, Boston Scientific Corporation, Natick, MA) is placed using the hemoclips as guidance for accurate distal placement. The preferred stent type is based on the type of neoadjuvant therapy that will be performed. If a patient is going to receive neoadjuvant chemotherapy alone, then we prefer a metal stent. If a patient is going to receive neoadjuvant chemotherapy with radiation therapy, then we prefer a silicone stent for ease of removal at the time of esophagogastrectomy [4]. It is essential that only the 120 mm or 150 mm length stents are used with only ≥18 mm OD, in order to reduce migration rates [4, 6]. The endoscope is then reintroduced into the esophagus to assess for correct placement and good apposition of the stent to the esophageal mucosa. Stents are left in place until planned resection, death, or the need for reintervention [7].

Stent placement has been shown to improve dysphagia scores immediately post-procedure, thus allowing patients to increase their oral nutritional intake. Over time, patients demonstrate weight gain [8], better tolerance of neoadjuvant therapy, and improvement in quality of life [9] (Table 17.2). In addition, a significant proportion of patients do not proceed with resection following neoadjuvant therapy due to progression of disease. Placement of a stent as opposed to a feeding tube in this population avoids a more invasive procedure while improving overall quality of life [6]. Complications of stent placement include migration, erosion, perforation, esophageal spasm, and obstruction. Reintervention rate has been sited to range from 20 to 60 % most often for stent migration, but this is highly dependent on the type of stent placed [9]. Our recently completed prospective trial demonstrated a reintervention rate of 6 %, thus proving that with adequate length and outer diameter, reintervention rates can be minimal [4]. Overall, esophageal stenting is effective, more efficient, less invasive, with improved quality of life tolerance, and is the optimal way to improve both nutritional measures and overall outcomes in the management of esophageal cancer.

Table 17.2 Outcomes for esophageal stents during neoadjuvant therapy

Author	Date published	Number of patients	Complication rate (%)	Stent migration (%)	Dysphagia relief (%)	Success of therapy
Langer et al. [9]	2009	38	16	26	97.40	Improved nutritional and dysphagia results
Bower et al. [6]	2009	25	4	24	100	Improved nutritional result, tolerance of neoadjuvant therapy
Siddiqui et al. [10]	2009	12	22	60	100	Improved dysphagia with similar nutrition outcomes
Pellen et al. [11]	2012	16	25	44	100	Improved symptoms, maintenance of nutrition
Brown et al. [4]	2011	32	3	31	100	Improved dysphagia, maintenance of performance status
Lopes and Eloubeidi [12]	2010	11	27	18	100	Improved dysphagia
Adler et al. [13]	2009	13	0	46	100	Improved dysphagia

Enteral Access

Enteral access can be gained by placing a jejunostomy tube in either a percutaneous, laparoscopic, or open technique.

Percutaneous endoscopic jejunostomy (PEJ) tubes are placed in the endoscopy suite by the attending surgeon or gastroenterologist under IV conscious sedation. A variable pediatric colonoscope is the best endoscope for this procedure given the ability to variably make the scope stiffer with the adequate length needed to reach the proximal jejunum. The stomach and duodenum are traversed and the jejunum is insufflated and the site for tube placement is identified using transillumination and/or direct finger compression. The ideal location for tube placement is approximately 4 fingerbreadths below the left subcostal margin near the midclavicular line. This area is then prepped and draped and anesthetized with lidocaine. A 1 cm incision is made at the site and a needle is advanced into the jejunum under direct visualization perpendicular to the abdominal wall. The guidewire is then introduced through the needle and snared by the endoscope, which is then pulled back out of the patient's mouth. The wire is disconnected from

the scope and the PEJ tube is advanced over the wire until the wire can again be snared from the opposite end by the endoscope. The entire apparatus is again advanced into the pharynx through the esophagus into the stomach.

PEJ tube placement offers the advantage of an endoscopic procedure under conscious sedation, since most patients will require nutritional support during treatment, even if they are able to eat prior to initiating therapy. Potential complications of this procedure include injury to the bowel vessels, bleeding, infection, erosion, and bowel injury. In only a small number of patients will the esophageal tumors be so obstructive as to not allow passage of the endoscope. Overall, PEJ tubes are an option for enteral support of esophageal cancer patients, but should be used with caution. The current reported PEJ failure rate based on the inability to access the proximal jejunum is approximately 15–20 %.

A laparoscopic jejunostomy tube is placed as an extension of the diagnostic laparoscopy with the use of one umbilical port and 2 additional 5 mm ports (Fig. 17.1). This procedure is performed under general anesthesia in the operating room (Table 17.3). Access to the abdomen is gained using a Hassan trocar in the midline with

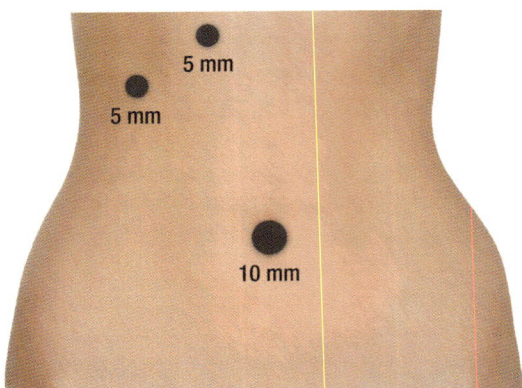

Fig. 17.1 Port sites for laparoscopic jejunostomy: 10 mm at umbilicus and two right upper quadrant 5 mm ports. *Mm* millimeter

Table 17.3 Outline of steps for placement of laparoscopic jejunostomy tube

Step	Action
1	Place 10 mm umbilical port
2	Place 5 mm RUQ ports ×2
3	Identify jejunum, adhesiolysis if necessary
4	Identify jejunum 30–40 cm distal to ligament of Treitz
5	Place purse string at chosen site
6	Place tube through abdominal wall
7	Make enterotomy and place tube through enterotomy. Secure purse string
8	Fix bowel to intraperitoneal abdominal wall with abdomen desufflated
9	Secure tube to skin

RUQ right upper quadrant, *Cm* centimeter, *Mm* millimeter

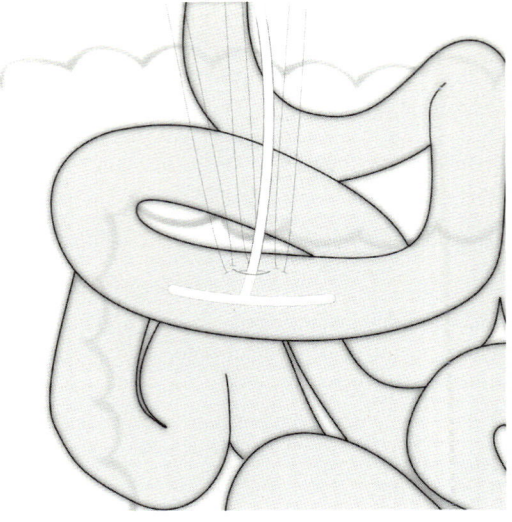

Fig. 17.2 Illustration of purse string suture in a laparoscopic jejunostomy tube located 30–40 cm distal to the ligament of Treitz

two more ports placed in the right upper quadrant under direct visualization. Visualization of the jejunum is achieved by adhesiolysis if needed and with the use of atraumatic bowel graspers to the location where the site for the J-tube placement is chosen. The jejunum is identified and followed backward to the ligament of Treitz, which commonly requires pulling the transverse colon caudally. A site for the jejunotomy is chosen 30–40 cm distal from the ligament of Treitz. The actual placement of the tube can be performed intracorporeally or extracorporeally. Three or four intracorporal 4-0 Vicryl or PDS sutures are placed circumferentially around the tube site using a laparoscopic suturing device (Fig. 17.2 and Video 17.3). A smaller catheter, 12–16 French, is passed through the abdominal wall using a stab incision and dissection with electrocautery. We prefer to use a T-tube. A jejunotomy is made, and the feeding tube is inserted into the enterotomy. The bowel is fixed to the abdominal wall at the site of the enterotomy using absorbable suture after the abdomen is desufflated. The tube is fixed to the skin with Nylon suture and all ports are closed [14]. An alternative method for laparoscopic feeding tube placement is demonstrated in Video 17.4.

The extracorporeal technique can also be performed in appropriate size patients (usually <35BMI), to which the site of the jejunostomy tube is brought out through the umbilical port site and a direct jejunal tube is placed in the same above technique, but just under direct visualization. Either technique is effective and obtains the same minimally invasive success of a jejunostomy tube placement. While laparoscopic feeding jejunostomy has been more frequently described, laparoscopic gastrostomy is also feasible.

Table 17.4 Outcomes for laparoscopic jejunostomy tube during neoadjuvant therapy

Author	Date published	Number of patients	Complication rate (%)	Tube exchange rate (%)	Success of therapy
Ben-David et al. [15]	2013	153	2.60	7.20	Provision of enteral therapy
Siddiqui et al. [10]	2009	24	4		Improvement in nutritional status
Jenkinson et al. [16]	2007	43	2.30	20.90	Optimization of nutrition

Laparoscopic enteral feeding tube placement is minimally invasive, although this approach does subject the patient to general anesthesia. Placement is under direct visualization, whether it is placed into the stomach or jejunum, and allows for avoidance of the greater curvature of the stomach, thus avoiding the gastroepiploic artery. In addition, laparoscopy can be used for complete visualization of the peritoneal contents, thus allowing for assessment of metastatic disease and completion of staging before neoadjuvant therapy.

Complications of both laparoscopic gastrostomy and jejunostomy include bleeding, infection, leakage of enteral contents, fistula formation, and injury to the small and large bowel. Gastrostomy tubes specifically may cause gastric outlet obstruction. Jejunostomy tubes may cause bowel obstruction or intestinal volvulus and are more likely to become blocked due to the smaller caliber of tube that may safely be placed into the jejunum. In a retrospective series, Ben-David et al. demonstrated that preoperative jejunostomy tube placement is a safe option for enteral access, citing dislodgment or blockage as the most frequent complication [15]. Refer to Table 17.4.

Conclusion

Nutritional status is an important part of the initial patient assessment and plays a role in pre- and postoperative outcomes. Patients should be cared for by a multidisciplinary team with experience in all types of feeding access. Overall, there are several methods of improving nutrition for esophageal cancer, and these methods must be individualized to each patient.

References

1. Miller KR, Bozeman MC. Nutrition therapy issues in esophageal cancer. Curr Gastroenterol Rep. 2012;14: 356–66.
2. Ryan AM, Hearty A, Prichard RS, et al. Association of hypoalbuminemia on the first postoperative day and complications following esophagectomy. J Gastrointest Surg. 2007;11:1355–60.
3. Kleinberg L. Therapy for locally advanced adenocarcinoma of the gastroesophageal junction: optimizing outcome. Semin Radiat Oncol. 2013;23:38–50.
4. Brown RE, Abbas AE, Ellis S, et al. A prospective phase II evaluation of esophageal stenting for neoadjuvant therapy for esophageal cancer: optimal performance and surgical safety. J Am Coll Surg. 2011; 212:582–8.
5. Poziomyck AK, Weston AC, Lameu EB, et al. Preoperative nutritional assessment and prognosis in patients with foregut tumors. Nutr Cancer. 2012;64: 1174–81.
6. Bower M, Jones W, Vessels B, et al. Nutritional support with endoluminal stenting during neoadjuvant therapy for esophageal malignancy. Ann Surg Oncol. 2009;16:3161–8.
7. Martin R, Duvall R, Ellis S, Scoggins CR. The use of self-expanding silicone stents in esophageal cancer care: optimal pre-, peri-, and postoperative care. Surg Endosc. 2009;23:615–21.
8. Bower M, Jones W, Vessels B, et al. Role of esophageal stents in the nutrition support of patients with esophageal malignancy. Nutr Clin Pract. 2010;25:244–9.
9. Langer FB, Schoppmann SF, Prager G, et al. Temporary placement of self-expanding oesophageal stents as bridging for neo-adjuvant therapy. Ann Surg Oncol. 2010;17:470–5.
10. Siddiqui AA, Glynn C, Loren D, Kowalski T. Self-expanding plastic esophageal stents versus jejunostomy tubes for the maintenance of nutrition during neoadjuvant chemoradiation therapy in patients with esophageal cancer: a retrospective study. Dis Esophagus. 2009;22: 216–22.
11. Pellen MG, Sabri S, Razack A, et al. Safety and efficacy of self-expanding removable metal esophageal stents during neoadjuvant chemotherapy for resectable esophageal cancer. Dis Esophagus. 2012;25:48–53.

12. Lopes TL, Eloubeidi MA. A pilot study of fully covered self-expandable metal stents prior to neoadjuvant therapy for locally advanced esophageal cancer. Dis Esophagus. 2010;23:309–15.

13. Adler DG, Fang J, Wong R, et al. Placement of Polyflex stents in patients with locally advanced esophageal cancer is safe and improves dysphagia during neoadjuvant therapy. Gastrointest Endosc. 2009;70:614–9.

14. Fischer JE. Fischer's mastery of surgery. Philadelphia: Wolters Kluwer Health/Lippincott Williams & Wilkins; 2012.

15. Ben-David K, Kim T, Caban AM, et al. Pre-therapy laparoscopic feeding jejunostomy is safe and effective in patients undergoing minimally invasive esophagectomy for cancer. J Gastrointest Surg. 2013;17:1352–8.

16. Jenkinson AD, Lim J, Agrawal N, Menzies D. Laparoscopic feeding jejunostomy in esophagogastric cancer. Surg Endosc. 2007;21:299–302.

Robotic Utilization in Esophageal Cancer Surgery

18

Richard van Hillegersberg, Roy J.J. Verhage,
Pieter C. van der Sluis, Jelle P.H. Ruurda,
and A. Christiaan Kroese

Introduction

Optimal treatment for esophageal cancer consists of transthoracic en bloc esophagectomy (TTE) with an extensive mediastinal lymph node dissection. This approach through thoracotomy is accompanied by significant morbidity, mainly consisting of cardiopulmonary complications.

To reduce surgical trauma and morbidity of open transthoracic esophagectomy, less invasive surgical techniques such as transhiatal esophagectomy (THE) and minimally invasive esophagectomy (MIE) have been introduced.

Recent analyses of the MIE to date have shown a decreased operative blood loss, reduced complication rate, and shorter hospital stay [1–3].

Electronic supplementary material Supplementary material is available in the online version of this chapter at 10.1007/978-3-319-09342-0_18. Videos can also be accessed at http://www.springerimages.com/videos/978-3-319-09341-3.

R. van Hillegersberg, MD, PhD (✉)
R.J.J. Verhage, MD, PhD • P.C. van der Sluis, MD, MSc
J.P.H. Ruurda, MD, PhD
Department of Surgery,
University Medical Center Utrecht,
Heidelberglaan 100, Utrecht 3584 CX,
The Netherlands
e-mail: r.vanhillegersberg@ucmutrecht.nl

A.C. Kroese, MD
Division of Anesthesiology,
Intensive Care and Emergency Medicine,
University Medical Center Utrecht,
Utrecht, The Netherlands

However, conventional endoscopic surgery has important limitations, such as a 2-dimensional view, a disturbed hand-eye-coordination, and limited degrees of freedom. Robotic systems have been developed to overcome these limitations [4]. During esophagectomy, the robotic platform enables the surgeon to perform an accurate mediastinal dissection of the esophagus *en bloc* with surrounding lymphatic tissue and mediastinal fat, often harboring metastatic disease. Robot-assisted thoracoscopic esophagectomy (RAMIE) in conjunction with conventional laparoscopy has shown to be technically feasible. Moreover, it provides sufficient oncological resection and is associated with low blood loss [5, 6]

Indications

Appropriate patient selection is essential to a successful esophageal surgery program. Approximately 30–40 % of esophageal cancer patients are eligible to undergo an esophagectomy at curative intent, taking into account tumor stage and comorbidity. The minimally invasive approach may offer a greater percentage of patients, a potentially curative surgical resection. Patients with stage I–IV disease, i.e., T1–T4a tumors, and no evidence of distant metastases are eligible to RAMIE. The ten times magnified 3-dimensional operative field, combined with an excellent manipulative freedom, allows radical resection even in advanced cases [7].

S.N. Hochwald, M. Kukar (eds.), *Minimally Invasive Foregut Surgery for Malignancy: Principles and Practice*,
DOI 10.1007/978-3-319-09342-0_18, © Springer International Publishing Switzerland 2015

In order to improve oncological outcome, multimodality treatment including neoadjuvant chemotherapy or chemoradiotherapy has become the standard of care in recent years [8]. A meta-analysis calculated hazard ratios for all-cause mortality comparing neoadjuvant chemotherapy (0.87 (0.79–0.96); $p=0.005$) or chemoradiotherapy (0.78 (95 % CI 0.70–0.88; $p<0.0001$) with surgery alone. These data suggest a survival benefit of neoadjuvant chemoradiotherapy or chemotherapy over surgery alone in patients with esophageal cancer. However, a clear advantage of neoadjuvant chemoradiotherapy over neoadjuvant chemotherapy has not been established [9].

Perioperative Management

Preoperative

All patients planning to undergo RAMIE are seen by an anaesthesiologist in the preoperative clinic. The physical status of the patient is assessed and preoperative testing is guided by institutional guidelines. Patients with the presence of and increased degree of perioperative complications (e.g., cardiovascular complications) will be referred for additional specialty care, as necessary, and treatment as directed by the anaesthesiologist.

Intraoperative

Thoracic epidural analgesia (TEA) most likely decreases the risk of postoperative respiratory failure and results in improved pain control [10]. Furthermore, TEA may increase the blood supply to the esophagogastric anastomosis area after esophagectomy [11]. Although there are no specific publications on the effects of TEA during minimally invasive esophagectomy, the advantages of TEA in the postoperative course of open esophagectomy can probably be extrapolated to thoracoscopic esophagectomy.

Normally, the epidural catheter is placed between the fifth and the eight thoracic vertebrae. Usually epidural sufentanil is used intraoperatively and a continuous infusion of bupivacaine and morphine is applied postoperatively. To enable selective deflation of the right lung during the thoracoscopic phase, patients are intubated with a left-sided double-lumen tube. Patients receive two large-bore peripheral cannulae, a central venous line in the right internal jugular vein, an arterial line, a urinary catheter, and a nasogastric tube. Antibiotic prophylaxis is provided by i.v. administration of 2,000 mg cefazolin and 500 mg metronidazole. Thirty minutes before incision, 10 mg/kg methylprednisolone is administered to minimize postoperative pulmonary complications [12].

Patients receive general anesthesia with either propofol or volatile anesthesia. During the thoracoscopic phase of the operation, patients are positioned in the left lateral decubitus position, and selective ventilation of the left lung is instituted. Continuous intravenous muscle relaxation is used to facilitate dissection of the esophagus along the trachea, azygos vein, aorta, and pulmonary veins as sudden, unexpected movements of the patient could have detrimental effects. The patient must be protected against inadvertent contact from the motions of the robotic arms. After the instruments are connected to the arms of the robot and are placed inside the patient, the body position cannot be modified unless the instruments are disengaged and removed from the body cavity.

When the robotic system is in place, access to the patient in case of emergency is limited. Therefore, the surgical team should be capable of rapidly removing the robot if required.

Management of One-Lung Ventilation in RAMIE

To install one-lung ventilation (OLV), a left-sided double-lumen tube (DLT) is used. Positioning of the DLT is most reliably achieved with a fiberoptic bronchoscope. It has been shown that left DLTs, when positioned only by inspection and auscultation, were in fact malpositioned in more than 33 % of the cases. After positioning the patient from supine to lateral, the position of the DLT is checked again routinely. Cuff pressure is measured to prevent high intracuff pressures and possible mucosal damage. During OLV both lungs are perfused. Perfusion of the nonventilated lung inevitably leads to transpulmonary shunting, impairment of oxygenation, and possible hypoxemia. During OLV a protective lung ventilation (PLV) protocol is applied, consisting of a pressure-controlled ventilation strategy with a maximum pressure of 20 cm H_2O. Tidal volume is reduced to 6 ml/kg predicted body weight. Furthermore, 5 cm H_2O PEEP is routinely used. Although hypoxemia is a constant threat, the lowest possible fraction of inspired oxygen (FiO_2) is delivered to prevent oxidative damage and postoperative acute lung injury.

In case of hypoxemia, the first treatment is an increase in FiO_2. If no improvement occurs, the surgeon is informed and the nonventilated lung is expanded with 100 % oxygen. Our clinical experience suggests that dislocation of the DLT, atelectasis, and bronchial occlusion of the ventilated lung with blood or secretions are the most occurring causes of hypoxemia. Therefore, immediate fiberoptic bronchoscopy is performed to rule out or even correct dislocation of the DLT and occluded bronchi. Once these are ruled out, a recruitment maneuver is performed to open possible atelectasis.

When hypoxemia persists, the administration of oxygen with or without CPAP to the nonventilated lung is a valuable option [13]. Clear communication with the surgeon is necessary in these circumstances as both maneuvers may have a negative impact on the surgical exposure during thoracoscopy. When applying CPAP, the nonventilated lung is first reinflated as CPAP alone does not inflate an atelectatic lung. At the end of the thoracoscopic phase, the nonventilated lung is reinflated under direct vision and extensive recruitment maneuvers are performed after which two-lung ventilation is restarted and 10 cm H_2O PEEP is added. There is no more need for lung separation during the rest of the operation and usually the DLT is exchanged for a single-lumen tube (SLT).

Fluid Management

Fluid strategy during RTE is aimed at a mildly positive fluid balance of approximately 500–1,000 ml at the end of the procedure. The use of central venous oxygen saturation may have additional value in particular in patients with decreased cardiac function. However, at the moment, no large-scale randomized trials are available.

Perioperative Complications

The most common complications encountered perioperatively include arrhythmias, most often seen as the result of manipulation of the heart during the thoracoscopic phase of the operation. Usually these arrhythmias are self-limited after interruption of the surgical manipulation. Another complication regularly seen is the development of a pneumomediastinum as a result of the opening of the hiatus during the laparoscopic phase of the operation. Hemodynamics may show the characteristics of a tension pneumothorax. Again the surgeon should be informed immediately and asked to lower the pressure of the pneumoperitoneum. If indicated, thoracic drains are inserted to relieve the pneumomediastinum.

Postoperative Care

Postoperatively all patients remain under general anesthesia and are intubated until they are transferred to the intensive care unit. Extubation is aimed for the same day. Although immediate extubation in the operating room has been described and considered safe, we consider it appropriate to ventilate patients postoperatively until chest X-ray is obtained and information on the actual respiratory status is available. When the X-ray shows no significant atelectasis, weaning from ventilation is started.

Robot-Assisted Thoracoscopic Dissection (Video 18.1)

Robotic Instruments

- Hook
- Cadiere
- Needle driver
- Long tip forceps
- Hem-o-lok® Ligation clips

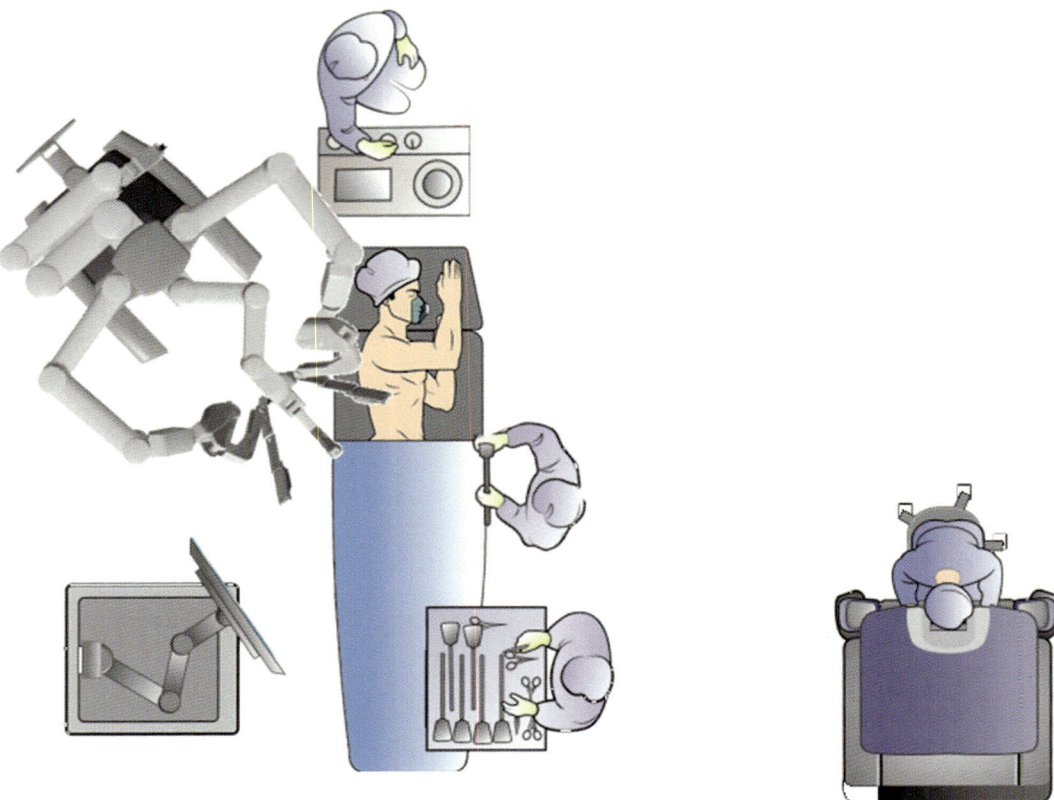

Fig. 18.1 OR setup. The patient is in left lateral position. The robot is docked from the dorsocranial side

Positioning

The patient is positioned in the left lateral decubitus position, tilted 45° toward the prone position.
The operating table is flexed, lowering the legs
and upper thorax (the patient is positioned with
the xiphoid above the pivoting point of the table).
This extends the thorax and widens intercostal
space for introducing trocars. The bedside cart is
brought into the operative field from the dorsocranial side of the patient (Fig. 18.1). Before incision, the right lung is desufflated. A 10-mm
camera port is placed at the sixth intercostal
space, posterior to the posterior axillary line. Two
8-mm ports are placed just anterior to the scapu-
lar rim in the fourth intercostal space and more
posterior in the ninth intercostal space. Two thoracoscopic ports are used in the fifth and seventh
intercostal spaces just posterior to the posterior
axillary line. These ports are used for conven-

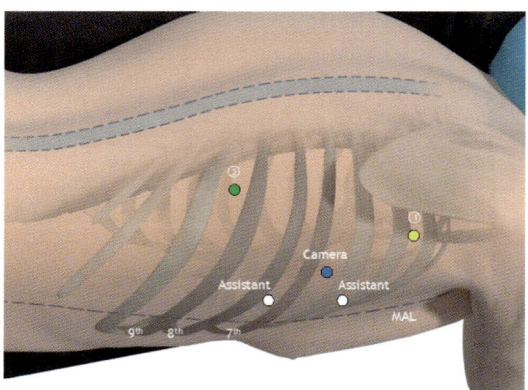

Fig. 18.2 Port position. Robotic arms 1 (*yellow*), 2
(*green*) and camera (*blue*). Two assisting ports (*white*)

tional thoracoscopic assistance such as suction,
traction, and clipping (Fig. 18.2). CO_2 insufflation of the thoracic cavity with 6 mmHg permits
excellent vision, without the need for retracting

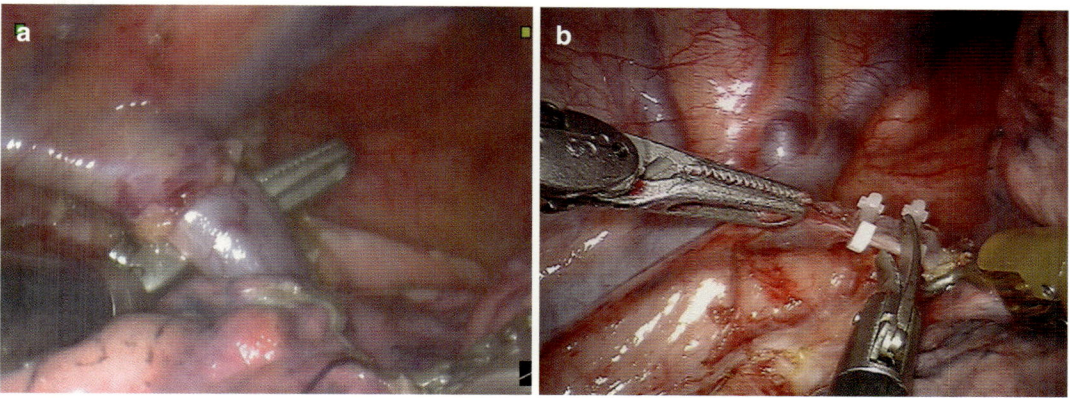

Fig. 18.3 (**a**) Identification of the azygos vein (AV). (**b**) Division of the azygos vein over the esophagus

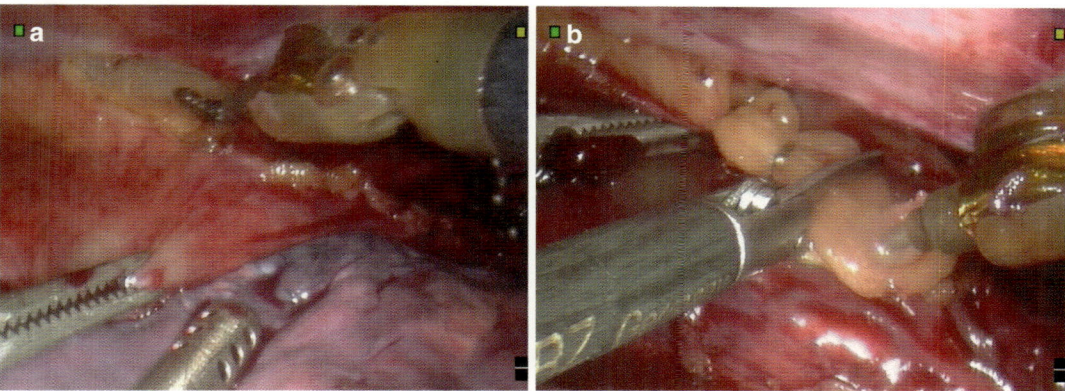

Fig. 18.4 (**a**) The thoracic duct (TD) is identified. (**b**) The thoracic duct (TD) is identified, clipped at the level of the diaphragm, and divided

the lung from the operative field. In case of a non-compliant lung, a retractor can be used.

Operative Steps

After division of any pulmonary adhesions and a proper overview of the operating field is achieved, the right pulmonary ligament is divided. The parietal pleura is dissected at the anterior side of the esophagus from the diaphragm up to the azygos arch. The azygos arch is carefully ligated with robotic hemoloc clips (Fig. 18.3a, b). Then dissection of the parietal pleura is continued above the aortic arch for a right paratracheal lymph node dissection. The right vagal nerve is dissected below the level of the carina.

Subsequently, the parietal pleura is dissected at the posterior side of the esophagus cranially to caudally along the azygos vein, including the thoracic duct. Paratracheally left, the left recurrent nerve is identified and carefully protected. At the level of the diaphragm, the thoracic duct is clipped with a 10-mm endoscopic clipping device (Endo Clip™ II; Covidien, Mansfield, Massachusetts, USA) to prevent postoperative chylous leakage (Fig. 18.4a, b).

At the level of the diaphragm, a Penrose drain is placed around the esophagus to provide traction, which facilitates esophageal mobilization (Fig. 18.5). The esophagus is then resected en bloc with the surrounding mediastinal lymph nodes and the thoracic duct from the diaphragm up to the thoracic inlet. Aortoesophageal vessels

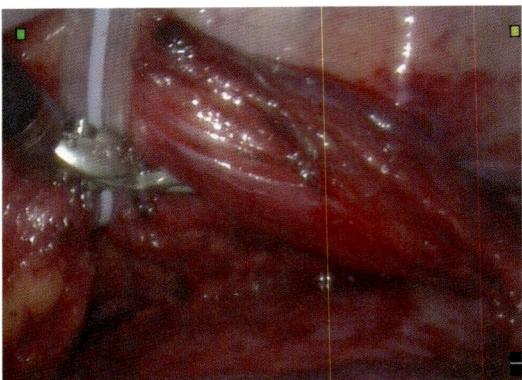

Fig. 18.5 A Penrose drain (PD) is placed around the esophagus (E) at the level of the pericardium to retract the esophagus anteriorly

are identified and clipped by the assisting surgeon. The extensive lymphadenectomy includes the right- and left-sided paratracheal (lymph node station 2R, 2L), tracheobronchial (lymph node station 4), aortopulmonary window (station 5), carinal (station 7), and periesophageal (station 8) lymph nodes. A 24-Fr chest tube is placed, and the lung is insufflated under direct vision.

Laparoscopic Dissection
(Video 18.1)

Instruments

- Harmonic scalpel
- 2× fenestrated bowel clamps
- Endopaddle
- Clipper
- Hem-o-lok® Ligation clips

Positioning

After completion of the robot-assisted thoracoscopic esophageal mobilization, the patient is put in supine position. An 11-mm camera port is introduced left paraumbilically, and an 11-mm working port is placed at the right midclavicular line at the umbilical level. A 5-mm working port is placed more cranially at the right midclavicular line. A 5-mm assisting port is placed in the left

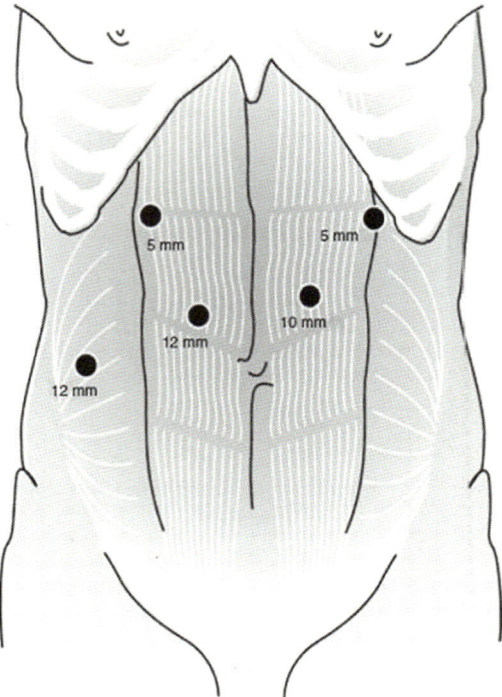

Fig. 18.6 Laparoscopic trocar placement

subcostal area, and a 12-mm port is placed pararectally right for the liver retractor (Fig. 18.6). The abdomen is insufflated to a carbon dioxide pressure level of 15 mmHg.

Operative Steps

The hepatogastric ligament is opened. The greater and lesser curvatures are dissected with ultrasonic harmonic scalpel (Harmonic Ace®, Ethicon Endo-Surgery, Johnson & Johnson, New Brunswick, New Jersey, USA). The hiatus is opened, and the distal esophagus is dissected from the right and left crus. The carbon dioxide pressure level is reduced to 6 mmHg to avoid excessive intrathoracic pressure, and a chest tube is placed in the left pleural sinus. Dissection and lymphadenectomy then continue around the celiac trunk. The left gastric artery and vein then are transected at their origin with Hem-o-lok® Ligation clips (Teleflex Medical, NC, USA). Abdominal lymphadenectomy includes lymph nodes surrounding the left gastric artery and the lesser omental lymph nodes.

The cervical esophagus is mobilized through a left-sided longitudinal neck incision along the sternocleidoid muscle. No formal cervical lymph node dissection is carried out, but cervical lymph nodes are dissected if lymph node metastases are suspected macroscopically during the cervical phase of esophagectomy. The esophagus is dissected and a cord is attached to the proximal part of the specimen to enable pull-up of the gastric conduit along the anatomical tract of the esophagus.

The esophagus and surrounding lymph nodes are pulled into the abdomen under laparoscopic vision. A 7-cm transverse incision is made at the level of the left paraumbilical port for extraction of the specimen and stomach using a wound protector.

Outside the abdomen, a 5-cm-wide gastric tube is constructed with staplers (GIA TM 80, 3·8 mm; Covidien, Dublin, Ireland), and the stapled line is oversewn with 3-0 polydioxanone. Routine extracorporal oversewing was reintroduced as two serious complications occurred when the staple line was not oversewn [14]. The specimen consisting of the esophagus and cardia of the stomach is sent for pathological examination. After the gastric tube has been pulled to the neck, a hand-sewn end-to-side esophagogastrostomy is performed in the neck using 3-0 polydioxanone single-layer running sutures. Excess gastric tubing is removed using a GIA stapler.

A feeding jejunostomy (Freka® FCJ-Set, Fresenius Kabi AG, Bad Homburg vd H., Germany) is placed at the level of the transverse incision.

Postoperative Care

Clinical Care

Postoperatively, patients are transferred to the intensive care unit (ICU). After leaving the operating room, mechanical ventilation is continued briefly usually extubating later that evening.

After 1 day in the ICU, patients are transferred to a medium care (MC) ward.

Important for postoperative care are a nasogastric tube, feeding jejunostomy, and an epidural catheter. The nasogastric tube is used for gastric decompression and to provide a splinting in case of anastomotic dehiscence. Fixation of the tube is imperative, as reintroduction can cause damage to the anastomosis.

No oral intake is allowed for 5 days minimum. During that first week, feeding is provided by the feeding jejunostomy. After 5 days without any indication of anastomotic dehiscence, sips of water are initiated. If there is no evidence of anastomotic leak, oral intake is gradually supplemented to solid foods under close supervision of a clinical nutritionist. The feeding jejunostomy is left *in situ* up to 6 weeks after discharge from the hospital. Only after sufficient intake is maintained, the jejunostomy is removed at the outpatient clinic.

Pain medication through the epidural catheter is required to improve postoperative ventilation and coughing. Other strategies to prevent postoperative pulmonary complications include elevation of the bed by 15–30°, physical respiratory therapy, and early mobilization.

Results of RAMIE

To overcome the limitations of conventional (thoraco)scopic surgery, the robot-assisted minimally invasive thoraco-laparoscopic esophagectomy was developed in the UMC Utrecht in 2003. From our first experience, it was concluded that RAMIE is a feasible and safe technique [5, 7]. It is associated with reduced blood loss, shorter intensive care unit stay, and a lower percentage of cardiopulmonary complications compared to literature reports of open transthoracic esophagectomy. Mortality, hospital stay, and lymph node retrieval were comparable. Short-term oncological outcomes were equivalent to results from open transthoracic surgery. Disadvantages of robot-assisted surgery compared to open surgery are a prolonged operative time, high costs associated with robot acquisition and maintenance, and the use of disposable tools.

Following our initial report of RAMIE in 2009, we analyzed the following consecutive series of 108 patients until 2011. We found a high percentage (95 %) of radical resections despite the high rate of T3 tumors (78 %) and only 64 % received neoadjuvant therapy. A median of 26 dissected lymph nodes was retrieved. Follow-up was at least 25 months with a median follow-up of 34 months. Median disease-free survival was 21 months and median overall survival was 29 months, with a 5-year overall survival of 40 months. The percentage of in-hospital pulmonary infections after RAMIE in our series was 34 % [15].

This percentage is higher than reported in the randomized trial comparing minimally invasive esophagectomy (MIE) to open transthoracic esophagectomy. Results from this trial showed a pulmonary complication rate in the MIE group of 12 % [1]. However, different definitions of postoperative pneumonia were used. Our definition of pneumonia was defined as the decision to treat suspected pneumonia (MCDC grade II) [16]. The definition of pneumonia used in the randomized controlled trial was more strict (i.e., infiltrate on pulmonary radiography combined with a positive sputum culture) leading to a lower percentage of pneumonia. Applying this definition on our cohort yields a pneumonia rate of 18 %, which is comparable to MIE.

Our results from robot-assisted esophagectomy are in concordance with a recently published systematic review [17]. This systematic review included nine articles (130 cases) describing robot-assisted esophagectomy. It was concluded that robot-assisted esophagectomy was a feasible and safe technique. In terms of short-term oncological outcomes, RAMIE was at least equivalent to the open transthoracic approach for esophageal cancer. The systematic review strongly emphasized the need for well-conducted randomized controlled trials and long-term survival to prove the superiority of robot-assisted minimally invasive thoraco-laparoscopic esophagectomy over open transthoracic esophagectomy. Therefore, we initiated the ROBOT trial (ClinicalTrial.gov Identifier: NCT01544790) to compare RAMIE with open transthoracic

esophagectomy. Results from this randomized controlled trial are to be expected in 2015 [18].

References

1. Biere SS, van Berge Henegouwen MI, Maas KW, et al. Minimally invasive versus open oesophagectomy for patients with oesophageal cancer: a multicentre, open-label, randomised controlled trial. Lancet. 2012;379: 1887–92.
2. Verhage RJ, Hazebroek EJ, Boone J, Van Hillegersberg R. Minimally invasive surgery compared to open procedures in esophagectomy for cancer: a systematic review of the literature. Minerva Chir. 2009;64:135–46.
3. Luketich JD, Pennathur A, Awais O, et al. Outcomes after minimally invasive esophagectomy: review of over 1000 patients. Ann Surg. 2012;256:95–103.
4. Ruurda JP, Draaisma WA, van Hillegersberg R, et al. Robot-assisted endoscopic surgery: a four-year single-center experience. Dig Surg. 2005;22:313–20.
5. van Hillegersberg R, Boone J, Draaisma WA, et al. First experience with robot-assisted thoracoscopic esophagolymphadenectomy for esophageal cancer. Surg Endosc. 2006;20:1435–9.
6. Kernstine KH. Robotics in thoracic surgery. Am J Surg. 2004;188:89S–97.
7. Boone J, Schipper ME, Moojen WA, et al. Robot-assisted thoracoscopic oesophagectomy for cancer. Br J Surg. 2009;96:878–86.
8. van Hagen P, Hulshof MC, van Lanschot JJ, et al. Preoperative chemoradiotherapy for esophageal or junctional cancer. N Engl J Med. 2012;366:2074–84.
9. Gebski V, Burmeister B, Smithers BM, et al. Survival benefits from neoadjuvant chemoradiotherapy or chemotherapy in oesophageal carcinoma: a meta-analysis. Lancet Oncol. 2007;8:226–34.
10. Block BM, Liu SS, Rowlingson AJ, et al. Efficacy of postoperative epidural analgesia: a meta-analysis. JAMA. 2003;290:2455–63.
11. Michelet P, Roch A, D'Journo XB, et al. Effect of thoracic epidural analgesia on gastric blood flow after oesophagectomy. Acta Anaesthesiol Scand. 2007;51:587–94.
12. Sato N, Koeda K, Ikeda K, et al. Randomized study of the benefits of preoperative corticosteroid administration on the postoperative morbidity and cytokine response in patients undergoing surgery for esophageal cancer. Ann Surg. 2002;236:184–90.
13. Verhage RJ, Boone J, Rijkers GT, Cromheecke GJ, Kroese AC, Weijs TJ, Borel Rinkes IH, van Hillegersberg R. Reduced local immune response with CPAP during single lung ventilation for oesophagectomy. Br J Anaesth. 2014;112(5):920–8.
14. Boone J, Rinkes IH, van Hillegersberg R. Gastric conduit staple line after esophagectomy: to oversew or not? J Thorac Cardiovasc Surg. 2006;132:1491–2.
15. van der Sluis PCR, JP, Verhage RJJ, van der Horst S, Haverkamp L, Siersema PD, Borel Rinkes IHM, ten

Kate FJW, van Hillegersberg R. Robot-assisted minimally invasive thoraco-laparoscopic esophagectomy with two-field lymphadenectomy for esophageal cancer: report of 108 consecutive procedures. 2014 (submitted).

16. Dindo D, Demartines N, Clavien PA. Classification of surgical complications: a new proposal with evaluation in a cohort of 6336 patients and results of a survey. Ann Surg. 2004;240:205–13.

17. Clark J, Sodergren MH, Purkayastha S, et al. The role of robotic assisted laparoscopy for oesophagogastric oncological resection; an appraisal of the literature. Dis Esophagus. 2011;24:240–50.

18. van der Sluis PC, Ruurda JP, van der Horst S, et al. Robot-assisted minimally invasive thoraco-laparoscopic esophagectomy versus open transthoracic esophagectomy for resectable esophageal cancer, a randomized controlled trial (ROBOT trial). Trials. 2012;13:230.

Minimally Invasive Intragastric Surgery

19

Didier Mutter and Marius Nedelcu

Introduction

Laparoscopic intragastric surgery (LIGS) represents a minimally invasive technique for lesions, which mainly exist in the gastric lumen or at the gastroesophageal junction. In 1995, Ohashi initially described this technique to resect early gastric cancer, which could not be treated by endoscopic mucosal resection (EMR) [1]. Since then, it has evolved with respect to both technological advances (e.g., the development of cuffed or single access ports) and tactical innovations by many teams (Table 19.1). The good results of this approach associated with our ever-increasing experience allowed us to propose it systematically as an option for the management of gastric lesions.

The aim of this chapter is to identify the indications and to describe the technical principles of this novel technique used in our current practice. The objective is also to expand the surgeon's armamentarium in order to safely address more complex intragastric processes while offering the benefits of minimal access surgery.

Indications

Indications for laparoscopic intragastric surgery (LIGS) can be found for all tumors, which may be resected without systematic gastrectomy or lymph node resection. It includes anecdotal foreign body removal [8, 9] and pancreatic pseudocyst drainage [10]. Typical indications include the resection of benign lesions [11–13], lesions with inconclusive pathological findings after biopsy, when malignancy cannot be ruled out [4, 14], and finally early malignancy especially at the level of the esophago-gastric region [2]. At present, these tumors can be detected by different modalities (upper endoscopy, abdominal CT scan). The most frequent tumors are gastrointestinal stromal tumors (GISTs). These are frequently located at the esophagogastric junction, not easily accessible for resection via an endoscopic retroflexed view. Upper endoscopy represents the standard tool for the diagnosis of such lesions, but in certain cases its therapeutic purpose

Electronic supplementary material Supplementary material is available in the online version of this chapter at 10.1007/978-3-319-09342-0_19. Videos can also be accessed at http://www.springerimages.com/videos/978-3-319-09341-3.

D. Mutter, MD, PhD, FACS (✉)
Department of Digestive and Endocrine Surgery,
IRCAD, IHU, University Hospital of Strasbourg,
Nouvel Hôpital Civil – Pôle Hépato-Digestif,
Hôpitaux Universitaires de Strasbourg,
1, Place de l'Hôpital, Strasbourg,
Alsace 67091, France
e-mail: didier.mutter@chru-strasbourg.fr;
didier.mutter@ircad.fr

M. Nedelcu, MD
Department of Digestive and Endocrine Surgery,
University Hospital of Strasbourg,
Nouvel Hôpital Civil – Pôle Hépato-Digestif,
Hôpitaux Universitaires de Strasbourg,
Strasbourg, Alsace, France

S.N. Hochwald, M. Kukar (eds.), *Minimally Invasive Foregut Surgery for Malignancy: Principles and Practice*,   199
DOI 10.1007/978-3-319-09342-0_19, © Springer International Publishing Switzerland 2015

Table 19.1 Review of the literature

Year	Authors	Journal	Number of cases	Particularities
1995	Ohashi [1]	*Surgical Endoscopy*	8 cases	6 early gastric cancer, 1 submucosal leiomyoma, 1 giant polyp
2000	Hiki et al. [2]	*Der Chirurg*	13 cases	1 case of conversion due to intraoperative hemorrhage
2011	Sahm et al. [3]	*Surg Laparosc Endosc Percutan Tech*	7 cases	6 gastrointestinal stromal tumors and 1 leiomyoma
2004	Uchikoshi et al. [4]	*Surg Laparosc Endosc Percutan Tech*	7 cases	4 cases of gastrointestinal stromal tumors, 2 leiomyomas, and 1 schwannoma
2012	Hara et al. [5]	*Surg Laparosc Endosc Percutan Tech*	10 cases	1 case of conversion due to technical difficulties
2011	Shim et al. [6]	*J Surg Oncol*	6 cases	5 leiomyomas, and one case GIST
2011	Na et al. [7]	*J Gastric Cancer*	7 cases	5 gastrointestinal stromal tumors and 2 leiomyomas

has obvious limitations. The main advantage of laparoscopic intragastric surgery is yielded by the direct approach to this region contrary to the retroflexed approach provided by endoscopy. Its limitation is not only due to the visualization of the lesion but also to the main shortcoming of the indirect endoscopic approach which is the inability to offer sufficient strength and precision to control dissection in a safe manner. Laparoscopic intragastric surgery completely overcomes such limitations and also offers an appropriate dissection angle using the basic "triangulation" principle of general laparoscopy.

Preoperative Workup

For preoperative diagnosis and surgical planning, preoperative upper endoscopy is a key step to ascertain the precise localization of the tumor. It is needed to define the anatomical landmarks of the lesions regarding the gastric curvatures, distance to the cardia, pylorus, and main vessels. The lesions are also examined by CT scan and endoscopic ultrasound (US) to determine the depth of invasion of the gastric wall. Endoscopic US is a major tool to identify contraindications represented by transmural tumors or local lymph node metastases. Finally, such data should be confirmed intraoperatively by the excellent vision provided by the laparoscopic exploration as well as by the endogastric approach.

Surgical Technique

The anatomical localization of the tumor is the most important factor to determine the ideal resection technique. When facing a tumor of the anterior gastric wall, the tumor is easy to visualize, and a tangential wedge resection through conventional transperitoneal laparoscopy is the method of choice [3]. Sometimes, the location of the tumor may be confirmed by simultaneous endoscopic exploration. If the tumor is located on the posterior gastric wall, proximal to the cardia or pylorus, a conventional wedge resection cannot be performed with appropriate margins. In this respect, intragastric surgery could well represent a valid option.

Different surgical techniques have been described for laparoscopic intragastric surgery. Our standard approach for a laparoscopic intragastric surgery is represented by a multiple intragastric port approach, as described in Video 19.1. A pneumoperitoneum is briefly established using an open access at the umbilical level. It allows to explore the abdomen and determine the ideal position of transgastric laparoscopic ports in relation to the anatomy of the stomach. Endoscopy aiming to localize the actual position of the tumor may be completed at this moment. The tumor can be located by a mark or a suture on the gastric wall. The location of the stomach wall incision is then identified. Two transparietal stitches are placed adjacent to this area and will be used to lift

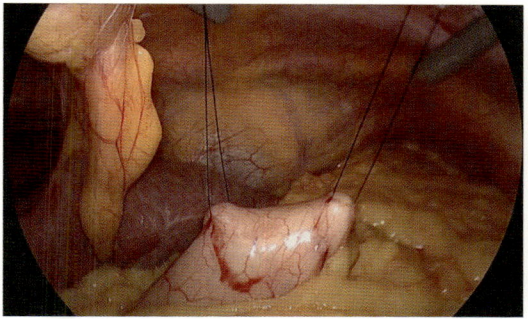

Fig. 19.1   Gastric exposure

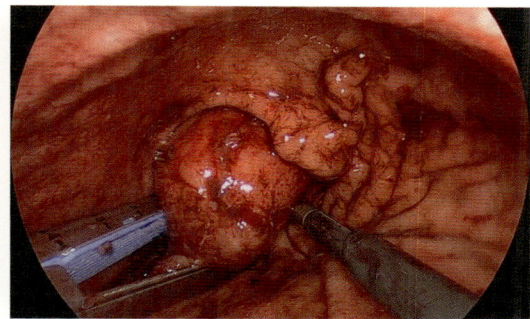

Fig. 19.4   Tumor resection

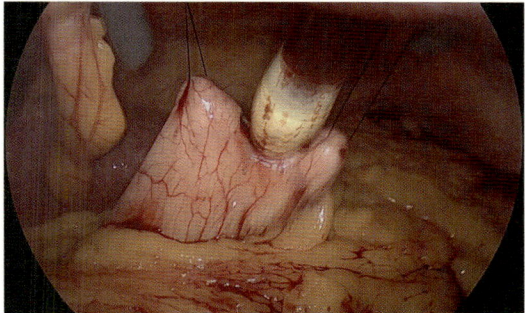

Fig. 19.2   Intragastric trocar insertion

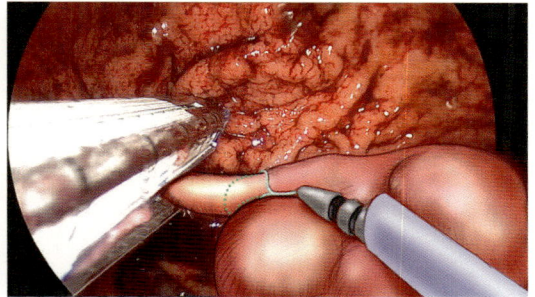

Fig. 19.5   Final stapling with suture assistance

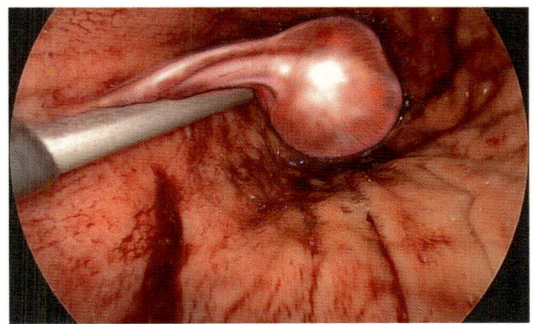

Fig. 19.3   Intragastric identification of the tumor

up the stomach and fix it to the parietal wall (Fig. 19.1). A 12 mm cuffed port is inserted into the stomach under laparoscopic guidance (Fig. 19.2). Two additional 5 mm ports are inserted and positioned to ensure triangulation in relation to the tumor's position. The two cuffed 5 mm ports are also introduced into the stomach under direct control after partial insufflation. The peritoneal cavity is desufflated, and the stomach is explored (Fig. 19.3). There is no need for a

high rate of insufflation of the stomach, as the anterior wall is lifted up by traction applied to the abdominal wall by means of stitches. Usually, no distal or proximal balloon blockage is required due to lower esophageal sphincter and pyloric resting tone. In order to achieve adequate access, multiple ports should be positioned according to general laparoscopic principles in order to achieve maximum triangulation for the dissection site. The cardioesophageal junction is a difficult location, which requires optimal visualization and triangulation of instruments for safe surgical maneuvers.

Resection and suture can be performed as a standard procedure, but most of the time, the use of stapling is preferred for many reasons, including speed, safety, and reliability as illustrated by this case (Figs. 19.4 and 19.5). It only requires the replacement of the 5 mm port by a 12 mm one. In well-selected cases (e.g., pedunculated tumors), the advantage of this technique is to obtain resection and hemostasis simultaneously, using the same instrument. However, achieving

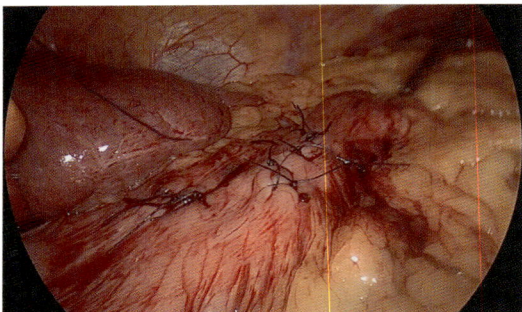

Fig. 19.6 Gastrotomy closure

Table 19.2 Key steps of intragastric surgery

1.	Gastric exposure
2.	Intragastric trocar insertion
3.	Intragastric identification of the tumor
4.	Tumor resection by transgastric stapling
5.	Final stapling with suture assistance
6.	Gastrotomy closure

adequate margins can be difficult, and the risk of tumor rupture might be increased, particularly in case of gastrointestinal stromal tumors. In such cases, tricks including traction on the parietal gastric wall assist in achieving a full-thickness resection of the stomach wall, preserving safety margins in case of malignant lesions. The port should be positioned so that stapling can be easily accomplished in the narrow space of the insufflated stomach, and the use of roticulating staplers is mandatory. Figure 19.6 depicts the closed gastrotomy.

In some cases, when tumors are located on the posterior and mobile part of the greater curvature, or if they have a long pedicle, they can be everted through the gastric incision and presented to the peritoneal cavity. This approach has first been described by Morinaga et al. [15] for a tumor located near the gastroesophageal junction. Ma et al. [16] have reported a series of 56 cases of gastric GIST in which 19 patients underwent laparoscopic transgastric tumor-everting resections. They have even extended the indications of this technique to posterior wall tumors near the greater curvature in 5 cases. The key steps of the procedure are described in Table 19.2.

Discussion

Increased screening of the upper gastrointestinal tract has led to the discovery of a greater number of intragastric lesions. Despite the frequent benign nature of such lesions, complete tumor removal for pathological examination is recommended in order to rule out any underlying malignancy. Whenever endoscopic resection is not feasible, the conventional transperitoneal laparoscopic approach represents the next least invasive approach.

Ohashi described laparoscopic "intragastric" or "intraluminal" surgery in eight patients: six with early gastric cancer, one with submucosal leiomyoma, and one with a giant gastric polyp [1]. The current literature on intragastric multiport surgery focuses on lesions of the gastroesophageal junction which have heterogeneous origins (leiomyoma, GIST, T1a gastric cancer, etc.). In this technically challenging location, the multiport approach can be extremely useful, offering the advantage of improved triangulation of instruments in order to facilitate the dissection of the submucosal layer and suturing of the mucosa. Presently, most manuscripts on intragastric resection describe the placement of several ports into the gastric lumen [6, 17–20]. The particular combined laparoscopic and endoscopic approach with one intragastric port has been described by Lippert et al. [3]. Gastroscopy helped to intragastrically localize, visualize, and mobilize the tumor with a polypectomy snare. Resection can be performed by means of stapling under laparoscopic control. In 2 out of 7 patients, an additional 5 mm port was used to remove the tumor. Resection can be performed oncologically; however, full parietal wall resection might allow safe margins for large-based tumors. In such cases, this approach could well represent an alternative method of treatment as shown by Pfau et al. [13]. They have described the successful resection of a giant pedunculated mid-esophageal lipoma using a laparoscopic stapler through one of the two trocars placed transabdominally and intragastrically. The tumor (3.5 cm in diameter) was retrieved via an Endopouch® specimen retrieval bag and extracted through the intragastric laparoscopic port.

The transgastric route also allows the performance of submucosal resections. A potential perforation will be easily controlled using a laparoscopic approach at the end of the procedure. The need to approximate the mucosa to facilitate the healing process remains debatable. Closure of the mucosal defect might promote rapid healing as demonstrated by Yumiba et al. and could prevent an esophagogastric junction stricture [21]. Other authors such as Uchikoshi et al. [4] do not usually close mucosal defects with sutures unless uncontrollable bleeding is encountered. We prefer the use of full-thickness resections made possible by relying heavily on laparoscopic staplers.

Malignancy is of critical importance when it comes to this approach. It can sometimes be difficult to preoperatively determine whether tumors are benign or malignant, even from intraoperative frozen sections [22]. Major surgical resections would be excessive for a benign tumor. Llorente reported a case of gastric leiomyoma subjected to laparoscopic gastric resection [23]. Consequently, enucleation or ideally atypical partial resection must be considered for these patients. If the final pathology modifies the initial diagnosis and reveals a malignant lesion, a second-look operation is necessary [24].

An experience of 27 cases with 3 surgical approaches (open laparotomy, laparoscopic partial gastrectomy, and laparoscopic intragastric surgery) was reported by Hara et al. [5]. In this retrospective review, all gastric submucosal tumors were adjacent to the esophagogastric junction. Globally, intragastric surgery was preferred for lesions with intragastric growth, a standard laparoscopic approach was used in cases with transgastric or exogastric growth, and the open approach was selected for bulky lesions. Their completion rates were 50 % in the laparoscopic group and 90 % in the transgastric group, respectively. Additionally, the overall rate of cardia preservation was 80 % in the laparoscopic group, 100 % in the transgastric group, and 29 % in the open group, respectively. Although selection of the surgical approach based on the surgeon's choice represents the major bias of this manuscript, it demonstrates a significant benefit

of this new minimally invasive approach. This confirms that laparoscopic intragastric surgery offers the greatest advantage over a conventional resection for lesions at the gastroesophageal junction, as gastric resections in this area usually necessitate resection of the gastroesophageal junction. The size of the tumor is not a limitation per se. Laparoscopic intragastric surgery can be applied to large tumors and to those located near the cardia and pylorus as well as on the posterior wall of the stomach, where a conservative laparoscopic wedge resection is frequently not feasible. However, LIGS has no application for tumors on the anterior wall or showing extragastric growth as they can easily be resected by wedge resection, using the principles of triangular stapling.

After resection, specimen removal can be achieved through different ways. It has to be placed into a bag and should be removed through the mouth or should be placed into the abdominal cavity in order to be taken out in the same way as any laparoscopic surgical specimen. Small-sized specimens can even be extracted through a 12 mm port.

The perioperative management of these patients is simple and can follow the principles of early recovery after surgery (ERAS) or the principles used in bariatric surgery. No drain is inserted into the abdominal cavity, and the nasogastric tube is removed at the end of the surgical procedure. Patients are administered proton pump inhibitors (PPIs) intravenously or orally for 7 days. Liquid intake is allowed the day after surgery, and patients have their first meal on postoperative day 2. Patients receive a single shot of perioperative antibiotic prophylaxis. Total hospital stay lasts between 2 and 5 days depending on the type of resection as well as on potential resection-related hazards.

Conclusions

Laparoscopic intragastric surgery offers and can enhance the typical benefits of laparoscopic surgery such as reduced pain, faster recovery, and shorter length of hospital stay. The intragastric approach has reached a wide acceptance from advanced laparoscopic teams and should be systematically proposed as an alternative to other new minimally invasive approaches, including single-port surgery and natural orifice transluminal endoscopic surgery (NOTES) [25]. Based on our experience, intragastric surgery is ideally suited to address lesions located at the posterior or superior aspect of the stomach. Such lesions are frequently difficult or impossible to access via an endoscopic approach and would therefore require resection of the esophagogastric junction if addressed via a conventional laparoscopic or open approach. An adequate preoperative workup to precisely determine the optimal indication and strategy, including adequate position of intragastric ports, is crucial.

References

1. Ohashi S. Laparoscopic intraluminal (intragastric) surgery for early gastric cancer. A new concept in laparoscopic surgery. Surg Endosc. 1995;9:169–71.
2. Hiki Y, Sakuramoto S, Katada N, et al. Combined laparoscopic- endoscopic procedure in stomach carcinoma. Chirurg. 2000;71:1193–201.
3. Sahm M, Pross M, Lippert H. Intraluminal resection of gastric tumors using intragastric trocar technique. Surg Laparosc Endosc Percutan Tech. 2011;21:169–72.
4. Uchikoshi F, Ito T, Nishida T, Kitagawa T, Endo S, Matsuda H. Laparoscopic intragastric resection of gastric stromal tumor located at the esophago-cardiac junction. Surg Laparosc Endosc Percutan Tech. 2004;14:1–4.
5. Hara J, Nakajima K, Takahashi T, et al. Laparoscopic intragastric surgery revisited: its role for submucosal tumors adjacent to the esophagogastric junction. Surg Laparosc Endosc Percutan Tech. 2012;22:251–4.
6. Shim JH, Lee HH, Yoo HM. Intragastric approach for submucosal tumors located near the Zline: a hybrid laparoscopic and endoscopic technique. J Surg Oncol. 2011;104:312–5.
7. Na JU, Lee SI, Noh SM. The single incision laparoscopic intragastric wedge resection of gastric submucosal tumor. J Gastric Cancer. 2011;11:225–9.
8. El-Hayek K, Timratana P, Brethauer SA, Chand B. Complete endoscopic/transgastric retrieval of eroded gastric band: description of a novel technique and review of the literature. Surg Endosc. 2013;27(8):2974–9.
9. Son T, Inaba K, Woo Y, Pak KH, Hyung WJ, Noh SH. New surgical approach for gastric bezoar: "hybrid access surgery" combined intragastric and single port surgery. J Gastric Cancer. 2011;11:230–3.
10. Holeczy P, Danis J. Laparoscopic transgastric pancreatic pseudocystogastrostomy — first experience with

extraluminal approach. Hepatogastroenterology. 1998; 45:2215–8.
11. Geis WP, Baxt R, Kim HC. Benign gastric tumors. Minimally invasive approach. Surg Endosc. 1996;10: 407–10.
12. Watson DI, Game PA, Devitt PG. Laparoscopic resection of benign tumors of the posterior gastric wall. Surg Endosc. 1996;10:540–1.
13. Weigel TL, Schwartz DC, Gould JC, Pfau PR. Transgastric laparoscopic resection of a giant esophageal lipoma. Surg Laparosc Endosc Percutan Tech. 2005;15:160–2.
14. Li VK, Hung WK, Chung CK, et al. Laparoscopic intragastric approach for stromal tumours located at the posterior gastric wall. Asian J Surg. 2008;31:6–10.
15. Morinaga N, Sano A, Katayama K. Laparoscopic transgastric tumor-everting resection of the gastric submucosal tumor located near the esophagogastric junction. Surg Laparosc Endosc Percutan Tech. 2004;14: 344–8.
16. Ma JJ, Hu WG, Zang L, et al. Laparoscopic gastric resection approaches for gastrointestinal stromal tumors of stomach. Surg Laparosc Endosc Percutan Tech. 2011;21(2):101–5.
17. Ghushe ND, Dulai PS, Trus TL. Laparoendoscopic transgastric resection of a submucosal mass at the gastroesophageal junction. J Gastrointest Surg. 2012; 16:2321.
18. Heniford BT, Arca MJ, Walsh RM. The mini-laparoscopic intragastric resection of a gastroesophageal stromal tumor: a novel approach. Surg Laparosc Endosc Percutan Tech. 2000;10:82–5.
19. Choi YB, Oh ST. Laparoscopy in the management of gastric submucosal tumors. Surg Endosc. 2000;14: 741–5.
20. Ridwelski K, Pross M, Schubert S, et al. Combined endoscopic intragastral resection of a posterior stromal gastric tumor using an original technique. Surg Endosc. 2002;16:537.
21. Yumiba T, Ito T, Ikushima H, et al. Effect of mucosal suture on the healing of mucosal defect in laparoscopic intragastric surgery. Gastric Cancer. 2003;6:96–9.
22. Schiu M, Farr G, Papachristou DN, Hajdu S. Myosarcoma of the stomach: natural history, prognostic factors and management. Cancer. 1982;49: 177–87.
23. Llorente J. Laparoscopic gastric resection for gastric leiomyoma. Surg Endosc. 1994;8:887–9.
24. Taniguchi E, Kamiike W, Yamanishi H, Ito T, Nezu R, Nishida T, Momiyama T, Ohashi S, Okada T, Matsuda H. Laparoscopic intragastric surgery for gastric leiomyoma. Surg Endosc. 1997;11(3):287–9.
25. Asakuma M, Perretta S, Allemann P, Cahill R, Con SA, Solano C, Pasupathy S, Mutter D, Dallemagne B, Marescaux J. Challenges and lessons learned from NOTES cholecystectomy initial experience: a stepwise approach from the laboratory to clinical application. J Hepatobiliary Pancreat Surg. 2009;16(3):249–54.

Georgios Rossidis

Introduction

Laparoscopic partial gastrectomy, also called wedge gastrectomy, refers to resection of part of the stomach without the subsequent need for a gastrojejunostomy, in a laparoscopic fashion. It is an approach that has gained popularity for resection of lesions that are either benign (ulcers, polyps, cysts, leiomyomas, heterotopic pancreas) or malignant (gastrointestinal stromal tumors). The surgical approach to all submucosal stromal tumors is similar, and we will attempt to describe the laparoscopic approach to the resection of these lesions and the challenges associated with the size and anatomic location. The chapter will describe the surgical management of GIST tumors, the most common submucosal lesion of the stomach.

Since the first description of a laparoscopic resection of a submucosal tumor by Lukaszczyk and Preletz in 1992 [1], advances in laparoscopic techniques, instruments, and stapling devices have made the laparoscopic approach to a wedge resection safe, with excellent outcomes [2, 3], and is now the accepted treatment. The extremely rare lymph node metastasis and the need for only a grossly negative margin make the laparoscopic approach even more attractive. A study by DeMatteo et al. showed no survival advantage

between microscopically negative and the microscopically positive resections in tumors with macroscopically negative margins [4]. A partial gastrectomy without gastrojejunostomy confers the same progression-free survival as a more formal gastrectomy, with the added benefit of far lower postoperative morbidity and mortality. Initially, the laparoscopic approach was reserved for smaller tumors, in order to minimize the risk of tumor spillage and peritoneal seeding. The GIST Consensus Conference recommended that laparoscopic resection for gastric GISTs should be limited to tumors smaller than 2 cm [5]. More recent studies challenge this concept and show that laparoscopic approaches can provide comparable oncologic outcomes and better postoperative recovery, regardless of tumor size or location, when compared to open resections, even at sizes bigger than 5 cm [6]. The size of the tumor is not the only challenge to a successful laparoscopic resection. The location of the tumor can also be a formidable challenge to a laparoscopic approach especially for lesions located on the lesser curve and very close to the gastroesophageal junction (GEJ) or in the prepyloric antrum. Many authors have described these challenges and approaches to resections of these challenging tumors. Privette et al. proposed a classification scheme (Fig. 20.1), dividing the tumors into three types based on the anatomic location and offered distinct approaches for each type [7]. Song et al. published successful outcomes of ten patients with lesions very near the GEJ proving that a tailored laparoscopic approach

G. Rossidis, MD
Department of Surgery, University of Florida,
100286, Gainesville, FL 32610, USA
e-mail: georgios.rossidis@surgery.ufl.edu

for lesions near the GEJ can be feasible and safe [8]. Japanese authors have published a tailored approach to resection of GISTs based on the lesion's size, anatomic location, and growth (Fig. 20.2) [9]. The different surgical approaches will be described in detail.

Symptomatology and Diagnosis

While GISTs are rare with an annual incidence in the United States of 1,000–2,500 cases per year, they are still the most common non-adenomatous

lesion requiring gastric resection. The symptoms are usually related to the size and location of the tumor. Larger lesions usually present as a palpable tumor with symptoms of pressure and abdominal pain. Smaller lesions may present with acute upper GI blood loss or anemia and fatigue. Dysphagia may be the main symptom in lesions occurring at the gastroesophageal junction or at the pylorus. Many GISTs are asymptomatic and may be diagnosed during upper endoscopy for the workup of other conditions. Computed tomography and upper endoscopy are diagnostic for GISTs. The classic findings are a submucosal mass with smooth borders or a rounded appearance or an exophytic lesion. On endoscopy GISTs are firm, smooth, distinct, rounded, or lobulated submucosal lesions. The above findings are so characteristic that they exclude the need for a needle biopsy. Percutaneous biopsy is contraindicated also because of the risk of tumor spillage. In the case of large lesions in need for neoadjuvant therapy or with associated liver lesions suggestive of metastatic disease, endoscopic ultrasound (EUS)-guided needle biopsy may be warranted.

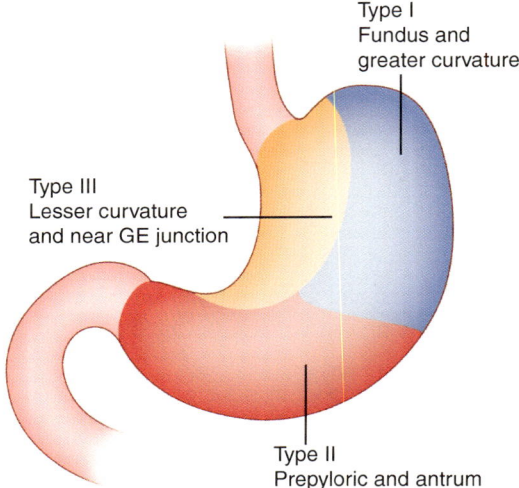

Fig. 20.1 Privette's anatomic classification of gastric lesions and the distinct surgical approach to them

Preoperative Planning

The patient's overall health status and medical conditions should be assessed, and cardiopulmonary comorbidities should be evaluated as for any other major abdominal procedure.

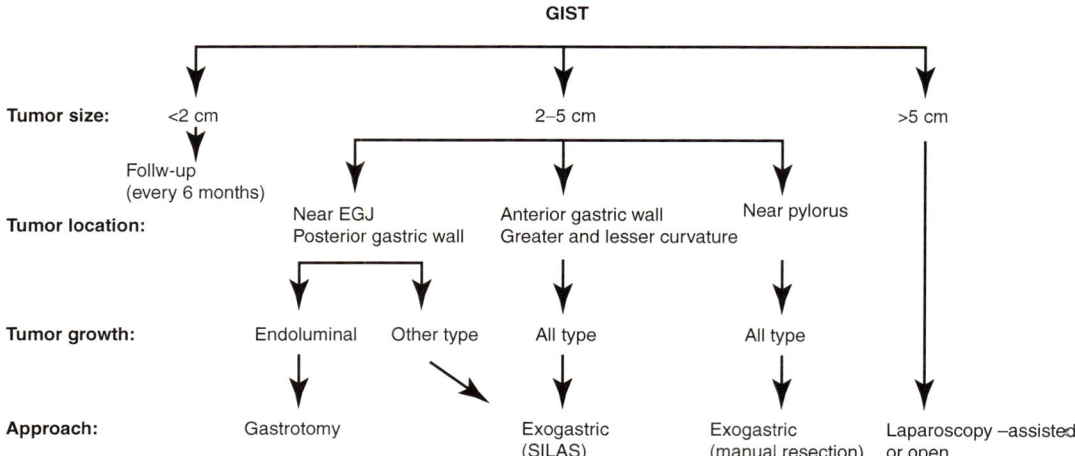

Fig. 20.2 Therapeutic strategy for suspected gastric GISTs (From Sasaki et al. [9], with permission)

Fig. 20.3 Patient positioning and position of primary and assistant surgeon

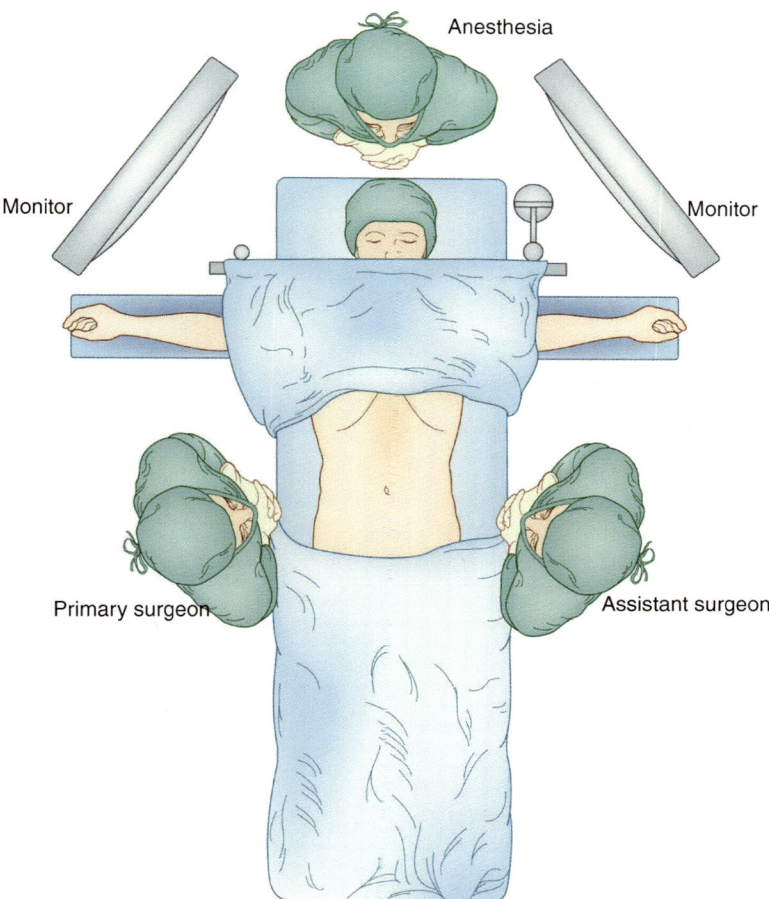

Previous abdominal procedures and operations should be noted, as intra-abdominal adhesions may make a laparoscopic approach far more challenging.

All the pertinent imaging and workup must be reviewed, and after a detailed discussion of all benefits, risks, and alternatives, an informed consent should be obtained.

Surgical Technique

The patient is placed in a supine position with both arms extended. The primary surgeon is positioned on the right side of the patient and the assistant surgery on the left side of the patient. Monitors are placed over the patient's shoulders bilaterally (Fig. 20.3). As with all foregut procedures, a footboard is placed at the patient's feet,

and the thighs and legs are strapped so as to support the patient during steep reverse Trendelenburg position (Fig. 20.4). A Foley catheter is inserted for precise urine output measurements, and an orogastric tube is inserted to decompress the stomach.

The different approaches shall be described based on the anatomic location of the lesion.

Fundus and Greater Curve

The trocar placement for lesions of the greater and lesser curve of the stomach is shown in Fig. 20.5. Access to the peritoneal cavity is obtained via the left subcostal incision with the use of an optical port under direct vision, and 15 mmHg of carbon dioxide is required to achieve pneumoperitoneum. The other ports are then

Fig. 20.4 A footboard and 2 straps support the patient during steep reverse Trendelenburg

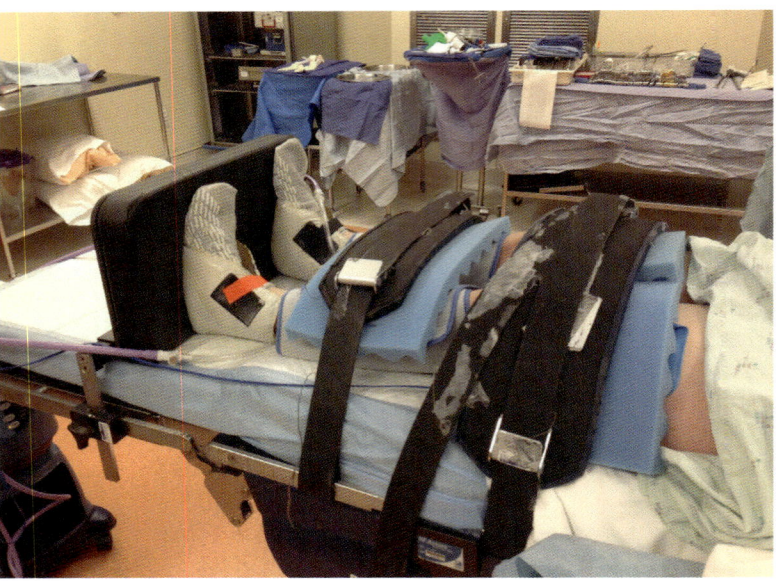

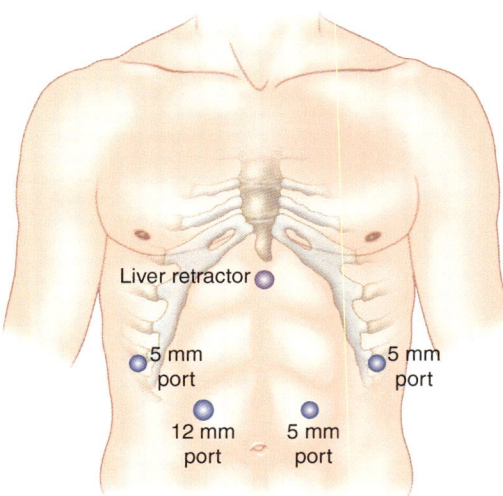

Fig. 20.5 Trocar placement for extragastric resection of lesions. The surgeon stands on the right side of the table and the assistant on the left

placed. The camera is inserted in the 5 mm port in the left upper quadrant. The peritoneal cavity is inspected, and the patient is placed in steep reverse Trendelenburg position to expose the stomach and the hiatus. A liver retractor is introduced in to the peritoneal cavity to elevate the left lobe of the liver to provide better visualization.

Intraoperative esophagogastroscopy is employed to identify the tumor and its exact location (especially for endophytic lesions) and also to ensure adequate margins. The short gastric vessels are divided with the use of a bipolar energy device with the surgeon retracting the stomach medially and the assistant retracting the omentum and the gastrosplenic ligament laterally. For an anterior wall lesion, the next step is to elevate the anterior wall with atraumatic graspers, and an endoscopic GIA stapler is passed under the tumor incorporating an adequate margin of normal gastric tissue to ensure negative margins (Fig. 20.6). The lesion is placed in a laparoscopic extraction bag. A non-touch lesion lifting method is described by Kiyozaki et al., where traction sutures are placed on the gastric wall over normal stomach 2 cm away from the lesion and are pulled out through the abdominal wall. Thus the tumor is lifted, and the GIA stapler is passed under the tumor to excise it [10]. This method allows the excision of the tumor with decreased risk of tumor spillage and also allows the resection the posterior gastric wall lesions. With adequate mobilization of the stomach, rotation of the stomach allows a posterior gastric wall lesion to face anteriorly and therefore to be removed as an anterior wall lesion.

Larger lesions that are endophytic, requiring more extensive resection, require the placement

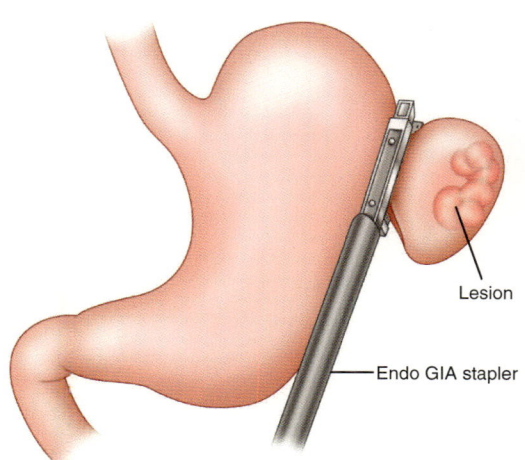

Fig. 20.6 Excision of greater curve lesion using an endoscopic GIA Stapler. Normal gastric tissue is incorporated to ensure negative margins

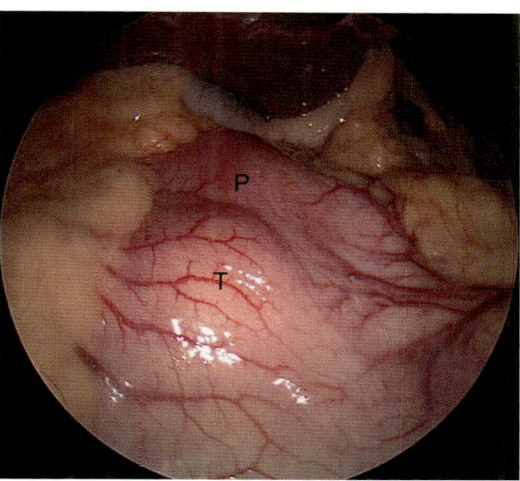

Fig. 20.7 A lesion located in close proximity to the pylorus. *T* tumor, *P* pylorus

of a bougie (40 Fr) to ensure luminal patency of the stomach post resection of the lesion.

Antrum/Prepyloric Region

While tumors in the distal stomach or prepyloric region can be excised with the method described above, tumors adjacent to the pylorus are more challenging, due to the difficulty in achieving negative margins without compromising the patency of the pylorus (Fig. 20.7). Posterior lesions limited to the mucosa or submucosa can be excised via an anterior gastrotomy. The access to the peritoneal cavity and port placement is as described above. Upper endoscopy can localize the lesion and assist with the location of the anterior gastrotomy. A horizontal anterior gastrotomy is performed with the use of electrocautery or ultrasonic shears and must be made no closer than 3–4 cm from the pylorus (Fig. 20.8). Traction sutures are placed proximal and distal to the mass, and the lesion is pulled out through the gastrotomy into the peritoneal cavity. The lesion is then removed with an endoscopic GIA stapler (Fig. 20.9). The horizontal incision is closed in a vertical fashion in order to not compromise the luminal diameter of the distal stomach. Traction

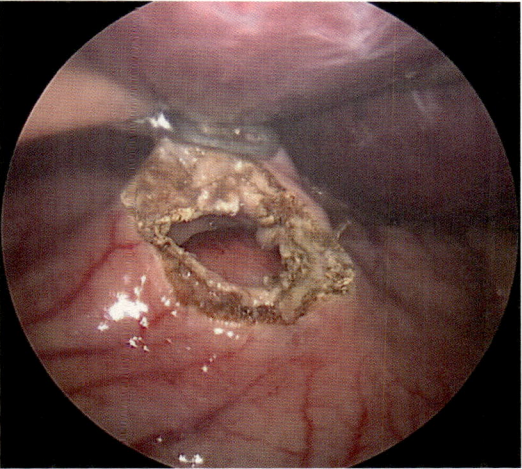

Fig. 20.8 Resection of prepyloric lesion. An anterior gastrotomy is created. The lesion can be seen in the gastric lumen

sutures are placed on the anterior gastric wall, and a GIA stapler is passed below them to staple the anterior defect (Fig. 20.10). The already placed endoscope is then utilized to assess the prepyloric area for bleeding, ensure the luminal patency, and rule out a staple line leak. Larger lesions or lesions that involve the pylorus may not be amenable to wedge gastrectomy, and a resection with reconstruction may be required to avoid stenosis of the gastric outlet.

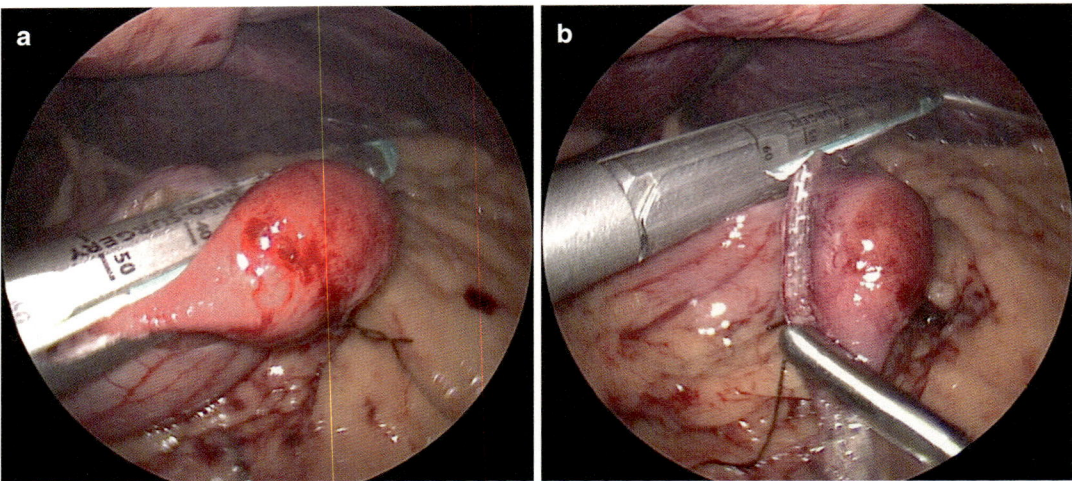

Fig. 20.9 (**a, b**) The lesion is pulled out through the gastrotomy into the peritoneal cavity and is then divided with an endoscopic GIA stapler

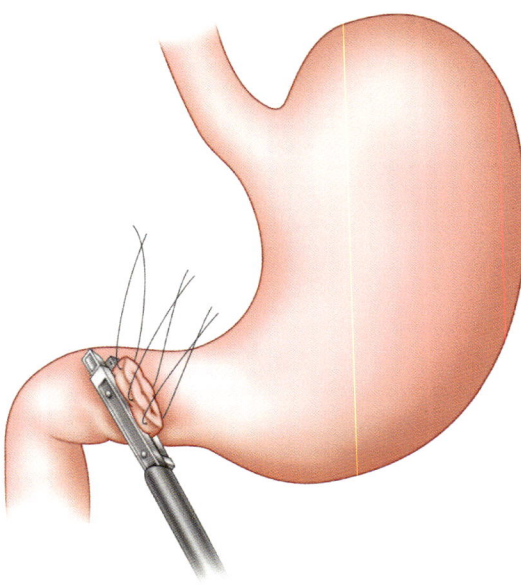

Fig. 20.10 The anterior gastrotomy is approximated with full-thickness sutures and is stapled off with the use of an endoscopic GIA staple

Lesser Curve/Gastroesophageal Junction

Lesser curvature lesions can be excised with the same method as described above for greater curve lesions. The hepatogastric ligament is divided with bipolar energy device, and branches of the left gastric artery and coronary vein are divided as well. Stay sutures placed proximal and distal to the lesion can lift the lesion, and an endoscopic GIA stapler is passed below the mass and the lesion is stapled off. The lesion is extracted in an extraction bag. Lesions near the GE junction can be managed in fashion similar to lesions near the pylorus, through a gastrotomy and subsequent resection [11]. Placement of a 40 Fr bougie during resection and closure will prevent narrowing of the gastric inlet. For lesions that are situated at the GE junction, laparoscopic resection becomes very challenging. Lesions that do not invade deep to the submucosa can be excised via enucleation through a combination of an endoscopic and transgastric laparoscopic approach. The lesion is first identified via upper endoscopy, and it is raised via endoscopic injection of dilute epinephrine. The stomach is then distended, and laparoscopic ports are inserted into the gastric lumen. A balloon tipped trocar is used to attach the stomach to the abdominal wall and allow the placement of the other trocars. With an angled laparoscope and electrocautery, the lesion is enucleated (Fig. 20.11) and retrieved via the mouth with the use of the endoscope. The mucosal defect is reapproximated with absorbable suture. The endoscope then confirms the

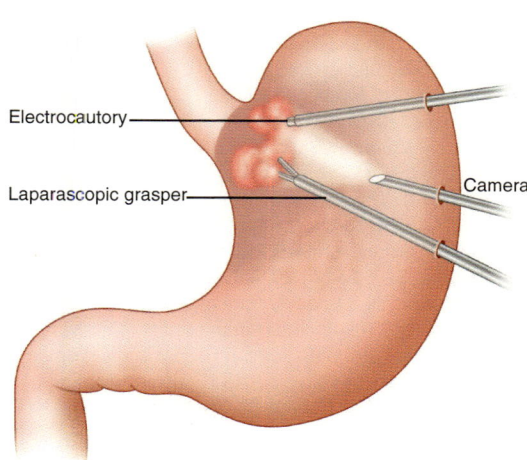

Electrocautory

Laparascopic grasper

Camera

Fig. 20.11 Lesions located at the GE junction can be excised via enucleation through transgastric ports and can be retrieved transorally with the use of an endoscope

patency of the gastroesophageal junction, hemostasis and rules out a leak at the area of resection.

Postoperative Care

Patients recover on the surgical ward unless comorbidities dictate a stay in an intermediate care or intensive care unit for better monitoring. The Foley catheter is removed, and the patient takes sips of water on postoperative day 1. For more complex resections at difficult anatomic locations or in the presence of larger lesions where extensive resection is required, an upper GI study to rule out a leak and to confirm luminal patency is performed. The patient is discharged on postoperative day 3 on full liquid diet, and the diet is advanced to a pure diet, to a soft diet, and ultimately to a regular diet at 2 weeks increments.

Outcomes

There is evidence to support that laparoscopic wedge gastrectomy can be performed safely and is reproducible. Novitsky et al. have published their outcomes showing no major postoperative complications or mortality, short hospitalization,

negative margins on all of their patients, and a long-term disease-free survival of 92 % [2]. Matsuhashi et al. published their experience and a literature review confirming the safety and reproducibility of laparoscopic wedge gastrectomy with sound oncologic outcomes [12]. A recent meta-analysis by Ohtani et al. including 644 patients showed that laparoscopic surgery for gastric GIST was associated with a reduction in intraoperative blood loss, shorter period to flatus, earlier resumption of oral intake, and shorter duration of hospital stay over the short term and with a significantly lower rate of overall recurrence, metastatic recurrence, and local recurrence in the long term compared to open surgery [13].

Conclusion

The recent technological strides in both laparoscopy and endoscopy allow surgeons to provide a minimally invasive approach for palliation and curative resection of gastric lesions. Advanced preoperative or intraoperative endoscopy allows the localization and characterization of gastric lesions at different locations. With the use of endoscopic, laparoscopic, and intragastric approaches, we can provide a minimally invasive approach for almost all gastric lesions amenable to a wedge resection. In combination with molecular targeted adjuvant therapy in the form of Imatinib, laparoscopic partial gastrectomy for GISTs can provide excellent outcomes and long-term survival.

References

1. Lukaszczyk JJ, Preletz RJ. Laparoscopic resection of benign stromal tumor of the stomach. J Laparoendosc Surg. 1992;2:331–4.
2. Novitsky YW, Kercher KW, Sing RF, Heniford BT. Long-term outcomes of laparoscopic resection of gastric gastrointestinal stromal tumors. Ann Surg. 2006;243:738–45; discussion 745–7.
3. Matthews BD, Walsh RM, Kercher KW, et al. Laparoscopic vs open resection of gastric stromal tumors. Surg Endosc. 2002;16:803–7.
4. DeMatteo RP, Lewis JJ, Leung D, Mudan SS, et al. Two hundred gastrointestinal stromal tumors:

recurrence patterns and prognostic factors for survival. Ann Surg. 2000;231:51–8.

5. Demetri GD, van Oosterom A, van Glabbeke M, et al. Consensus meeting for the management of gastrointestinal stromal tumors. Report of the GIST Consensus Conference of 20-21 March 2004, under the auspices of ESMO. Ann Oncol. 2005;16:566–78.

6. Lee HH, Hur H, Jung H, Park CH, et al. Laparoscopic wedge resection for gastric submucosal tumors: a size-location matched case–control study. J Am Coll Surg. 2011;212(2):195–9.

7. Privette A, McCahill L, Borrazzo E, et al. Laparoscopic approaches to resection of suspected gastric gastrointestinal stromal tumors based on tumor location. Surg Endosc. 2008;22:487–94.

8. Song KY, Kim SN, Park CH. Tailored-approach of laparoscopic wedge resection for treatment of submucosal tumor near the esophagogastric junction. Surg Endosc. 2007;21:2272–6.

9. Sasaki A, Koeda K, Obuchi T, Nakajima J, et al. Tailored laparoscopic resection for suspected gastric gastrointestinal stromal tumors. Surgery. 2010;147(4):516–20.

10. Kiyozaki H, Saito M, Chiba H, Takata O, et al. Laparoscopic wedge resection of the stomach for gastrointestinal stromal tumor (GIST): non-touch lesion lifting method. Gastric Cancer. 2014;17:337–40.

11. Sakamoto Y, Sakaguchi Y, Akimoto H, Chinen Y, et al. Safe laparoscopic resection of a gastric gastrointestinal stromal tumor close to the esophagogastric junction. Surg Today. 2012;42(7):708–11.

12. Matsuhashi N, Osada S, Yamaguchi K, Okumura N, et al. Long-term outcomes of treatment of gastric gastrointestinal stromal tumor by laparoscopic surgery. Hepatogastroenterology. 2013 [Epub ahead of print].

13. Ohtani H, Maeda K, Noda E, Nagahara H, et al. Meta-analysis of laparoscopic and open surgery for gastric gastrointestinal stromal tumor. Anticancer Res. 2013; 33(11):5031–41.

Principles and Practice of Laparoscopic Gastrectomy with Gastroduodenostomy (Billroth I)

21

Sang-Hoon Ahn and Hyung-Ho Kim

Introduction

Since Kitano first performed laparoscopic distal gastrectomy (LDG) for early gastric cancer in 1991, it has become a popular procedure for gastric cancer resection. However, LDG is a complex, technically demanding procedure, and the learning curve for its use on early gastric cancer is thought to require experiences with more than 40–50 cases [1, 2]. In addition to an experience, a surgeon would require an excellent surgical team, proper equipment, and a good facility to obtain a consistently good result from LDG.

Because it restores normal bowel continuity, Billroth I gastroduodenostomy is the most physiologic type of gastric resection. It is one of the most common types of reconstruction after distal gastrectomy. The advantages of Billroth I over Billroth II or Roux-en-Y gastrojejunostomy are the short surgical time, preservation of the physiologic passage

of food, and avoidance of gastrojejunostomy-related postgastrectomy syndrome (e.g., the afferent loop syndrome). According to the Korean Laparoscopic Gastrointestinal Surgery Study Group (KLASS) survey, 63.4 % of all distal gastrectomies performed in 2009 were Billroth I reconstructions [3].

Using LDG, Billroth I gastroduodenostomy can be performed extracorporeally or intracorporeally. Recently, LDG with intracorporeal anastomosis, such as intracorporeal Billroth I anastomosis (delta-shaped anastomosis) and intracorporeal uncut Roux-en-Y gastrojejunostomy, has become a popular procedure [4, 5]. We call this procedure a totally laparoscopic distal gastrectomy (TLDG). In this chapter, the current techniques of LDG with Billroth I anastomosis, including the details and advantages and disadvantages of each technique, are discussed.

Indications

LDG is usually indicated for gastric cancer, which requires lymphadenectomy, and for peptic ulcer disease and submucosal gastric tumors, which do not require lymphadenectomy. Billroth I anastomosis is usually performed for gastric cancer with negative proximal margins in the distal third of the stomach, indicating complete tumor excision. It is also indicated for type I gastric ulcer.

Electronic supplementary material Supplementary material is available in the online version of this chapter at 10.1007/978-3-319-09342-0_21. Videos can also be accessed at http://www.springerimages.com/videos/978-3-319-09341-3.

S.-H. Ahn, MD • H.-H. Kim, MD, PhD (✉)
Department of Surgery, Seoul National University
Bundang Hospital,
300 Gumi-dong, Bundang-gu, Seongnam, Gyeonggi
463-708, Republic of Korea
e-mail: viscaria@snubh.org; hhkim@snubh.org

Contraindication

Contraindications include severe cardiopulmonary disease, hemodynamically unstable patients, and detection of advanced gastric cancer during the preoperative workup. Relative contraindications include duodenal ulcer, duodenal ulcer scar, and tumor invasion into the pylorus.

Preoperative Preparation

In general, preoperative nasogastric tube insertion and preoperative bowel preparation are not mandatory.

Anesthesia and Antibiotic Coverage

General anesthesia with endotracheal intubation and muscle relaxants are usually used. Spinal or epidural anesthesia can be used; however, supplementation with intravenous sedative may be indicated to prevent nausea during bowel manipulation. A first-generation cephalosporin is administered for 24 h as prophylactic antibiotic coverage.

Position

The patient is placed in the supine position with the right arm at a right angle and the left arm placed alongside the body. The patient is then moved into a reverse Trendelenburg position with a 10–30° tilt. In some cases, a lithotomy position with reverse Trendelenburg is preferable, especially for single-incision laparoscopic distal gastrectomy.

Generally, the operator and scopist sit on the patient's right side, and the first assistant sits on the patient's left side. Sitting during the operation is recommended to reduce surgeon fatigue and to allow for more stable movement of equipment with reduced tremor.

Operative Equipment

- 10-mm, 30° or 45° rigid scope or flexible high-definition (HD) scope

  – An HD camera is mandatory in laparoscopic gastrectomy, and a flexible HD scope is preferred because it can visualize the entire intra-abdominal space, especially during suprapancreatic lymph node dissection.
- 5–12 mm trocars
- Video system
- Energy device (e.g., harmonic scalpel and LigaSure)
- Hemoclips
- Linear (45 and 60 mm) or circular staplers (29 or 31 mm)
- The skin is prepared in a routine manner.

Incision and Exposure

To introduce the first trocar, Hasson's open technique, which involves direct open visualization of the tissues, is the safest. With a No. 11 blade, the infraumbilical incision, including the half below the umbilicus, is created. The subcutaneous fat tissue is then dissected with a mosquito clamp. The rectus fascia is clamped with mosquito clamps and lifted. The fascia is divided using an electrocautery without exposing the rectus muscle because the incision is close to the umbilicus. Finally, a Kelly clamp is gently introduced along the anterior peritoneum until some resistance is felt, but the peritoneum is easily opened. An 11- or 12-mm trocar can be inserted after confirming that the peritoneal cavity is opened. At this point, there should be no resistance while inserting the trocar.

The peritoneal cavity is insufflated with carbon dioxide at a pressure of 10–13 mmHg. Tilting the operation table to the right or left side 10–20° may help exposure if necessary. A laparoscope is inserted through the port, and four more 5–12-mm trocars are placed on the upper abdominal wall under direct visualization. All trocars are inserted a fist's distance apart to avoid interference, and they are positioned on the lateral side of the rectus muscle so laparoscopic instruments cannot to be manipulated vertically or in mirror image. The left hand 5-mm trocar is inserted on the lateral portion of the rectus muscle. It is positioned between the rectus muscle's lateral border and the anterior axillary line according to the preference of the

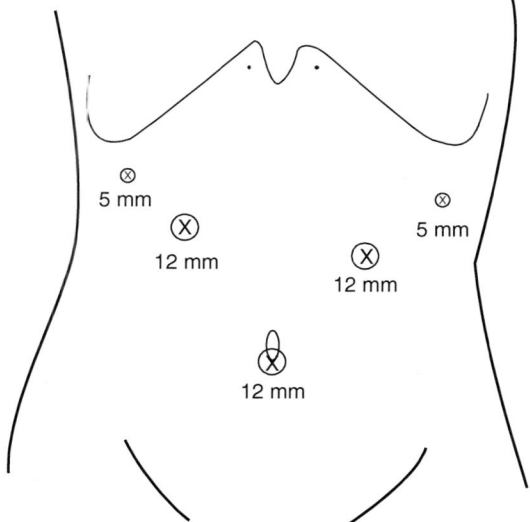

Fig. 21.1 Ports placement. Three 12-mm trocars are used for ports

operator. When an intracorporeal Billroth I anastomosis is performed, a 12-mm trocar is needed in the assistant's left hand to introduce a linear stapler for the duodenum transection and anastomosis (Fig. 21.1).

Detailed Procedure: Intracorporeal Delta-Shaped Anastomosis (Video 21.1)

Due to advances in technology and surgical techniques, the use of extracorporeal anastomosis is gradually shifting toward intracorporeal anastomosis. Several techniques for intracorporeal Billroth I anastomosis using a linear stapler, circular stapler, or hand-sewing technique have been reported in the literature. Among them, a linear stapler has several advantages over the other methods. It requires only a 12-mm trocar, which is easy to handle, and has three staple lines, which is thought to be more secure than the two staple lines created by a circular stapler.

There are several linear stapler techniques: the delta-shaped anastomosis [6], the triangulating-stapling technique [7], the bookbinding technique [8], and the linear gastroduodenostomy [9]. The delta-shaped anastomosis is a representative

of intracorporeal Billroth I anastomosis, which is a functional end-to-end gastroduodenostomy technique using linear staplers [6, 7, 9, 10]. Here, we describe the delta-shaped Billroth I anastomosis because it is the most popular and is easier technically (Table 21.1):

1. *Liver retraction*
    A. Because the left lobe of the liver overlies most of the lesser curvature of the stomach and the lesser omentum, liver retraction is absolutely necessary for a TLDG and intracorporeal anastomosis.
    B. Begin by penetrating a 2-0 straight Prolene needle into the abdomen just below the xiphoid in the midline (on the left side of the falciform ligament). Then, insert the needle from the peritoneal cavity to the outside of the body at the right upper epigastrium (on the right side of the falciform ligament). Clip the middle portion of the suture twice with a mid pars condensa. A gauze is placed between the liver and the suture to protect the liver. Both ends of the suture are pulled and are grasped snugly over the skin of the anterior abdominal wall with a mosquito clamp. This results in a V-shaped sling that retracts the liver cranially and anteriorly (Fig. 21.2) [20].

2. *Duodenum transection* (Fig. 21.3)
    A. After mobilization of the gastroduodenum, the duodenum is transected just below the pylorus using a linear stapler (blue or purple cartridge). A sufficient length of duodenum is required. To make the duodenal stump, a Kocher maneuver is sometimes required prior to the anastomosis to minimize tension on the anastomosis. Clearing adhesions on the transverse colon, hepatoduodenal ligament, gallbladder, and pancreas head is recommended
    B. The stapler is introduced through the left lower 12-mm port with the stapler directed posteroanteriorly instead of the usual craniocaudal direction. (Its direction is rotated 90° compared to the usual position. This can facilitate a favorable blood supply to the anastomosis and provides a wider space for the manipulation of the anvil side of a 45-mm linear stapler.

Table 21.1 Brief summary of published reports on intracorporeal Billroth I anastomosis

Author	Year	Staplers	The details of Billroth I anastomosis	Number of cases	Complications	Conclusions
Kanaya et al. [6]	2002	Linear	Delta shaped	9	No complications as a result of the anastomosis	Safe and feasible
Kim et al. [11]	2008	Linear	Delta shaped	25	12 % ($n=3$) 1 anastomotic leakage, 1 anastomotic stenosis, and 1 delayed gastric emptying	Safe and feasible
Tanimura et al. [12]	2008	Linear	Triangulating stapling	81	1 anastomotic leakage	Safe and feasible
Song et al. [13]	2008	Linear	Delta shaped	20	1 intra-abdominal bleeding	Shorter bowel recovery than extracorporeal anastomosis
Kinoshita et al. [14]	2011	Linear	Delta shaped	42	14.3 % ($n=6$) No leakage	Faster recovery than extracorporeal
Kim et al. [15, 16]	2011	Linear	Delta shaped	339/239	3.9 % ($n=9$) 2 anastomotic leakage, 1 anastomotic bleeding 3.5 % ($n=12$) 1 anastomotic leakage, 1 anastomotic bleeding	Better early surgical outcomes than extracorporeal anastomosis, especially in obese patients
Kanaya et al. [17]	2011	Linear	Delta shaped	100	1 minor anastomotic leakage	Mean follow-up 54.9 months, satisfactory outcomes
Lee et al. [18]	2011	Linear	Delta shaped	26	3.9 % ($n=1$) 1 anastomotic bleeding	Feasible and safe
Omori et al. [19]	2012	Circular	Delta shaped (single-incision laparoscopic distal gastrectomy)	20	No postoperative complications	Safe and feasible
Ikeda et al. [8]	2013	Linear	Bookbinding technique	10	No complications	Feasible and safe
Omori et al. [10]	2013	Linear	Triangulating stapling (single-incision laparoscopic distal gastrectomy)	45	No anastomotic complications	Safe and feasible

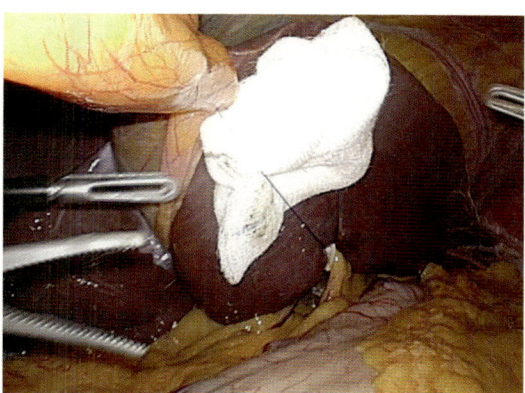

Fig. 21.2 Combined retraction of the falciform ligament and the left lateral lobe of the liver

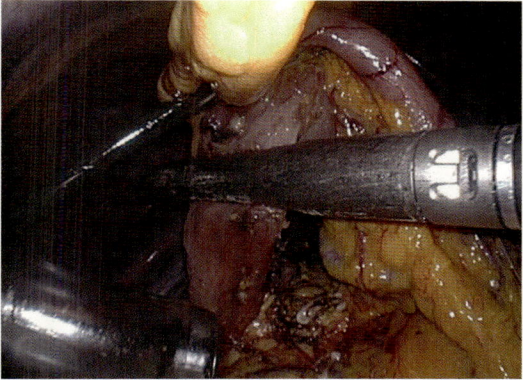

Fig. 21.3 Duodenum transection in a vertical direction through the 12 mm port of assistant

C. Check the color of the duodenal stump. If the blood supply to the duodenal stump is poor, immediately convert to a Billroth II or Roux-en-Y gastrojejunostomy after using an additional linear stapler to transect the duodenal portion receiving the poor blood supply.

3. *Tumor localization and stomach transection*
   A. After complete D1+ or D2 lymphadenectomy is performed, the stomach is transected. If the tumor is located below the angle, the proximal stomach is transected immediately above the angle without checking the location of tumor.
   B. If the tumor is located above the angle of the stomach, it is difficult to make an accurate proximal resection line because the lesion cannot be palpated or visualized. In this case, the location of lesion can be confirmed by intraoperative endoscopy or comparing the location between the endoscopic clips and the laparoscopic clips using intraoperative X-ray [21, 22].
   C. The proximal stomach is transected from the greater curvature by linear stapler (blue or gold or purple cartridge). Two linear staplers are enough to transect the stomach in most cases.

4. *Specimen delivery and check of the resection margins*
   A. The specimen is removed through the extension of the umbilical port after placing it in a plastic bag. The plastic bag allows the prevention of wound infection and potential implantation of tumor cells. In most cases, a 3–4-cm-long skin incision with a wound protector is sufficient to deliver the specimen.

5. *Stomach opening* (Fig. 21.4)
   A. A small opening on the greater curvature side of the remnant stomach is made using a laparoscopic electrocautery or harmonic scalpel. We recommend a harmonic scalpel to open the stomach because one full bite of a harmonic scalpel is appropriately the length of the opening, does not cause any bleeding, and leaves a "dog ear" that can be subsequently used for pulling the stomach.
   B. After the formation of the stomach opening, aspirate the intraluminal contents of the stomach using a suction device to prevent a spillage of the bowel contents. Sometimes, irrigation of the remnant stomach is recommended to reduce the potentially existing cancer free cells.

6. *Duodenum opening* (Fig. 21.4)
   A. The small opening on the posterior side of the duodenal stump is made using a laparoscopic electrocautery. We recommend hook or endo-shear with electrocautery to make a sharp incision on the duodenal edge, which is important to avoid creating a large opening. This is an important tip for creating the delta-shaped anastomosis.

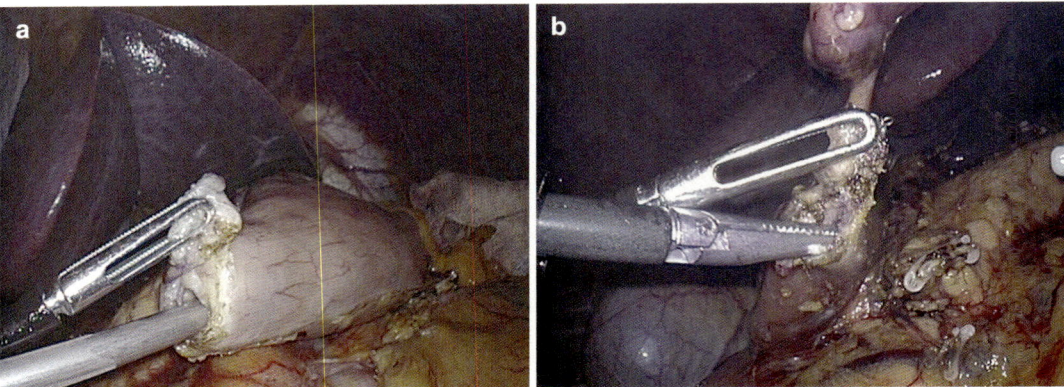

Fig. 21.4 (**a**) Formation of the stomach opening, (**b**) Formation of the duodenal opening

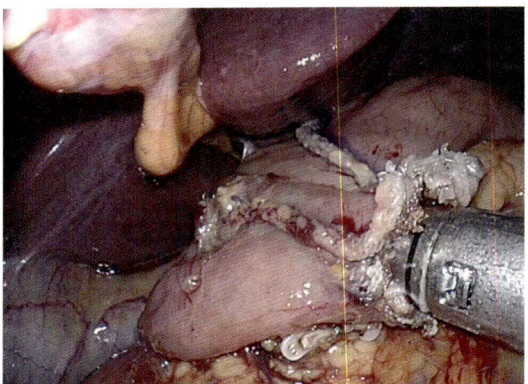

Fig. 21.5 Side-to-side gastroduodenostomy between the posterior wall of the stomach and the posterosuperior wall of the duodenum

7. *Linear stapler insertion* (Fig. 21.5)
   A. A 45-mm linear stapler (blue or purple cartridge) is inserted through the left lower 12-mm trocar.
   B. After open the linear stapler, the stapler side is inserted into the opening in the stomach in a manner similar to pulling up socks.
      (i) Place the end of the staple side into the opening of the stomach:
      (ii) Pull the dog ear of the stomach hole with the grasper.
      (iii) After full insertion of stapler, the staple line on the stomach is rotated to the left side by the operator's two graspers, and then the assistant grasps and pulls the midportion of the staple line to maintain the position of insertion and rotation.

C. The jaw of the linear stapler is then closed to avoid slipping of the stomach. The linear stapler is moved close to the duodenal hole with the stapler closed.
   (i) Place the end of the anvil of the stapler into the opening of the duodenum.
   (ii) Both the distal part and the staple side of the duodenum are grasped by the operator, and then the duodenum is pulled to the anvil. The anvil should not be pushed or thrust to the duodenum.
D. Before firing, the operator rotates the staple line of the duodenal stump to the right side, and the assistant rotates the staple line of the stomach to the left side to form a side-to-side gastroduodenostomy between the posterior wall of the remnant stomach and the posterosuperior wall of the duodenum.
E. The linear stapler is fired by the assistant after waiting for 15 s.
8. *Common entry hole closure* (Fig. 21.6)
   A. After firing the stapler, a common entry hole is made. Check the staple line for anastomotic bleeding through this hole.
   B. The operator retracts both ends of the previous stapling. The common entry hole is then closed with one or two consecutive firings of 60-mm linear staplers. There is another method. After transient approximation of the entry hole using 3 stay sutures (on both ends of the previous stapling and the midportion), the operator retracts two sutures, and the assistant retracts one suture.

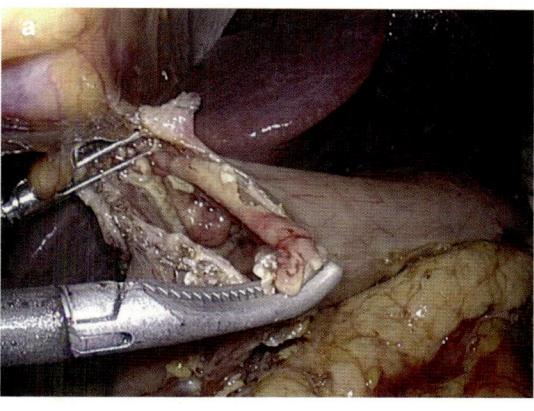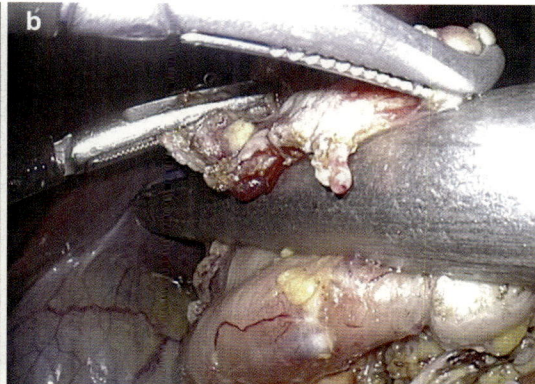

Fig. 21.6 (**a**) Retraction of both ends of the previous stapling by the operator's grasper. (**b**) Closure of the common entry hole using a 60 mm linear stapler

This retraction of the stay sutures allows horizontal alignment of the common entry hole.

C. We recommend placement of reinforcement sutures on the greater curvature side where there is maximum anastomotic tension.

Brief Description: Extracorporeal Billroth I Reconstruction

Extracorporeal Billroth I anastomosis has several advantages over intracorporeal anastomosis. It allows the proximal stomach to be accurately transected because the lesion can be palpated or visualized through the gastrotomy, and it requires fewer staples than an intracorporeal anastomosis. It is disadvantageous because it has to be performed in a narrow space, is technically difficult in obese patients, and sometimes causes severe postoperative pain at the mini-laparotomy site. We briefly discuss the extracorporeal end-to-side posterior wall anastomosis [1]:

1. *Mini-laparotomy*
   A. A 4–5-cm upper transverse incision is made at the right epigastrium. A plastic wound retractor is recommended to prevent wound infection.
2. *Duodenum transection*
   A. After complete retrieval of the duodenum from the abdominal cavity, a purse-string clamp is applied to the duodenum 1 or

2 cm distal to the pylorus, and a 2-0 straight Prolene needle is inserted through the purse-string clamp. A nylon tape is tied just proximal to the purse-string clamp to prevent spillage from the stomach, and the duodenum is divided.

3. *Anvil placement into the duodenal stump*
   A. After the division of the duodenum, the proximal gastroduodenum is placed into the abdominal cavity. This procedure provides a large working space without interference from the gastroduodenum. The anvil of a circular stapler is inserted into the duodenal stump, and a purse-string suture is tied over the anvil. Endoloop reinforcement is sometimes useful to secure the purse-string suture.
4. *Tumor localization and stomach transection*
   A. The proper line for the proximal resection is confirmed by palpation or direct visualization of the endoscopic intragastric clip, which was placed preoperatively.
   B. The stomach is transected from the greater curvature to the midpoint of the section line using a Kelly clamp and an Allen clamp. The remaining proximal stomach (the lesser curvature side) is divided using a linear stapler.
5. *Extracorporeal end to posterior wall of the stomach Billroth I*
   A. After the resected stomach and lymph nodes are removed, the body of a circular stapler (29 or 31 mm) is inserted into the

remnant stomach through the opening, which was previously closed with an Allen clamp.

B. The central rod is advanced to penetrate the posterior-greater curvature side wall of the stomach and then connected to the anvil previously placed in the duodenum. At least 3 cm in length is needed from the proposed closure line of the opening.

C. After the circular stapler is closed and fired, the anastomotic staple line through the opening of the stomach is checked for bleeding.

6. *Closure of the stomach opening*

A. After the opening of the remnant stomach is roughly closed with three Allis clamps, it is completely closed using additional linear staplers.

References

1. Lee SI, Choi Y-S, Park DJ, Kim HH, Yang H-K, Kim MC. Comparative study of laparoscopy-assisted distal gastrectomy and open distal gastrectomy. J Am Coll Surg. 2006;202:874–80. doi:10.1016/j.jamcollsurg.2006.02.028.

2. Kim MC, Jung G-J, Kim HH. Learning curve of laparoscopy-assisted distal gastrectomy with systemic lymphadenectomy for early gastric cancer. World J Gastroenterol. 2005;11:7508–11.

3. Jeong O, Park Y-K. Clinicopathological features and surgical treatment of gastric cancer in South Korea: the results of 2009 nationwide survey on surgically treated gastric cancer patients. J Gastric Cancer. 2011;11:69–77. doi:10.5230/jgc.2011.11.2.69.

4. Ahn S-H, Son S-Y, Lee C-M, Jung H, Park DJ, Kim HH. Intracorporeal uncut Roux-en-Y gastrojejunostomy reconstruction in pure single-incision laparoscopic distal gastrectomy for early gastric cancer: unaided stapling closure. J Am Coll Surg. 2014;218:e17–21. doi:10.1016/j.jamcollsurg.2013.09.009.

5. Hosogi H, Kanaya S. Intracorporeal anastomosis in laparoscopic gastric cancer surgery. J Gastric Cancer. 2012;12:133–9. doi:10.5230/jgc.2012.12.3.133.

6. Kanaya S, Gomi T, Momoi H, Tamaki N, Isobe H, Katayama T, Wada Y, Ohtoshi M. Delta-shaped anastomosis in totally laparoscopic Billroth I gastrectomy: new technique of intraabdominal gastroduodenostomy. J Am Coll Surg. 2002;195:284–7.

7. Tanimura S, Higashino M, Fukunaga Y, Kishida S, Nishikawa M, Ogata A, Osugi H. Laparoscopic distal gastrectomy with regional lymph node dissection for gastric cancer. Surg Endosc. 2005;19:1177–81. doi:10.1007/s00464-004-8936-4.

8. Ikeda T, Kawano H, Hisamatsu Y, Ando K, Saeki H, Oki E, Ohga T, Kakeji Y, Tsujitani S, Kohnoe S, Maehara Y. Progression from laparoscopic-assisted to totally laparoscopic distal gastrectomy: comparison of circular stapler (i-DST) and linear stapler (BBT) for intracorporeal anastomosis. Surg Endosc. 2013;27:325–32. doi:10.1007/s00464-012-2433-y.

9. Song HM, Lee SL, Hur H, Cho YK, Han SU. Linear-shaped gastroduodenostomy in totally laparoscopic distal gastrectomy. J Gastric Cancer. 2010;10:69–74. doi:10.5230/jgc.2010.10.2.69.

10. Omori T, Masuzawa T, Akamatsu H, Nishida T. A simple and safe method for Billroth I reconstruction in single-incision laparoscopic gastrectomy using a novel intracorporeal triangular anastomotic technique. J Gastrointest Surg. 2013;18:1–4. doi:10.1007/s11605-013-2419-7.

11. Kim J-J, Song KY, Chin HM, Kim W, Jeon HM, Park CH, Park SM. Totally laparoscopic gastrectomy with various types of intracorporeal anastomosis using laparoscopic linear staplers: preliminary experience. Surg Endosc. 2008;22:436–42. doi:10.1007/s00464-007-9446-y.

12. Tanimura S, Higashino M, Fukunaga Y, Takemura M, Nishikawa T, Tanaka Y, Fujiwara Y, Osugi H. Intracorporeal Billroth 1 reconstruction by triangulating stapling technique after laparoscopic distal gastrectomy for gastric cancer. Surg Laparosc Endosc Percutan Tech. 2008;18:54–8. doi:10.1097/SLE.0b013e3181568e63.

13. Song KY, Park CH, Kang HC, Kim J-J, Park SM, Jun KH, Chin HM, Hur H. Is totally laparoscopic gastrectomy less invasive than laparoscopic-assisted gastrectomy?: prospective, multicenter study. J Gastrointest Surg. 2008;12:1015–21. doi:10.1007/s11605-008-0484-0.

14. Kinoshita T, Shibasaki H, Oshiro T, Ooshiro M, Okazumi S, Katoh R. Comparison of laparoscopy-assisted and total laparoscopic Billroth-I gastrectomy for gastric cancer: a report of short-term outcomes. Surg Endosc. 2011;25:1395–401. doi:10.1007/s00464-010-1402-6.

15. Kim MG, Kawada H, Kim BS, Kim TH, Kim KC, Yook JH, Kim BS. A totally laparoscopic distal gastrectomy with gastroduodenostomy (TLDG) for improvement of the early surgical outcomes in high BMI patients. Surg Endosc. 2011;25:1076–82. doi:10.1007/s00464-010-1319-0.

16. Kim MG, Kim KC, Kim BS, Kim TH, Kim HS, Yook JH, Kim BS. A totally laparoscopic distal gastrectomy can be an effective way of performing laparoscopic gastrectomy in obese patients (body mass index ≥ 30). World J Surg. 2011;35:1327–32. doi:10.1007/s00268-011-1034-6.

17. Kanaya S, Kawamura Y, Kawada H, Iwasaki H, Gomi T, Satoh S, Uyama I. The delta-shaped anastomosis in laparoscopic distal gastrectomy: analysis of the initial 100 consecutive procedures of intracorporeal gastroduodenostomy. Gastric Cancer. 2011;14:365–71. doi:10.1007/s10120-011-0054-0.

18. Lee HW, Kim H-I, An JY, Cheong J-H, Lee KY, Hyung WJ, Noh SH. Intracorporeal anastomosis using linear stapler in laparoscopic distal gastrectomy: comparison between gastroduodenostomy and gastrojejunostomy. J Gastric Cancer. 2011;11:212–8. doi:10.5230/jgc.2011.11.4.212.

19. Omori T, Tanaka K, Tori M, Ueshima S, Akamatsu H, Nishida T. Intracorporeal circular-stapled Billroth I anastomosis in single-incision laparoscopic distal gastrectomy. Surg Endosc. 2012;26:1490–4. doi:10.1007/s00464-011-2034-1.

20. Shabbir A, Lee JH, Lee M-S, Park do J, Kim HH. Combined suture retraction of the falciform ligament and the left lobe of the liver during laparoscopic total gastrectomy. Surg Endosc. 2010;24:3237–40. doi:10.1007/s00464-010-1118-7.

21. Kim H-I, Hyung WJ, Lee CR, Lim JS, An JY, Cheong J-H Choi SH, Noh SH. Intraoperative portable abdominal radiograph for tumor localization: a simple and accurate method for laparoscopic gastrectomy. Surg Endosc. 2011;25:958–63. doi:10.1007/s00464-010-1288-3.

22. Park DJ, Lee HJ, Kim SG, Jung HC, Song IS, Lee KU, Choe EJ, Yang HK. Intraoperative gastroscopy for gastric surgery. Surg Endosc. 2005;19:1358–61. doi:10.1007/s00464-004-2217-0.

Joshua Ellenhorn

Clinical Studies

Laparoscopic surgical procedures have been successfully adopted for abdominal surgery because of their favorable effects on pain, postoperative recovery, pulmonary function, and incision-related complications [1, 2]. Laparoscopic resection for colorectal cancer has become a standard of care based on the positive results of several randomized trials [3–5]. Despite early concerns about the adequacy of resection for oncologic indications, clinical studies have demonstrated that laparoscopic resections for abdominal malignancy can be performed with equivalent extent of resection compared to open resection. Clinical studies in pancreatic [6], cervical [7], endometrial [8], colorectal [2], prostate [9], and renal carcinoma [10] have demonstrated that the laparoscopic approach yields similar margins and nodal clearance to open surgery. Survival rates are also similar to that seen in traditional open surgery.

For gastric adenocarcinoma, minimally invasive techniques have been adopted relatively slowly. Kitano et al. reported the first laparoscopic-assisted gastrectomy with lymphadenectomy over two decades ago [11]. However, despite encouraging results, laparoscopic resection for gastric cancer is only now gaining acceptance in North America. Concerns about technical difficulty, completeness of resection and adequacy of lymphadenectomy have limited enthusiasm for laparoscopic gastrectomy.

The first and only prospective randomized trial comparing laparoscopic to open gastrectomy in a Western country was published in 2005 [12]. In the small trial, Huscher et al. randomized 59 patients with gastric cancer to laparoscopic or open gastrectomy. The laparoscopic approach was associated with a decreased estimated blood loss, earlier oral intake, and a shorter hospital stay. There was no difference in lymph node count suggesting that the laparoscopic approach did not compromise the adequacy of resection. There was no difference in 5-year disease-free or overall survival [12].

Several prospective randomized trials comparing laparoscopic to open resection have been conducted in Asia. The largest of these is the Korean Laparoscopic Gastrointestinal Surgery Study (KLASS) Group trial with over 1,400 patients recruited [13]. The main endpoint of the trial is survival which has not yet been published. Interim analysis revealed no difference in morbidity or mortality between the groups [14]. In another Korean study, 82 patients were randomized to open gastrectomy and 82 to laparoscopic resection

Electronic supplementary material Supplementary material is available in the online version of this chapter at 10.1007/978-3-319-09342-0_22. Videos can also be accessed at http://www.springerimages.com/videos/978-3-319-09341-3.

J. Ellenhorn, MD
Department of Surgery, Cedars-Sinai Medical Center, 8635 West Third Street, Suite 880 West, Los Angeles, CA 90048, USA
e-mail: dr@ellenhornmd.com

Table 22.1 Summary of randomized trials

Author	Year	Lap	Open	Adequacy of resection	Results for lap group	Survival
Kitano et al. [11]	2002	14[a]	14	Identical	Less EBL and pain, earlier recovery of bowel function	na
Hayashi et al. [16]	2005	14[a]	14	Equally radical	Shorter epidural use	na
Lee et al. [17]	2005	24[a]	23	No significant difference	Fewer pulmonary complications	No difference at 14 months
Huscher et al. [12]	2005	30	29	No significant difference	No difference	No difference at 5 years
Kim et al. [15]	2008	82[a]	82	na	Less EBL and pain medicine, shorter hospital stay, improved QOL	na
Kim et al. [14]	2010	179[a]	161	na	No difference in morbidity or mortality	na
Cai et al. [18]	2011	61[a]	62	No difference	Less pulmonary infection	No difference at 2 years

[a]Laparoscopic assisted with an open component
EBL estimated blood loss, *Lap* laparoscopic, *na* not available

[15]. Laparoscopic resection was associated with longer operative times but lower blood loss, a shorter hospital stay, and an improvement in quality of life [15]. Seven randomized trials comparing laparoscopic to open resection have completed accrual (Table 22.1). The results of the trials suggest that laparoscopic resection takes longer and has a similar morbidity and mortality to open resection but is associated with a faster return of bowel function, less blood loss, and reduced postoperative pain.

Several meta-analyses of randomized and nonrandomized trials have been published. A recent meta-analysis of laparoscopic versus open distal gastrectomy concluded that laparoscopic gastrectomy was associated with lower blood loss, faster return of bowel function, and a shorter hospital stay but a slight reduction in lymph node yield [19]. Although there was no difference in the proportion of patients with 15 or more lymph nodes in their specimen, the laparoscopic group had a median of 3.9 fewer lymph nodes than the open group. The implications of this small difference in lymph node yield is unclear [19]. A meta-analysis of laparoscopic versus open gastrectomy for early stage gastric cancer concluded that the laparoscopic approach was associated with

longer operative times, less blood loss, earlier return of bowel activity, and shorter hospital. They also found that laparoscopic resection yielded slightly fewer lymph nodes [20]. Two meta-analyses focusing on patients with locally advanced gastric cancer had similar conclusions except that the lymph node yields of the laparoscopic groups in these meta-analyses were similar to the open groups [21, 22].

In most of the Asian studies, the laparoscopic groups included a large proportion of patients undergoing open intestinal transection and gastrojejunal or gastroduodenal anastomoses. In Western series, the procedures almost always include intracorporeal anastomoses and are therefore considered laparoscopic as opposed to laparoscopic-assisted resections. Compared to laparoscopic-assisted gastrectomy, totally laparoscopic gastrectomy is associated with less blood loss, shorter time to first flatus, and shorter postoperative hospital stay [23]. There is no significant difference in operative time, mean number of lymph nodes retrieved, and postoperative complications [23]. An evaluation of the largely nonrandomized Western data is therefore warranted (Table 22.2). Western series support the conclusions that, compared to open distal gastrectomy,

Table 22.2 Summary of Western distal gastrectomy studies

Author	Year	Country	Laparoscopic group (n)	Open group (n)	Laparoscopic lymph node harvest – mean	Open lymph node harvest – mean	Laparoscopic length of stay	Open LOS (days)	Laparoscopic 30-day morbidity	Open 30-day morbidity	Laparoscopic 30-day mortality	Open 30-day mortality
Reyes et al. [24]	2001	USA	18	18	8	11	6.3	8.6	na	na		
Huscher et al. [12]	2005	Italy	30	29	30	33	10.3	14.5	23.3	27.6	3.3	6.7
Dulucq et al. [28]	2005	France	14	15	17	15	16	25	12.5	17.5	0	0
Pugliese et al. [29]	2007	Italy	43		32	36	9.8	16.7	10	14	2	3
Strong et al. [25]	2009	USA	30	30	18	21	5	7	26	63	0	0
Guzman et al. [26]	2009	USA	30	48	24	26	7	10	30	46	0	0
Scatizzi et al. [27]	2011	Italy	30	30	31	37	7	9	7	26	0	0
Chouillard et al. [30]	2010	France	51	79	19	22	8	11.5	12	16	0	2.5

laparoscopic distal gastrectomy takes longer [24–27] but yields a similar lymph node count [12, 26, 28–30] with less blood loss [12, 24, 26, 29], shorter hospital stay [12, 26–30], and lower postoperative morbidity [25–28]. Short-term [25, 27, 29, 30] and 5-year [12] survivals of laparoscopic distal gastrectomy are similar to those following open gastrectomy.

Patient Selection

The decision to perform a laparoscopic versus an open gastrectomy depends on several factors. The most important consideration is the skill and experience of the operating surgeon. Laparoscopic gastrectomy is an operation requiring advanced laparoscopic skills to perform an adequate lymphadenectomy and an intestinal anastomosis. The procedure also requires an operating room team equipped with appropriate laparoscopic atraumatic graspers, an energy device, liver retractor, wound protector, and laparoscopic reticulating staplers. The procedure is particularly demanding in obese patients. Challenges in laparoscopic resection in obese patients include decreased surgical visibility, dissection hindered by adipose tissue, and difficulty with anastomoses. Higher BMI is an independent risk factor for pancreatic fistula following laparoscopic distal gastrectomy [31].

Prior upper abdominal surgery can make laparoscopic gastrectomy technically difficult. Laparoscopic or open cholecystectomy often results in adhesion of the first portion of the duodenum to the gallbladder bed. Careful dissection can usually allow full mobilization of the duodenum off the liver bed. An adequate lymphadenectomy can be performed following an open or laparoscopic cholecystectomy as long as the patient did not undergo an open common bile duct exploration. Prior right hemicolectomy or splenectomy can complicate laparoscopic distal gastrectomy. Prior gastric resection or transverse colectomy is a relative contraindication to laparoscopic gastrectomy because the plane of dissection for lymphadenectomy will have been altered or obliterated. In general, adequate resection

with lymphadenectomy can be accomplished following neoadjuvant chemotherapy but may be technically demanding in some patients who have had prior radiation therapy. As with any laparoscopic procedure, it is incumbent on the operating surgeon to be cognizant of their own surgical limitations and have a low threshold to convert any case to open if it cannot be performed thoroughly and safely laparoscopically. Poor cardiopulmonary reserve is a relative contraindication to laparoscopic gastrectomy because of the decrease in venous return and increase in pulmonary resistance associated with prolonged pneumoperitoneum.

Hand-assisted laparoscopic gastrectomy has been advocated by some surgeons in an attempt to overcome the technical challenges associated with a totally laparoscopic approach [32]. Although a hand assist approach may enable a surgeon early in their learning curve to complete a laparoscopic-assisted distal gastrectomy, it will inevitably require an incision significantly larger than that required for specimen extraction with a totally laparoscopic approach. Routine reliance on the use of a hand port might also limit the surgeon's own technical development and proficiency.

Patient Positioning and Room Setup

The patient is placed in the supine position with both arms tucked. General endotracheal anesthesia is administered. A nasogastric tube is placed to decompress the stomach, and a Foley catheter is inserted into the bladder. Intravenous antibiotics are administered within 1 h of the incision and redosed as necessary. Deep venous thrombosis prophylaxis is accomplished with sequential pneumatic compression stockings on the lower extremities. In addition, all patients are administered 5,000 units of subcutaneous unfractionated heparin in the immediate preoperative period.

Eggcrate foam is secured to the operating room with wide tape, and the patient is placed on the eggcrate without an intervening bedsheet. This secures the patient to the surgical bed and prevents shifting during maximum reverse Trendelenburg position [33]. The video monitors

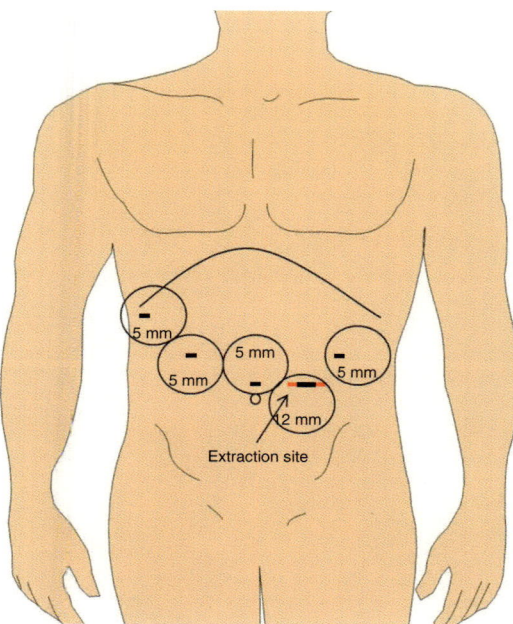

Fig. 22.1 Laparoscopic port site placement. A 5 mm supra-umbilical camera port is flanked by the right and left upper quadrant 5 mm dissection ports. A 12 mm left-sided stapling port is later enlarged for specimen extraction. A 5 mm right lateral subcostal port site is used for placement of a liver retractor

Table 22.3 Sequence of laparoscopic subtotal gastrectomy with gastrojejunostomy and D2 lymphadenectomy

1	Omentectomy
2	Transection of right gastroepiploic vessels
3	Transection of postpyloric duodenum
4	Division of lesser omentum
5	Dissection of capsule over superior boarder of pancreatic neck
6	Dissection of hepatic artery and portal vein nodes
7	Division of origin of the left gastric artery
8	Dissection of proximal splenic artery nodes
9	Stripping of lesser curvature of proximal stomach
10	Transection of stomach
11	Stapled side-to-side gastrojejunostomy

are positioned near the shoulders on each side of the operating table. The procedure is performed with a surgeon and an assistant. The surgeon begins on the right side of the table with the assistant on the left side of the table. The scrub nurse is positioned on the right side of the table.

Operative Procedure (Video 22.1)

The procedure is performed with four 5 mm ports and a single 12 mm port for laparoscopic stapling (Fig. 22.1). The peritoneal cavity is entered and insufflated with a Veress needle after a stab wound is made in the left subcostal space at Palmer's point. A 5 mm camera trocar is placed in the supra-umbilical region. A left upper quadrant 5 mm dissection port is placed. This port should be placed laterally enough to allow for placement of a 12 mm stapling port midway between the left upper quadrant and supra-umbilical ports. The abdomen is thoroughly explored for evidence of

liver or peritoneal metastatic disease. If metastatic disease is identified, the operation can be aborted or converted to a gastrojejunal bypass, if clinically indicated. If distant metastatic disease is not identified, an extreme right lateral subcostal port is then placed. A snake retractor placed through the right lateral port is triangulated closed and used to elevate the left lobe of the liver. The snake retractor is fixed in place with an adjustable robot arm-type retractor system. A right upper quadrant 5 mm dissecting port is placed. A 5 mm 30° angled camera is used for the entire operation. With some equipment, the 5 mm camera does not allow enough light to accomplish advanced laparoscopy. If the operation cannot be performed safely with a 5 mm camera, the supra-umbilical 5 mm port can be exchanged for a 10–12 mm port for a 30° angled 10 mm camera.

The omentum is reflected into the upper abdomen and dissected off of the transverse colon using a 5 mm energy device (Table 22.3). Dissection is conducted from the right side of the table, beginning at the midline and extending up to the lowest short gastric vessels. For this dissection, the camera can be moved to the left 12 mm port to allow the surgeon to work with both hands through the right upper quadrant and supra-umbilical port. The omental dissection is then carried up to the greater curvature. The camera is moved from the left to the supra-umbilical port, and the right side of the omentum is dissected from the transverse colon. This is best performed from the left side of the patient. After the

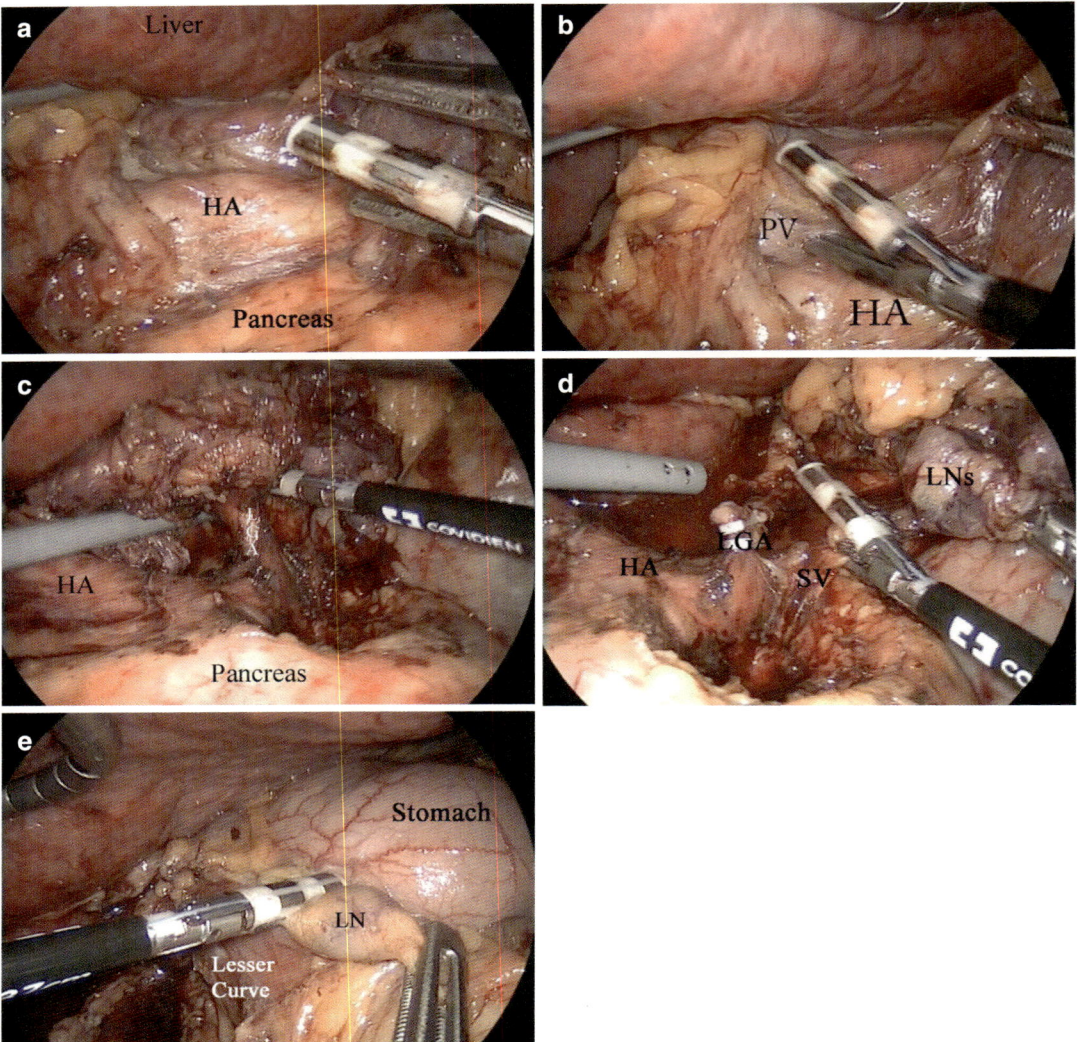

Fig. 22.2 Lymph node dissection. (**a**) The lymph node-bearing tissues are lifted off the hepatic artery and (**b**) lymph nodes along the portal vein and reflected to the left. (**c**) The origin of the left gastric artery is skeletonized, and (**d**) the lymph nodes along the proximal splenic artery are reflected on to the specimen. (**e**) Lymph nodes are dissected off the lesser curvature of the stomach. Hepatic artery (*HA*), portal vein (*PV*), left gastric artery (*LGA*), left gastric vein (*SV*), lymph node (*LN*)

complete separation of the omentum from the transverse colon, the base of the right gastroepiploic vessels are dissected at the level of the inferior border of the pancreas. The right gastroepiploic vessels are transected using an energy device. Attention is then turned to the supra-duodenal region, and the lesser omentum is opened. The first portion of the duodenum is surrounded and transected using a 60 mm endoscopic stapler using 3.5 mm (blue) staples or Tri-Staple™ 2.0, 2.5, and 3.0 mm (tan) staples. Staple line buttressing material is not used for any of the stapling in the procedure. None of the staple lines are imbricated with sutures, and sutures are not generally used to take tension off the staple lines.

The lymph node dissection is accomplished by clearing the fat over the portal hepatitis and proximal hepatic artery (Fig. 22.2). The fat is reflected to the left. Dissection is carried along the common hepatic artery up to the porta hepatis reflecting the nodal tissues to the left. The portal dissection is carried up reflecting the nodal tissues from the left side of the portal vein. With the nodal packet reflected to the left, dissection is then carried onto the proximal proper hepatic artery. The left gastric vein is transected at the upper border of the pancreas. The base of the left gastric artery is dissected and controlled with Hem-o-lok clips and transected. The nodal tissue along the proximal splenic artery is dissected, reflecting the nodes off of the body of the pancreas, exposing the splenic artery. This nodal packet is then reflected to the left. The entire nodal packet is reflected off of the retroperitoneum.

A gastroscopy is performed using an upper GI endoscope. The exact location of the tumor is noted by endoscopy, while the corresponding serosal area is identified by laparoscopy. This is best accomplished by pressing on the stomach in the region of the tumor with a laparoscopic dissector. A proximal gastric transection region is chosen and can be marked with sutures or clips.

The lesser omentum is transected close to the liver. The nodal tissues along the lesser curvature of the stomach are then dissected. This is performed by stripping the lymph node-bearing fat from the lesser curvature from proximal to distal. Following the node stripping, the lesser curvature often appears somewhat dark or ecchymotic in color, even though its blood supply remains robust. The stomach is then transected with an endoscopic stapler, taking an appropriate margin proximal to the tumor. The stomach is transected using sequential firings of a 60 mm endoscopic stapler using 4.1 mm (green) staples or Tri-StapleTM 3.0, 3.5, and 4.0 mm (purple) staples. The specimen is then grasped with a laparoscopic instrument.

The 12 mm stapling port is enlarged, and a wound protector is placed. The specimen is withdrawn through the wound protector and immediately opened by the pathologist to assess margins. The wound protector is loosened and turned around a 12 mm port. A moist laparotomy pad can be wrapped around the wound protector and secured with a Kocher clamp. After insufflating

the abdomen, the ligament of Treitz is identified. The proximal jejunum is carefully followed and reflected over the transverse colon. An area in the proximal jejunum, which approximates the stomach without tension, is chosen for the anastomosis. The anastomosis is best accomplished from the right side of the patient. The jejunum is laid next to the stomach such that the proximal end of the jejunum is to the right and the distal end is to the left (Fig. 22.3). This is done so that the stapling defect following formation of the anastomosis is on the afferent limb of the small bowel. Any difficulty with closure of this defect will not affect to the efferent limb of the gastrojejunostomy. A long 3-0 Vicryl traction suture is used to approximate the small bowel to the proximal gastric pouch just superior to the gastric staple line. This traction suture is brought through the 12 mm port (Fig. 22.3). An enterotomy is made with the energy device or hook electrocautery, in the small bowel and in the stomach just beyond the traction suture. A side-to-side anastomosis is performed using a 60 mm endoscopic stapler using 3.5 mm (blue) staples or Tri-Staple™ 2.0, 2.5, and 3.0 mm (tan) staples. It is important to place the stapler into position in the jejunum and stomach and then rotated it in a counterclockwise way, so that the anastomosis will be on the anterior wall of the stomach and not cross the gastric transection staple line. The stapling enterotomy defect is closed using two layers of running 3-0 Vicryl™ suture. Lapra-Tys™ can be used to secure the sutures.

A feeding jejunostomy tube is generally not necessary. The nasogastric tube is left in place in the gastric pouch and removed on the first postoperative morning. The patient is advanced from a clear liquid diet on the first and second postoperative days to a regular diet by postoperative days number three and four. Patients are discharged when they are able to tolerate a regular diet.

Reconstruction

Reconstruction following distal gastrectomy can take several forms [34, 35]. Billroth I gastroduodenostomy is not commonly performed in the United

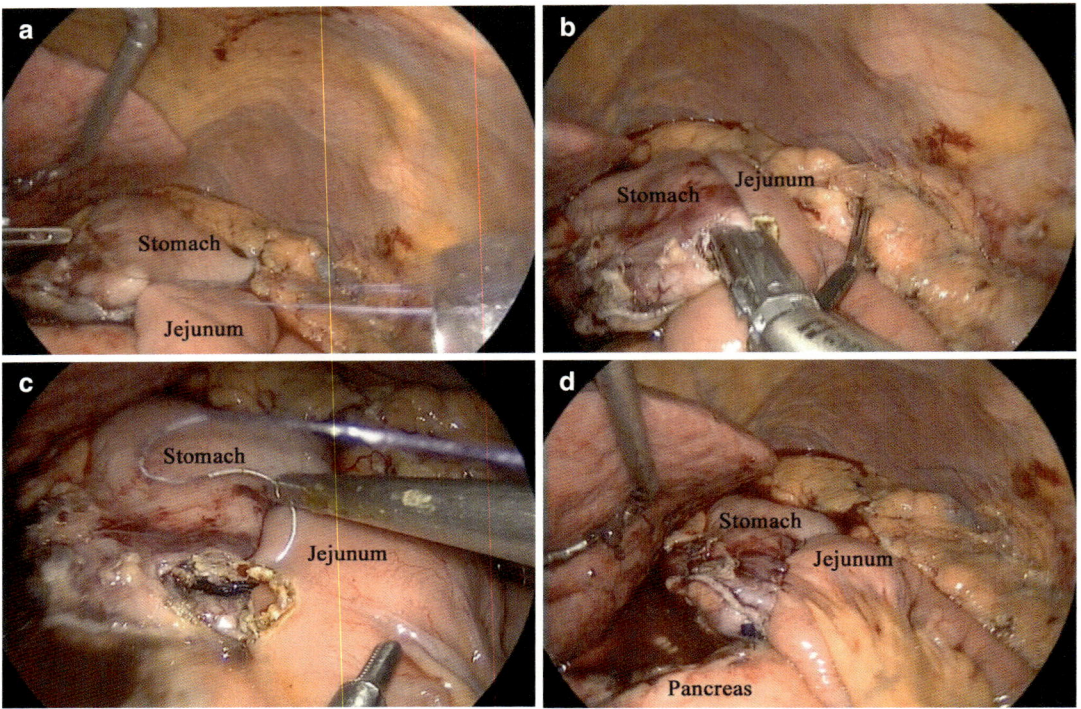

Fig. 22.3 Gastrojejunal anastomosis. (**a**)The proximal jejunum is approximated to the proximal gastric pouch with a traction suture, and (**b**) a 60 mm stapler is inserted

through enterotomies in the jejunum and stomach. (**c, d**) The stapling defect is closed with two layers of running suture

States and can be difficult to construct in patients for whom over 50 % of the stomach has been resected. Roux-en-Y gastrojejunostomy is commonly performed but requires two enteric anastomoses. Billroth II (BII) loop gastrojejunostomy requires only one anastomosis and is straightforward and easily performed using laparoscopic techniques. Because BII reconstruction involves fewer anastomoses, there is a reduced likelihood of anastomotic leak and internal hernia formation than are known to associate with a Roux-en-Y reconstruction. Unfortunately, concern for bile reflux gastritis severely limits its use by most gastrointestinal surgeons. Instead, Roux-en-Y reconstruction is favored after gastrectomy and has been recommended in the United States [36–39]. In my practice, all patients undergoing laparoscopic distal gastrectomy are reconstructed with a BII gastrojejunostomy because it is straightforward to perform laparoscopically [26, 40].

We compare quality of life of patients at least 6 months after laparoscopic partial gastrectomy with BII reconstruction with a small versus

larger gastric remnant. Patients were allocated into two groups based on the size of their remnant gastric pouch, one having at least 70 % of their stomach resected (small pouch) and the other having less than 70 % of their stomach resected (large pouch). Thirty patients consented to participate and completed the EORTC QOL-STO22 instrument. In general, patients expressed few symptoms. There was no significant difference between the large and small remnant pouch cohorts in overall symptoms or specific symptoms (Table 22.4).

Laparoscopic Versus Robotic Gastrectomy

Robotic surgery systems have been introduced as a solution to minimize the shortcomings of laparoscopy. Robotics provides definite technical advantages over conventional laparoscopy [41], but its role for gastric cancer is still unclear [41–44]. Since robotic gastrectomy was first reported [41, 45], its

Table 22.4 Quality of life measurement

Symptoms	Entire cohort mean score[a] (±STD)	Large pouch (16 patients) mean score (±STD)	Small pouch (14 patients) mean score (±STD)	p-value
Overall	1.47 (±0.44)	1.42 (±0.44)	1.53 (±0.46)	0.54

[a]Score scale: 1, not at all; 2, a little; 3, quite a bit; 4, very much

use has been expanding, primarily in high-volume centers. There have been very few studies and no randomized studies comparing laparoscopic gastrectomy to robotic gastrectomy. A recent meta-analysis of studies compared robotic to open gastrectomy for gastric cancer [46]. Only six articles compared robotic gastrectomy to laparoscopic gastrectomy [47–52]. The operative time for robotic gastrectomy was significantly longer than that for laparoscopic gastrectomy. There was no difference in the number of lymph nodes retrieved. The amount of blood loss was significantly less for robotic gastrectomy than for laparoscopic gastrectomy, and the length of hospital stay was significantly longer with laparoscopic gastrectomy. Five of the six series were not truly laparoscopic or robotic, utilizing an open incision for the gastric transaction and reconstruction. In addition, the robotic procedures were likely performed when the surgeons were more accomplished minimally invasive surgeons. These confounding variables might limit the validity of the conclusions favoring the robotic approach. While there may be real benefits to the use of robotics for gastrectomy and lymphadenectomy, downsides include significant costs and issues of availability of the technology. It remains to be seen whether the use of the surgical robot can facilitate an oncologically sound minimally invasive gastrectomy by a surgeon who lacks the skills to perform a straight laparoscopic approach.

References

1. Abraham NS, Young JM, Solomon MJ. Meta-analysis of short-term outcomes after laparoscopic resection for colorectal cancer. Br J Surg. 2004;91(9):1111–24. PubMed PMID: 15449261.
2. Schwenk W, Haase O, Neudecker J, Muller JM. Short term benefits for laparoscopic colorectal resection. Cochrane Database Syst Rev. 2005;(3):CD003145. PubMed PMID: 16034888.
3. Jayne DG, Thorpe HC, Copeland J, Quirke P, Brown JM, Guillou PJ. Five-year follow-up of the Medical Research Council CLASICC trial of laparoscopically assisted versus open surgery for colorectal cancer. Br J Surg. 2010;97(11) 1638–45. PubMed PMID: 20629110.
4. Lacy AM, Garcia-Valdecasas JC, Delgado S, Castells A, Taura P, Pique JM, et al. Laparoscopy-assisted colectomy versus open colectomy for treatment of nonmetastatic colon cancer: a randomised trial. Lancet. 2002;359(9325):2224–9. PubMed PMID: 12103285.
5. Janson M, Bjorholt I, Carlsson P, Haglind E, Henriksson M, Lindholm E, et al. Randomized clinical trial of the costs of open and laparoscopic surgery for colonic cancer. Br J Surg. 2004;91(4):409–17. PubMed PMID: 15048739.
6. Kendrick ML. Laparoscopic and robotic resection for pancreatic cancer. Cancer J. 2012;18(6):571–6. PubMed PMID: 23187844.
7. Kucukmetin A, Biliatis I, Naik R, Bryant A. Laparoscopically assisted radical vaginal hysterectomy versus radical abdominal hysterectomy for the treatment of early cervical cancer. Cochrane Database Syst Rev. 2013;10:CD006651. PubMed PMID: 24085528.
8. He H, Zeng D, Ou H, Tang Y, Li J, Zhong H. Laparoscopic treatment of endometrial cancer: systematic review. J Minim Invasive Gynecol. 2013;20(4):413–23. PubMed PMID: 23506718.
9. Sandhu GS, Nepple KG, Tanagho YS, Andriole GL. Laparoscopic prostatectomy for prostate cancer: continued role in urology. Surg Oncol Clin N Am. 2013;22(1):125–41, vii. PubMed PMID: 23158089.
10. Ni S, Tao W, Chen Q, Liu L, Jiang H, Hu H, et al. Laparoscopic versus open nephroureterectomy for the treatment of upper urinary tract urothelial carcinoma: a systematic review and cumulative analysis of comparative studies. Eur Urol. 2012;61(6):1142–53. PubMed PMID: 22349569.
11. Kitano S, Iso Y, Moriyama M, Sugimachi K. Laparoscopy-assisted Billroth I gastrectomy. Surg Laparosc Endosc. 1994;4(2):146–8. PubMed PMID: 8180768.
12. Huscher CG, Mingoli A, Sgarzini G, Sansonetti A, Di Paola M, Recher A, et al. Laparoscopic versus open subtotal gastrectomy for distal gastric cancer: five-year results of a randomized prospective trial. Ann Surg. 2005;241(2):232–7. PubMed PMID: 15650632. Pubmed Central PMCID: 1356907.
13. Kim HH, Han SU, Kim MC, Hyung WJ, Kim W, Lee HJ et al. Prospective randomized controlled trial (phase III) to comparing laparoscopic distal gastrectomy with open distal gastrectomy for gastric adenocarcinoma (KLASS 01). J Korean Surg Soc. 2013;84(2):123–30. PubMed PMID: 23396494. Pubmed Central PMCID: 3566471.
14. Kim HH, Hyung WJ, Cho GS, Kim MC, Han SU, Kim W, et al. Morbidity and mortality of laparoscopic gastrectomy versus open gastrectomy for gastric cancer:

an interim report – a phase III multicenter, prospective, randomized Trial (KLASS Trial). Ann Surg. 2010;251(3):417–20. PubMed PMID: 20160637.

15. Kim YW, Baik YH, Yun YH, Nam BH, Kim DH, Choi IJ, et al. Improved quality of life outcomes after laparoscopy-assisted distal gastrectomy for early gastric cancer: results of a prospective randomized clinical trial. Ann Surg. 2008;248(5):721–7. PubMed PMID: 18948798.

16. Hayashi H, Ochiai T, Shimada H, Gunji Y. Prospective randomized study of open versus laparoscopy-assisted distal gastrectomy with extraperigastric lymph node dissection for early gastric cancer. Surg Endosc. 2005;19(9):1172–6. PubMed PMID: 16132323.

17. Lee JH, Han HS, Lee JH. A prospective randomized study comparing open vs laparoscopy-assisted distal gastrectomy in early gastric cancer: early results. Surg Endosc. 2005;19(2):168–73. PubMed PMID: 15580441.

18. Cai J, Wei D, Gao CF, Zhang CS, Zhang H, Zhao T. A prospective randomized study comparing open versus laparoscopy-assisted D2 radical gastrectomy in advanced gastric cancer. Dig Surg. 2011;28(5–6):331–7. PubMed PMID: 21934308.

19. Vinuela EF, Gonen M, Brennan MF, Coit DG, Strong VE. Laparoscopic versus open distal gastrectomy for gastric cancer: a meta-analysis of randomized controlled trials and high-quality nonrandomized studies. Ann Surg. 2012;255(3):446–56. PubMed PMID: 22330034.

20. Peng JS, Song H, Yang ZL, Xiang J, Diao DC, Liu ZH. Meta-analysis of laparoscopy-assisted distal gastrectomy and conventional open distal gastrectomy for early gastric cancer. Chin J Cancer. 2010;29(4):349–54. PubMed PMID: 20346206.

21. Martinez-Ramos D, Miralles-Tena JM, Cuesta MA, Escrig-Sos J, Van der Peet D, Hoashi JS, et al. Laparoscopy versus open surgery for advanced and resectable gastric cancer: a meta-analysis. Rev Esp Enferm Dig. 2011;103(3):133–41. PubMed PMID: 21434716.

22. Qiu J, Pankaj P, Jiang H, Zeng Y, Wu H. Laparoscopy versus open distal gastrectomy for advanced gastric cancer: a systematic review and meta-analysis. Surg Laparosc Endosc Percutan Tech. 2013;23(1):1–7. PubMed PMID: 23386142.

23. Gao J, Li P, Li QG, Chen J, Wang DR, Tang D. Comparison between totally laparoscopic and laparoscopically assisted distal gastrectomy for gastric cancer with a short follow-up: a meta-analysis. J Laparoendosc Adv Surg Tech A. 2013;23(8):693–7. PubMed PMID: 23678885.

24. Reyes CD, Weber KJ, Gagner M, Divino CM. Laparoscopic vs open gastrectomy. A retrospective review. Surg Endosc. 2001;15(9):928–31. PubMed PMID: 11605108.

25. Strong VE, Devaud N, Allen PJ, Gonen M, Brennan MF, Coit D. Laparoscopic versus open subtotal gastrectomy for adenocarcinoma: a case-control study. Ann Surg Oncol. 2009;16(6):1507–13. PubMed PMID: 19347407.

26. Guzman EA, Pigazzi A, Lee B, Soriano PA, Nelson RA, Benjamin Paz I, et al. Totally laparoscopic gastric resection with extended lymphadenectomy for gastric adenocarcinoma. Ann Surg Oncol. 2009;16(8):2218–23. PubMed PMID: 19444523.

27. Scatizzi M, Kroning KC, Lenzi E, Moraldi L, Cantafio S, Feroci F. Laparoscopic versus open distal gastrectomy for locally advanced gastric cancer: a case-control study. Updates Surg. 2011;63(1):17–23. PubMed PMID: 21286896.

28. Dulucq JL, Wintringer P, Stabilini C, Solinas L, Perissat J, Mahajna A. Laparoscopic and open gastric resections for malignant lesions: a prospective comparative study. Surg Endosc. 2005;19(7):933–8. PubMed PMID: 15920691.

29. Pugliese R, Maggioni D, Sansonna F, Scandroglio I, Ferrari GC, Di Lernia S, et al. Total and subtotal laparoscopic gastrectomy for adenocarcinoma. Surg Endosc. 2007;21(1):21–7. PubMed PMID: 17031743.

30. Chouillard E, Gumbs AA, Meyer F, Torcivia A, Helmy N, Toubal M, et al. Laparoscopic versus open gastrectomy for adenocarcinoma: a prospective comparative analysis. Minerva Chir. 2010;65(3):243–50. PubMed PMID: 20668413.

31. Jiang X, Hiki N, Nunobe S, Kumagai K, Nohara K, Sano T, et al. Postoperative pancreatic fistula and the risk factors of laparoscopy-assisted distal gastrectomy for early gastric cancer. Ann Surg Oncol. 2012;19(1):115–21. PubMed PMID: 21739317.

32. Tanimura S, Higashino M, Fukunaga Y, Osugi H. Hand-assisted laparoscopic distal gastrectomy with regional lymph node dissection for gastric cancer. Surg Laparosc Endosc Percutan Tech. 2001;11(3):155–60. PubMed PMID: 11444743.

33. Klauschie J, Wechter ME, Jacob K, Zanagnolo V, Montero R, Magrina J, et al. Use of anti-skid material and patient-positioning to prevent patient shifting during robotic-assisted gynecologic procedures. J Minim Invasive Gynecol. 2010;17(4):504–7. PubMed PMID: 20471916.

34. Hoya Y, Mitsumori N, Yanaga K. The advantages and disadvantages of a Roux-en-Y reconstruction after a distal gastrectomy for gastric cancer. Surg Today. 2009;39(8):647–51. PubMed PMID: 19639429. Epub 2009/07/30. eng.

35. Nomura S, Kaminishi M. Surgical treatment of early gastric cancer. Dig Surg. 2007;24(2):96–100. PubMed PMID: 17460412. Epub 2007/04/27. eng.

36. Burden WR, Hodges RP, Hsu M, O'Leary JP. Alkaline reflux gastritis. Surg Clin North Am. 1991;71(1):33–44. PubMed PMID: 1989108. Epub 1991/02/01. eng.

37. Sugiyama Y, Sohma H, Ozawa M, Hada R, Mikami Y, Konn M, et al. Regurgitant bile acids and mucosal injury of the gastric remnant after partial gastrectomy. Am J Surg. 1987;153(4):399–403. PubMed PMID: 3565686. Epub 1987/04/01. eng.

38. Osugi H, Fukuhara K, Takada N, Takemura M, Kinoshita H. Reconstructive procedure after distal gastrectomy to prevent remnant gastritis. Hepatogastroenterology.

2004;51(58):1215–8. PubMed PMID: 15239282. Epub 2004/07/09. eng.

39. Csendes A, Burgos AM, Smok G, Burdiles P, Braghetto I, Diaz JC. Latest results (12-21 years) of a prospective randomized study comparing Billroth II and Roux-en-Y anastomosis after a partial gastrectomy plus vagotomy in patients with duodenal ulcers. Ann Surg. 2009;249(2):189–94. PubMed PMID: 19212169. Epub 2009/02/13. eng.

40. Pigazzi A, Ellenhorn JD, Ballantyne GH, Paz IB. Robotic-assisted laparoscopic low anterior resection with total mesorectal excision for rectal cancer. Surg Endosc. 2006;20(10):1521–5. PubMed PMID: 16897284. Epub 2006/08/10. eng.

41. Giulianotti PC, Coratti A, Angelini M, Sbrana F, Cecconi S, Balestracci T, et al. Robotics in general surgery: personal experience in a large community hospital. Arch Surg. 2003;138(7):777–84. PubMed PMID: 12860761.

42. Hyung WJ. Robotic surgery in gastrointestinal surgery. Korean J Gastroenterol. 2007;50(4):256–9.

43. Gutt CN, Oniu T, Mehrabi A, Kashfi A, Schemmer P, Buchler MW. Robot-assisted abdominal surgery. Br J Surg. 2004;91(11):1390–7. PubMed PMID: 15386325.

44. Baek SJ, Lee DW, Park SS, Kim SH. Current status of robot-assisted gastric surgery. World J Gastrointest Oncol. 2011;3(10):137–43. PubMed PMID: 22046490. Pubmed Central PMCID: 3205112.

45. Hashizume M, Sugimachi K. Robot-assisted gastric surgery. Surg Clin North Am. 2003;83(6):1429–44. PubMed PMID: 14712877.

46. Marano A, Choi YY, Hyung WJ, Kim YM, Kim J, Noh SH. Robotic versus laparoscopic versus open gastrectomy: a meta-analysis. J Gastric Cancer. 2013;13(3): 36–48. PubMed PMID: 24156033. Pubmed Central PMCID: 3804672.

47. Kim MC, Heo GU, Jung GJ. Robotic gastrectomy for gastric cancer: surgical techniques and clinical merits. Surg Endosc. 2010;24(3):610–5. PubMed PMID: 19688399.

48. Pugliese R, Maggioni D, Sansonna F, Costanzi A, Ferrari GC, Di Lernia S, et al. Subtotal gastrectomy with D2 dissection by minimally invasive surgery for distal adenocarcinoma of the stomach: results and 5-year survival. Surg Endosc. 2010;24(10):2594–602. PubMed PMID: 20414682.

49. Yoon HM, Kim YW, Lee JH, Ryu KW, Eom BW, Park JY, et al. Robot-assisted total gastrectomy is comparable with laparoscopically assisted total gastrectomy for early gastric cancer. Surg Endosc. 2012;26(5):1377–81. PubMed PMID: 22083338.

50. Woo Y, Hyung WJ, Pak KH, Inaba K, Obama K, Choi SH, et al. Robotic gastrectomy as an oncologically sound alternative to laparoscopic resections for the treatment of early-stage gastric cancers. Arch Surg. 2011;146(9):1086–92. PubMed PMID: 21576595.

51. Eom BW, Yoon HM, Ryu KW, Lee JH, Cho SJ, Lee JY, et al. Comparison of surgical performance and short-term clinical outcomes between laparoscopic and robotic surgery in distal gastric cancer. Eur J Surg Oncol. 2012;38(1):57–63. PubMed PMID: 21945625.

52. Huang KH, Lan YT, Fang WL, Chen JH, Lo SS, Hsieh MC, et al. Initial experience of robotic gastrectomy and comparison with open and laparoscopic gastrectomy for gastric cancer. J Gastrointest Surg. 2012;16(7):1303–10. PubMed PMID: 22450954.

Laparoscopic Proximal Gastrectomy with Double Tract Anastomosis

23

Yukinori Kurokawa, Noriko Wada, Shuji Takiguchi, and Yuichiro Doki

Introduction

Proximal gastrectomy is one of the modified surgical approaches for early gastric cancer located in the upper stomach without lymph node metastasis. It allows for storage, digestion, and absorption of food and prevents agastric anemia. Important things in proximal gastrectomy are the curability and postoperative quality of life. As for the curability, the range of dissected lymph nodes should follow the Japanese Gastric Cancer Treatment Guidelines (ver. 3) in principle [1], and the distance of tumor from the gastric stump is also important. As for quality of life, it is necessary to consider the reconstruction method that reduces reflux esophagitis. Recently, the development of instruments and techniques has enabled the performance of laparoscopic or laparoscopy-assisted proximal gastrectomy. The important points of the surgical technique of laparoscopic proximal gastrectomy with double tract anastomosis are described in this section.

Electronic supplementary material Supplementary material is available in the online version of this chapter at 10.1007/978-3-319-09342-0_23. Videos can also be accessed at http://www.springerimages.com/videos/978-3-319-09341-3.

Y. Kurokawa, MD (✉) • N. Wada, MD
S. Takiguchi, MD • Y. Doki, MD
Department of Gastroenterological Surgery,
Osaka University Graduate School of Medicine,
2-2-E2 Yamadaoka, Suita, Osaka 565-0871, Japan
e-mail: ykurokawa@gesurg.med.osaka-u.ac.jp

Operative Indication

Laparoscopic proximal gastrectomy is performed for clinical T1 tumors (within the submucosal layer) located in the upper stomach without lymph node metastasis in the preoperative assessment. Two clips to mark the distal side of the lesion and negative biopsy are recommended preoperatively to determine the transection line of the stomach. The extent of lymph node dissection should be D1+ (station Nos. 1, 2, 3a, 4sa, 4sb, 7, 8a, 9, 11p) according to the Japanese Gastric Cancer Treatment Guidelines (ver. 3) [1].

Surgical Procedures

Trocar Insertion

The patient is placed in the supine Trendelenburg position with legs apart. Five trocars are used as shown in Fig. 23.1. The surgeon stands on the patient's right, the assistant stands on the patient's left, and the camera operator stands between the patient's legs. The trocar for camera is inserted through the umbilical region. Under a 10 mmHg CO_2 pneumoperitoneum, the other four trocars are inserted. After an inspection of the abdominal cavity, the round ligament of liver is hung with string. A retractor is inserted through a pinhole incision at the epigastrium to retract the left lobe of the liver.

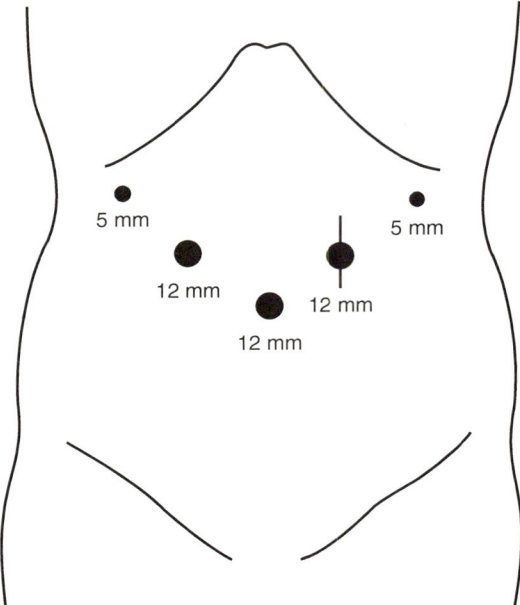

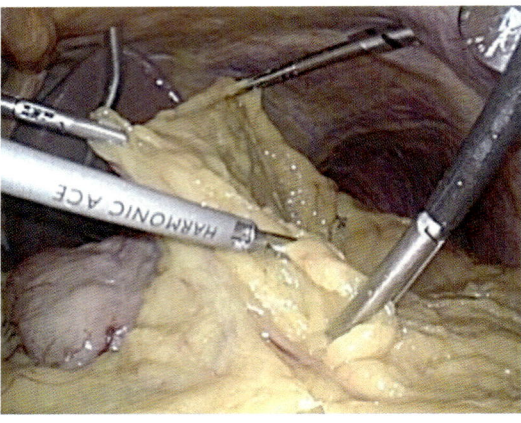

Fig. 23.2 An avascular area of the omentum approximately 3 cm apart from the gastroepiploic arcade is dissected toward the inferior pole of the spleen

Fig. 23.1 Trocar placement and a mini-laparotomy site for laparoscopic proximal gastrectomy. Five trocars are placed in the abdominal wall. The trocar site on the left rectus muscle is extended to 5 cm when the stomach is pulled out of the abdominal cavity

Dissection of the Left Gastrocolic Ligament (Video 23.1)

The assistant holds the left side of the gastroepiploic arcade in the right hand and holds the gastrocolic ligament and stretches it to caudal in the left hand. The surgeon holds the right side of the gastroepiploic arcade in the left hand and dissects an avascular area of the omentum approximately 3 cm apart from the gastroepiploic arcade toward the inferior pole of the spleen using a laparoscopic coagulating shears (LCS) in the right hand (Fig. 23.2). In order to mobilize the stomach freely, the physiological adhesions between the pancreas and the posterior wall of the stomach should be separated properly.

To dissect the right gastrocolic ligament, the standing position of the surgeon and the assistant is changed. The assistant holds the gastroepiploic arcade in both hands. The surgeon holds the gastrocolic ligament and stretches the gastrocolic ligament in a caudal direction in the left hand. The surgeon dissects the gastrocolic ligament toward the descending portion of duodenum with

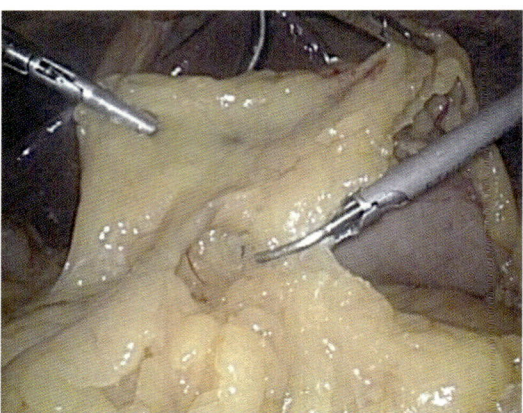

Fig. 23.3 The gastrocolic ligament is dissected toward the descending portion of duodenum

the LCS in the right hand (Fig. 23.3). The right gastroepiploic vessels are carefully preserved. If there are abnormally enlarged lymph nodes along the right gastroepiploic vessels or infrapyloric lymph nodes, the operative method needs to be changed to a total gastrectomy, considering the possibility of lymph node metastasis.

Lymph Node Dissection Along the Left Gastroepiploic Artery and the Short Gastric Artery (Video 23.2)

The assistant grips and lifts the posterior wall of the upper stomach in the right hand and draws

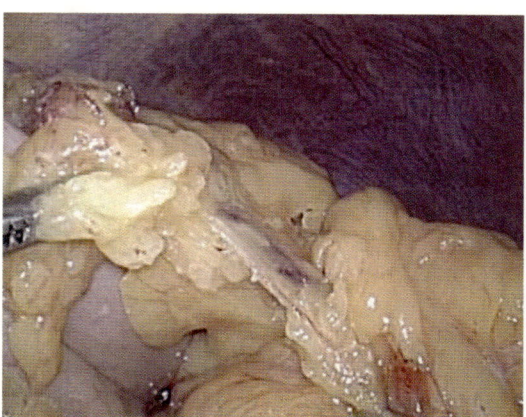

Fig. 23.4 The fat tissue around the inferior pole of the spleen is drawn to identify the left gastroepiploic vessels

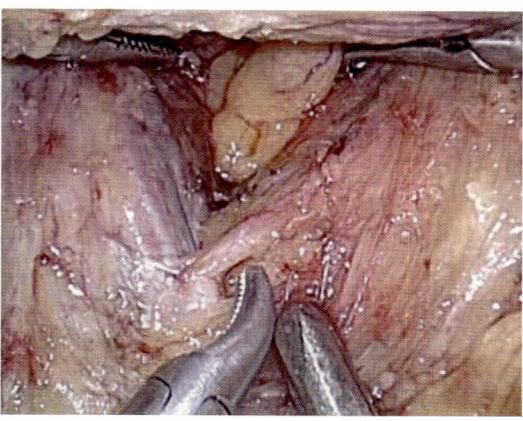

Fig. 23.6 The base of the esophageal cardiac branch of the left inferior phrenic artery is dissected

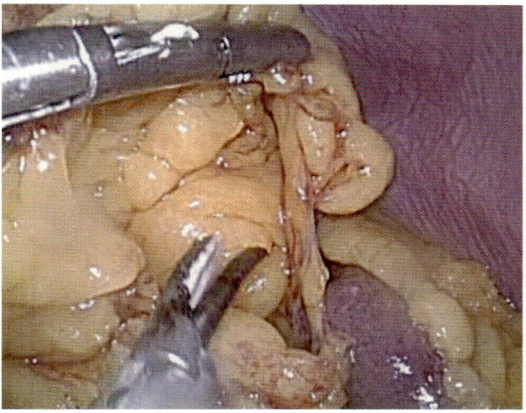

Fig. 23.5 The gastrosplenic ligaments is divided upward toward the superior pole of the spleen

the fat tissue near the inferior pole of the spleen to the left and expands the field of view in the left hand. The surgeon identifies the left gastro-epiploic artery rising from the tail of the pan-creas, peels off the surrounding fat tissue, and dissects the artery distal to the omental branch using the LCS after clipping the artery (Fig. 23.4).

The surgeon divides the gastrosplenic liga-ments upward toward the superior pole of the spleen with the LCS (Fig. 23.5). It is of particular concern to avoid injury to the spleen or the short gastric vessels by strong traction when the assistant expands the field of view. The short gas-tric vessels are dissected using the LCS with or without clipping these vessels. Because the

gastrosplenic ligaments around the superior pole of the spleen are short, complete dissection should be performed during resection of the esophagus.

Resection of the Abdominal Esophagus (Video 23.3)

The assistant grips and stretches the lesser curvature in both hands. If there are enlarged suprapyloric lymph nodes, the operative method needs to be changed to the total gastrectomy. The surgeon dissects an avascular area of the lesser curvature along the hepatic branch of the vagus nerve toward the abdominal esophagus. The operating surgeon dissects the esophageal diaphragmatic ligament and exposes the right crus and the front wall of the abdominal esopha-gus. The fat tissue surrounding the abdominal esophagus is peeled off, and the anterior and posterior branches of the vagus nerves are tran-sected using the LCS. The base of the esopha-geal cardiac branch of the left inferior phrenic artery is dissected using the LCS after clipping the vessel (Fig. 23.6). After a detachable vessel forceps are applied to the abdominal esophagus, the abdominal esophagus is divided above the esophagogastric junction using the LCS (Fig. 23.7). The residual gastrosplenic ligaments are dissected downward using the LCS with or without clipping of vessels.

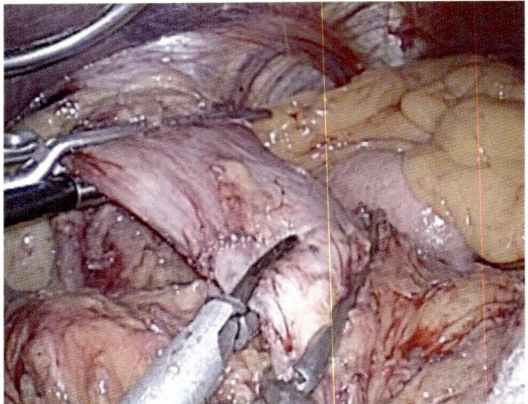

Fig. 23.7 The abdominal esophagus is divided above the esophagogastric junction after a detachable vessel forceps are applied

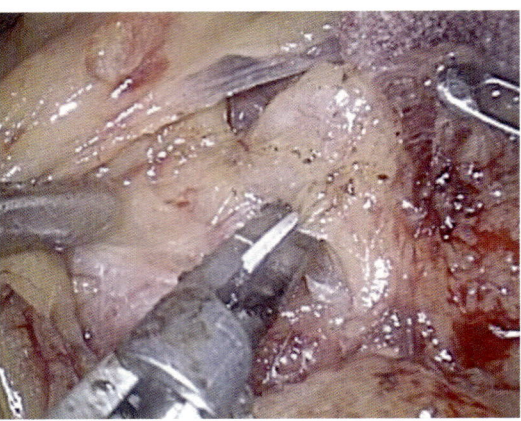

Fig. 23.9 The lymph nodes along the common hepatic artery are dissected just above the nerve plexus along the artery

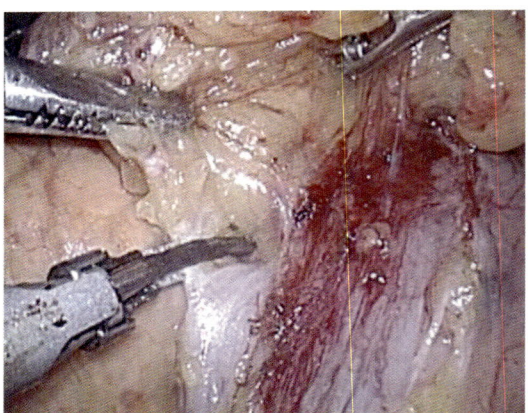

Fig. 23.8 The fat tissues including the lesser curvature lymph nodes are dissected upward to clear the stomach at the line of transection

Dissection of the Lesser Curvature
(Video 23.4)

The lesser curvature is completely dissected between the terminal branches of the left gastric artery and right gastric artery. The fat tissues including the lesser curvature lymph nodes are dissected upward carefully using the LCS to clear the stomach at the line of transection of the lesser curvature of the stomach (Fig. 23.8).

Lymph Node Dissection Along the Common Hepatic Artery
(Video 23.5)

The assistant grips and lifts the fat tissue on the upper border of the pancreas including the left gastric artery and stretches the gastropancreatic ligament in the right hand. The assistant gently pushes down the pancreatic body in the left hand holding gauze to show the superior border of the pancreas. The surgeon dissects the peritoneum along the upper border of the pancreas from the right to the left side of the abdomen. If the left gastric vein appears, it is clipped and dissected.

The surgeon holds and lifts the lymph nodes along the common hepatic artery in the left hand and dissects it just above the nerve plexus along the common hepatic artery using the LCS (Fig. 23.9). The surgeon identifies and exposes the base of the left gastric artery and transects it using the LCS after double clipping the vessel (Fig. 23.10). The surgeon dissects the lymph nodes along the common hepatic artery from the front of the common hepatic artery in a cephalad direction including the lymph nodes along the celiac artery.

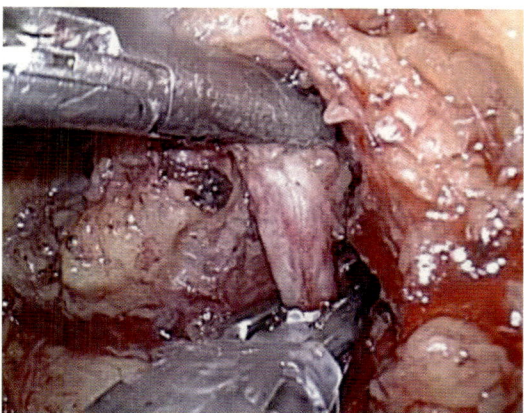

Fig. 23.10 The base of the left gastric artery is exposed and transected after double clipping the vessel

Lymph Node Dissection Along the Splenic Artery (Video 23.6)

First, the surgeon dissects the retroperitoneum from the crus to the pancreas body. The operator holds and lifts the lymph nodes along the splenic artery in the left hand and dissects the nodes just above the nerve plexus along the splenic artery toward the pancreatic tail using the LCS. The surgeon identifies the base of the posterior artery and dissects it using the LCS after clipping the vessel. The extent of dissection along the splenic artery is from its origin to halfway of the splenic artery. Then, the whole stomach can be mobilized freely.

Resection of the Stomach

A skin incision (5 cm) is made at the trocar site on the left rectus muscle of abdomen, and the stomach is pulled out of the abdominal cavity through the mini-laparotomy site. Confirming the clips which marked the lesion by palpation, the stomach is cut at the distal side of the clips with the autosuture linear stapler. Then, the stomach is removed. In case of intracorporeal resection, the marking clips should be confirmed by intraoperative esophagogastroduodenoscopy before cutting the esophagus.

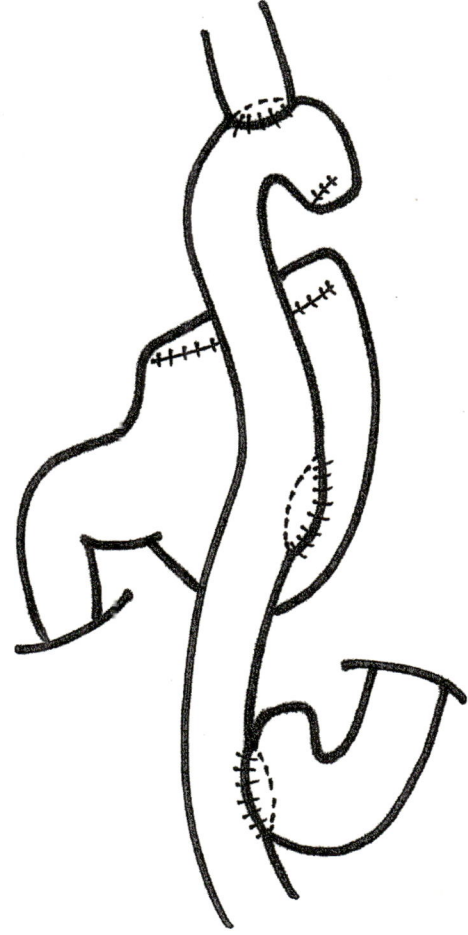

Fig. 23.11 Schema of double tract anastomosis

Reconstruction (Video 23.7)

There are mainly three reconstruction methods, esophagogastric anastomosis, jejunal interposition [2], and double tract anastomosis [3]. The optimal method has not been established. We prefer a double tract anastomosis method due to the reasons as follows: the anastomosis can be performed even if the remnant stomach is small; part of food passes the duodenum; and the remnant stomach can be checked postoperatively using esophagogastroduodenoscopy (Fig. 23.11).

For the double tract anastomosis, esophagojejunostomy is performed with the purse-string

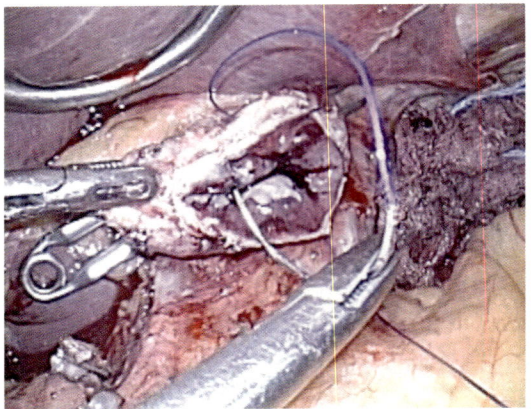

Fig. 23.12 The esophageal stump is sewn over with interrupted sutures laparoscopically to fix the anvil of a circular stapler

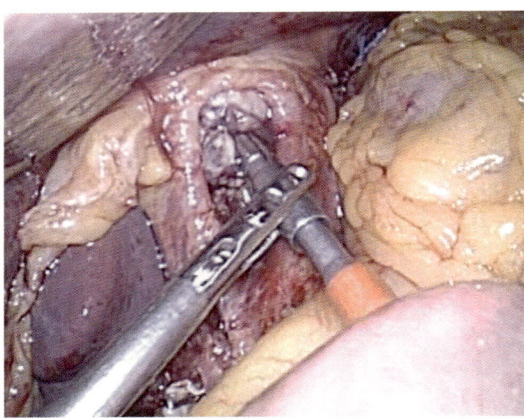

Fig. 23.14 Esophagojejunostomy is performed using a circular stapler introduced into the abdominal cavity through the mini-laparotomy site

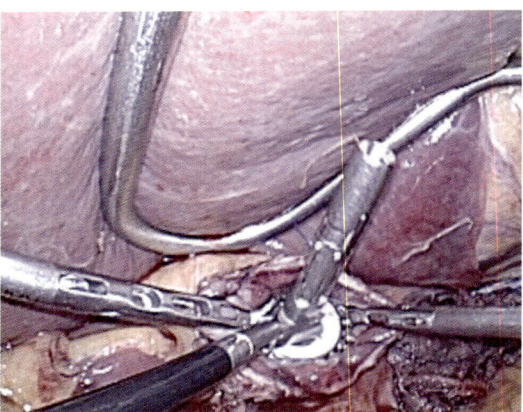

Fig. 23.13 The anvil of a circular stapler is inserted into the esophageal stump

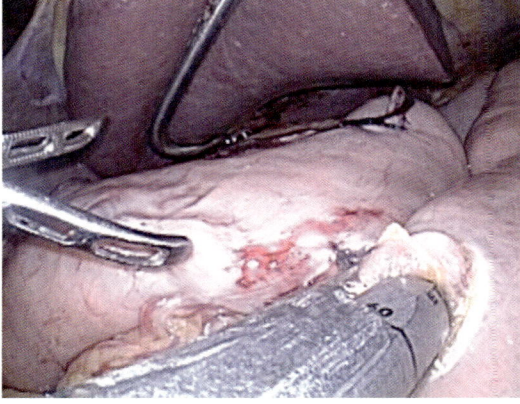

Fig. 23.15 A side-to-side gastrojejunostomy is performed using a linear stapler of which the forks are inserted into the holes in the anterior wall of the greater curvature of the remnant stomach and the jejunal limb

suture method as previously reported [4, 5]. The esophageal stump is sewn over with interrupted sutures laparoscopically or by using a device called the Endostitch (Fig. 23.12), and the anvil of a circular stapler is inserted into the esophageal stump (Fig. 23.13). The purse-string suture is tied and reinforced with a monofilament pretied loop. The jejunum is transected at a point about 20 cm from the ligament of Treitz. A circular stapler is inserted into the distal side of jejunum and is introduced into the abdominal cavity through the mini-laparotomy site, and esophagojejunostomy is performed (Fig. 23.14). Anastomotic leaks are evaluated using air insufflation.

Gastrojejunostomy is performed at a site 25 cm below the esophagojejunostomy. Small enterotomies are made in the anterior wall of the greater curvature of the remnant stomach and the jejunal limb. A linear stapler is introduced into the abdominal cavity, the forks are inserted into the holes, and a side-to-side gastrojejunostomy is performed (Fig. 23.15). The entry hole is closed by laparoscopic hand-sewn technique or standard hand-sewn through the mini-laparotomy site. Finally, jejunojejunostomy is performed at a site of 20 cm below the gastrojejunostomy.

Drain Insertion

The abdominal cavity is washed with saline. After confirmation of no bleeding under a pneumoperitoneum, a drain is inserted near the upper part of the pancreas through the right subcostal trocar.

Short-Term Outcomes in Our Institute

Between November 2011 and November 2013, we have performed laparoscopic proximal gastrectomy with double tract anastomosis for 13 patients with clinical T1 gastric cancer at the Osaka University Hospital. The mean operation time was 274 min, and the mean blood loss was 127 mL. According to the Clavien-Dindo classification, there were one grade II pancreatic fistula and one grade III anastomotic leakage complications. There were no treatment-related deaths or grade IV complications.

References

1. Japanese Gastric Cancer Association. Japanese classification of gastric carcinoma – 3rd English edition. Gastric Cancer. 2011;14:101–12.
2. Katai H, Sano T, Fukagawa T, Shinohara H, Sasako M. Prospective study of proximal gastrectomy for early gastric cancer in the upper third of the stomach. Br J Surg. 2003;90:850–3.
3. Ahn SH, Jung DH, Son SY, Lee CM, Park DJ, Kim HH. Laparoscopic double-tract proximal gastrectomy for proximal early gastric cancer. Gastric Cancer. 2014;17:562–70.
4. Takiguchi S, Sekimoto M, Fujiwara Y, Miyata H, Yasuda T, Doki Y, Yano M, Monden M. A simple technique for performing laparoscopic purse-string suturing during circular stapling anastomosis. Surg Today. 2005;35:896–9.
5. Wada N, Kurokawa Y, Takiguchi S, Takahashi T, Yamasaki M, Miyata H, Nakajima K, Mori M, Doki Y. Feasibility of laparoscopy-assisted total gastrectomy in patients with clinical stage I gastric cancer. Gastric Cancer. 2014;17:137–40.

Laparoscopy-Assisted Total Gastrectomy

24

Nobuhiko Tanigawa, Sang-Woong Lee, and George Bouras

Patient Positioning

The patient is positioned supine on a Maquet operating table (Maquet, Germany), with the right arm adducted and the left arm abducted to 90°. Pneumatic compressors are attached, and legs are bandaged to the lower limb supports, which are abducted and hyperextended to make space for the primary surgeon who stands in between the patient's legs. The patient is tilted head-up in a reverse-Trendelenburg position. Cardiac monitor electrodes are placed away from the ventral abdomen so that they don't get in the

Electronic supplementary material Supplementary material is available in the online version of this chapter at 10.1007/978-3-319-09342-0_24. Videos can also be accessed at http://www.springerimages.com/videos/978-3-319-09341-3.

N. Tanigawa, MD, FACS (✉)
Department of Surgery,
Tanigawa Memorial Hospital,
16-59, Kasuga 1-Chome, Ibaraki,
Osaka 567-0031, Japan
e-mail: tangiawa@tanigawa-hp.or.jp

S.-W. Lee, MD, PhD
Department of General and Gastroenterological Surgery, Osaka Medical College,
Takatsuki, Osaka, Japan

G. Bouras, BMBS, BMedSci, FRCS
Department of Surgery and Cancer,
Imperial College London, London, UK

way of the ports. Two seats are placed on either side of the patient for the assistants. Two video monitors are positioned on either side of the patient's head facing inward toward the primary operator (Figs. 24.1 and 24.2) [1].

Port Placement

Entry into the abdomen is gained through a 2 cm vertical skin incision that is made just above the umbilicus and a 12 mm Ethicon Excel blunt port is inserted. The supraumbilical optical port serves as a reference point for insertion of all other ports, two on either side of patient's abdomen. Both operative ports are placed 2 cm above the umbilical port and at a handbreadths distance laterally (12 mm right-hand and 5 mm left-hand port). Two further ports (both 5 mm) for the assistants are placed further superiorly near the costal margins, between the mid-clavicular and anterior axillary lines on the patient's right and more laterally on the mid-axillary line on the patient's left ensuring that the ports don't clash with the operative ports [2–4]. The umbilical wound is extended 3 cm superiorly along the midline for proximal procedures such as total and proximal gastrectomy that require esophagojejunal anastomosis and insertion of the circular stapler through a wound protector in the umbilical wound (Fig. 24.3) [5].

Fig. 24.1 Patient positioning

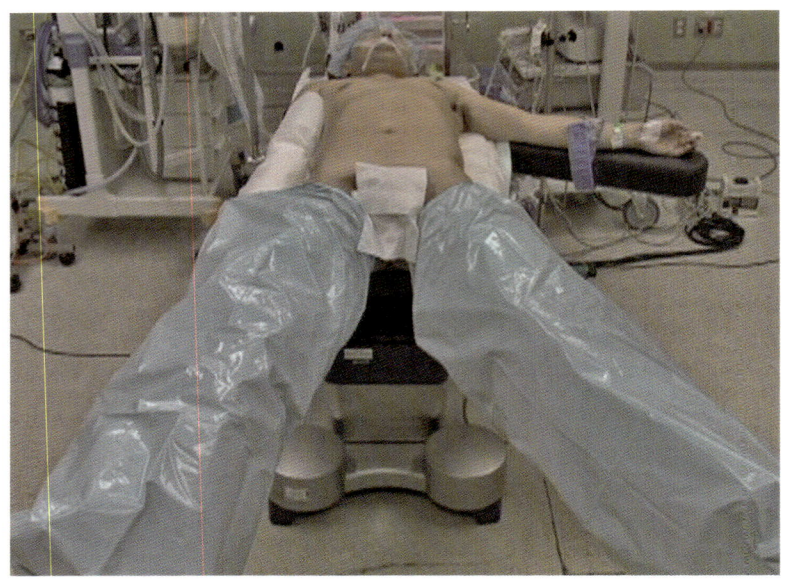

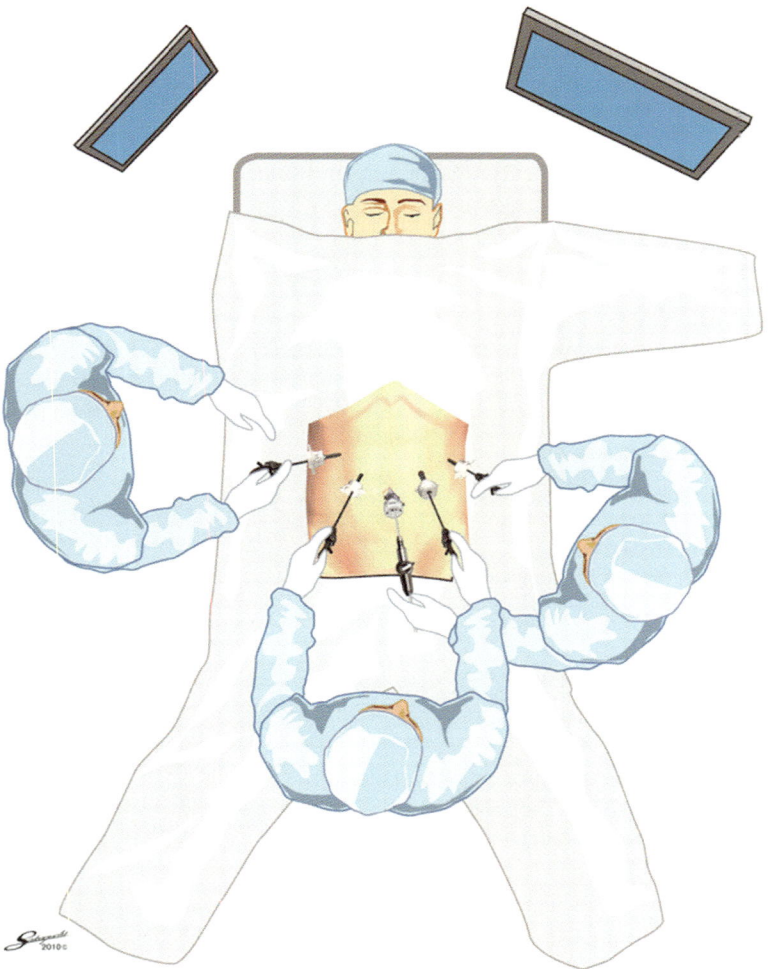

Fig. 24.2 Operating room setup (From Tanigawa [1] with permission)

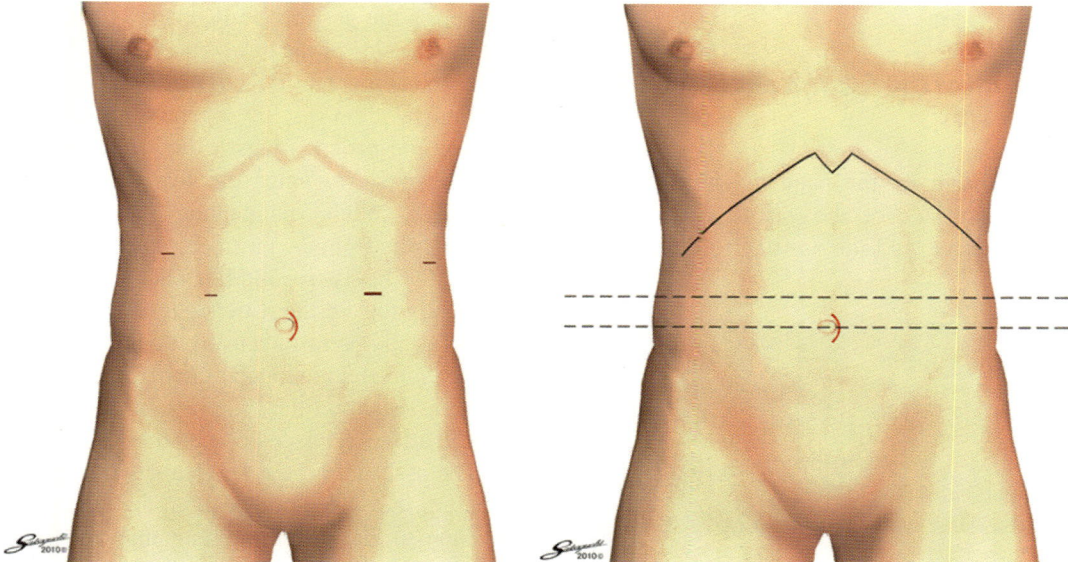

Fig. 24.3 Port positioning (From Tanigawa [1]) with permission)

Ports are first inserted into the right side of the abdomen (5 mm upper lateral port then 5 mm lower operative port) followed by the left side (5 mm upper lateral port then 12 mm lower operative port). The long needle is inserted through the skin at the marked site and peritoneal entry in the correct position and direction is confirmed. The needle is then withdrawn, and the skin is incised to accommodate the trocar. Artery forceps are used to separate the muscle before inserting the trocar in the desirable direction while avoiding visceral injury.

Liver Retraction

A 6 mm Penrose drain is prepared outside the body with colored sutures placed through it to provide ties for liver retractions. An incision is made on the superior leaf of the left triangular ligament above the left lobe of the liver with the Opti 2 while the assistants hold down the liver to apply tension. A space is created behind between the liver and the diaphragm with atraumatic graspers for passage of the middle part of the Penrose drain. The left lobe is then lifted to identify the corresponding space from below and the

middle portion of the Penrose drain passed from beneath mounted on a curved Karl-Storz grasper facing upward. Occasionally (especially with large left lobe of liver), the Penrose drain cannot be passed easily, and the black tie needs to be mounted on the tip of an Endo-Mini retractor to bring it through.

Once the middle portion is delivered over the liver, the white tie is placed to the right and the dye-stained tie to the left of the patient. Three small punctures are made in the epigastric skin with a number 11 blade for retrieval of each of the sutures. The Endo Close is inserted into the middle hole first and confirmed to enter the abdomen just to the left of the falciform ligament. The black tie is grasped and brought out to the skin where it is clipped secure with a mosquito. The white tie is brought through the right side skin hole and similarly the dye-stained tie through the left. The ties are then pulled laterally to lift the left lobe of the liver. Fine adjustments are made to achieve adequate exposure for the procedure. Ties are usually tightened in the order of white tie, dye-stained tie, and finally the black tie to complete the liver retraction (Figs. 24.4, 24.5, 24.6, 24.7, 24.8, and 24.9) [1]. There are other alternative techniques, but this is our preference.

Dissection

Division of the Gastrocolic Ligament to the Left

The assistant on the patient's right grasps the anterior surface of the gastric body near the greater curve, and the assistant on the patient's

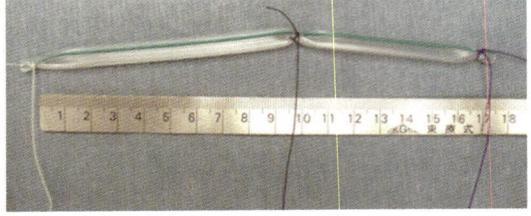

Fig. 24.4 Technique utilized for liver retraction

left grasps the gastrocolic ligament at the same level on the side of the transverse colon. The two assistants apply tension on the fatty tissue in between to allow for the operator standing in between the patient's legs to divide the gastrocolic ligament to enter the lesser sac (bursa omentalis). While maintaining a distance of 3–4 cm away from the gastroepiploic arcade, the division of the gastrocolic ligament is continued proximally toward the patient's left. Tissue division is usually performed using a combination of the LigaSure and monopolar diathermy.

The assistant on the right retracts the greater curve in a 10 o'clock position on the video monitor. The assistant on the left retracts the greater omentum in a 4 o'clock position and adjusts in real time so that the appropriate amount of tension is applied on the tissues that are being

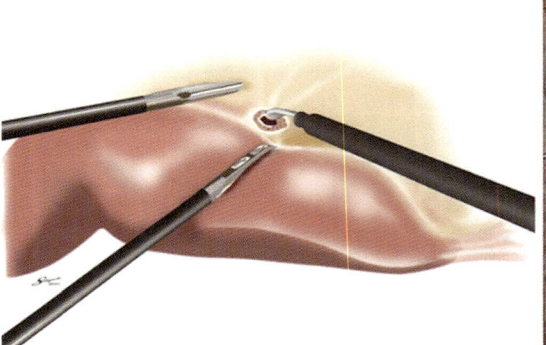
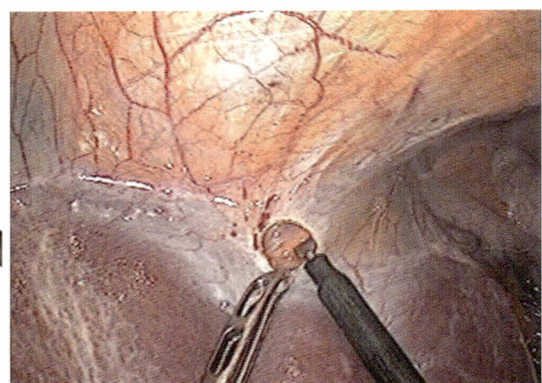

Fig. 24.5 Technique utilized for liver retraction (From Tanigawa [1] with permission)

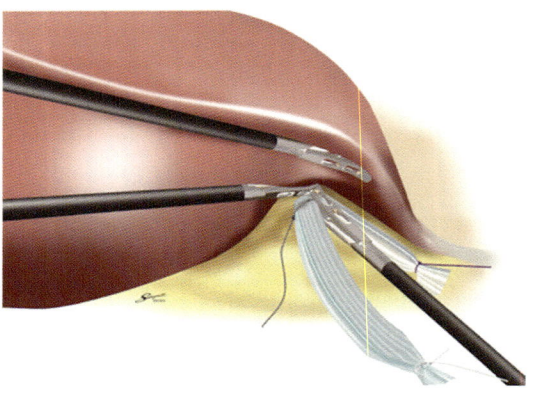
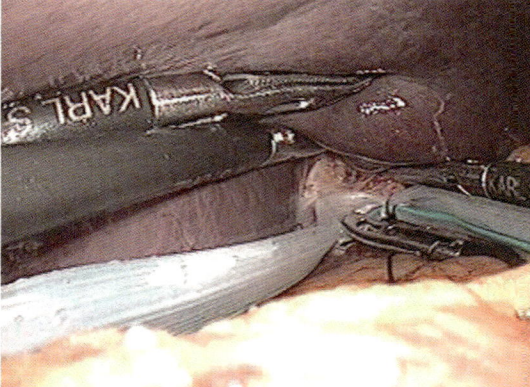

Fig. 24.6 Technique utilized for liver retraction (From Tanigawa [1] with permission)

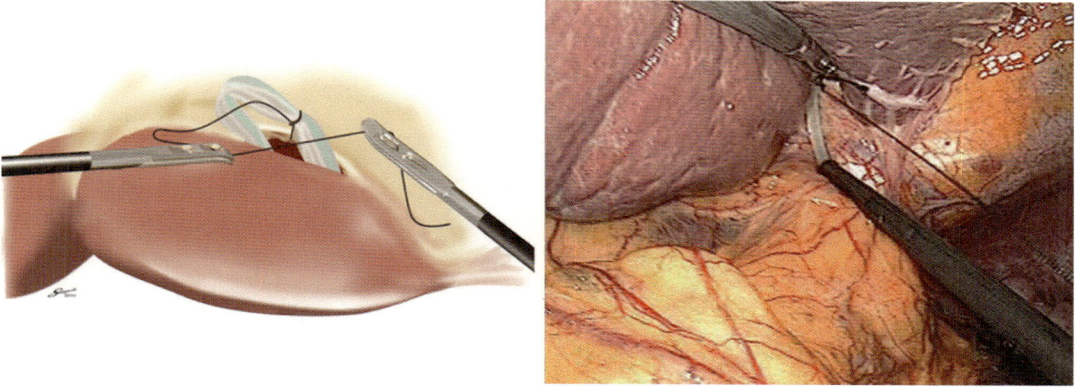

Fig. 24.7 Technique utilized for liver retraction (From Tanigawa [1] with permission)

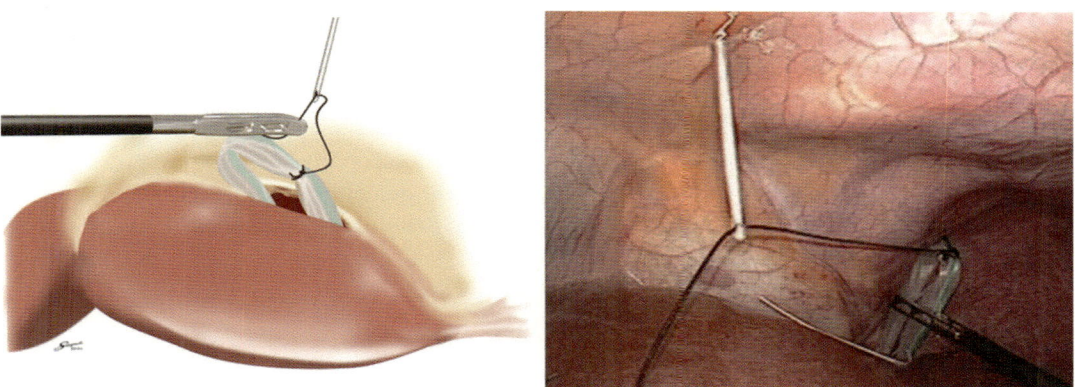

Fig. 24.8 Technique utilized for liver retraction (From Tanigawa [1] with permission)

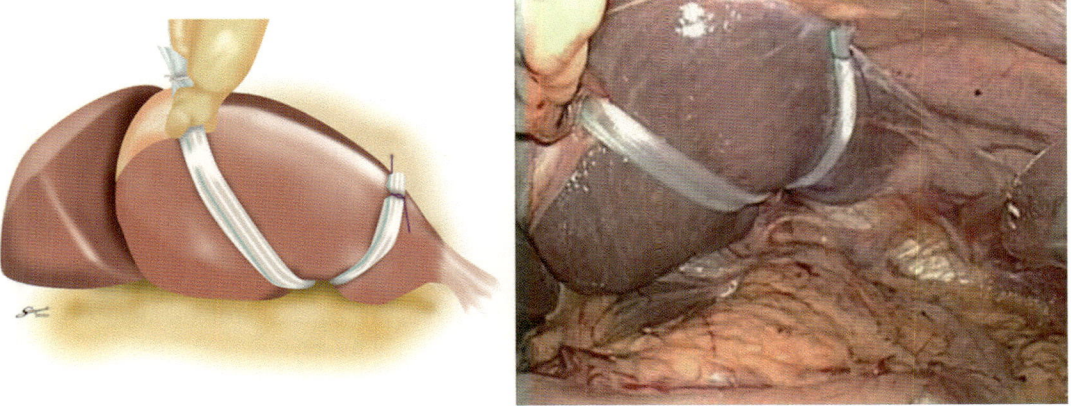

Fig. 24.9 Technique utilized for liver retraction (From Tanigawa [1] with permission)

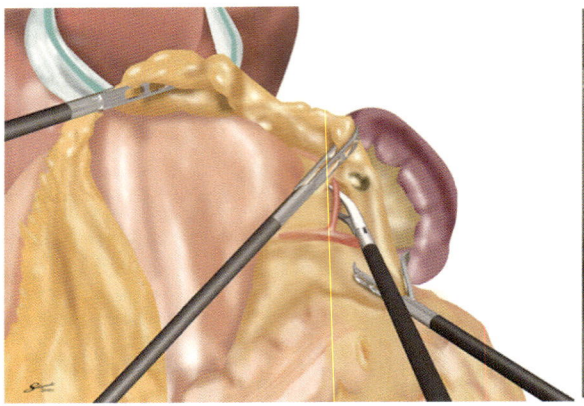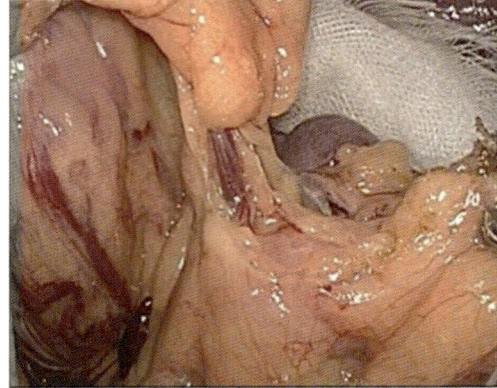

Fig. 24.10 Division of left gastroepiploic vessels (From Tanigawa [1] with permission)

divided. Care must be taken not to injure the transverse colon; the assistant on the left can grasp the tissues close to the colon while protecting the bowel wall with the grasper as the dissection is progressed toward the spleen.

Division of the Left Gastroepiploic Vessels and Dissection of Number 4sb Lymph Nodes

As the left gastroepiploic pedicle is approached, the assistant on the right grasps the posterior wall of the stomach near the greater curve and lifts in a 10 o'clock position to apply tension to the pedicle and gastrosplenic ligament. This helps clarify the anatomy and facilitates dissection around the root of the left gastroepiploic pedicle. Care must be taken not to apply too much tension to avoid traction injury to the spleen. Adhesions to the posterior gastric wall or the gastrocolic ligament are often present and need to be divided sharply with the diathermy or bipolar scissors to improve the exposure. The position of the root of the left gastroepiploic pedicle is determined from the inferomedial side (inside the lesser sac) from where the pedicle can be seen arising vertically from the retroperitoneum and running into the lifted greater curve of the stomach. The peritoneal layer is incised, and the vessels are skeletonized using the Marylands or dissecting forceps. The vessels are then clipped at their roots and divided by coagulation above the clips with the

4sb lymph nodes dissected on the side of the specimen (Fig. 24.10), [1]. The space beneath the gastrosplenic ligament is then entered and an avascular plane on the greater curve identified. Tissues are divided to reach the gastric wall at this point to complete the mobilization from this approach. According to the 13th edition of cancer treatment guidelines, 4sb lymph nodes are considered as 3rd-tier lymph nodes for gastric antrum lesions, and therefore resection is not mandatory in all cases.

Division of the Gastrosplenic Ligament and Dissection of Number 4sa Lymph Nodes

Beyond the left gastroepiploic vessels, the gastrocolic ligament fuses with the gastrosplenic ligament. The gastrosplenic ligament together with short gastric vessels is divided proximally close to the spleen until the fundus of the stomach is disconnected from the spleen (Fig. 24.11). Occasionally, large short gastric arteries are encountered that need to be clipped and coagulated with the LigaSure. Adhesions between the stomach, spleen, and omentum need to be carefully divided with monopolar diathermy or the LigaSure. Any parenchymal bleeding from the spleen caused by traction needs to be avoided as this can be difficult to control. Assistants must take care not to retract on the stomach omentum too strongly as there may be adhesions to the spleen.

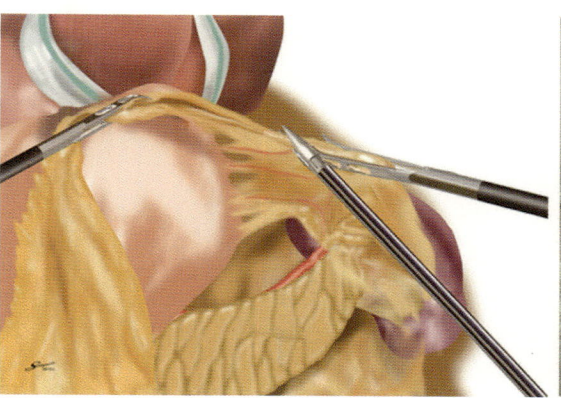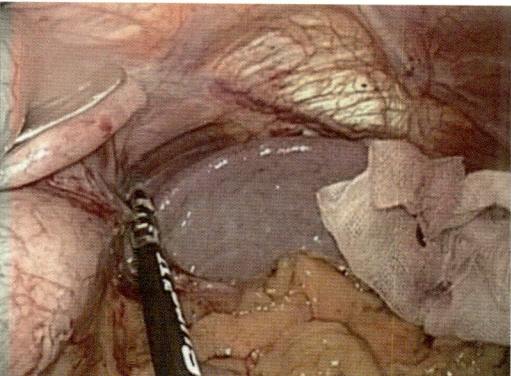

Fig. 24.11 Division of short gastric vessels (From Tanigawa [1] with permission)

Posterior Mobilization of the Proximal Stomach

Adhesions between the retroperitoneum and the posterior wall of proximal stomach are divided to free the stomach and expose the left gastric pedicle from the left side. Gastrodiaphragmatic attachments including those to the left crus of diaphragm are divided. The posterior gastric artery and the left inferior lateral diaphragmatic artery need to be identified and clipped prior to division with the LigaSure [6].

Dissection of 4d Lymph Nodes

Division of the gastrocolic ligament in the same plane parallel to the gastroepiploic arcade is continued distally toward the patient's right. The assistant on the right grasps the greater curve of the stomach and lifts in a 12 o'clock direction to create space behind the stomach and apply tension on the undivided distal part of the gastrocolic ligament. Adhesions to the anterior surface of the pancreas are divided to allow further lifting of the stomach and dissection toward the duodenum. As the gastrocolic ligament is divided, the plane between the transverse mesocolon and the greater omentum is identified, and any adhesions across this space are divided. The peritoneal reflection at the right lower limit of the lesser sac is then reached, and the fat is separated beyond this laterally in the plane anterior to the transverse

mesocolon. The right side assistant adjusts the ventral retraction to apply the right amount of tension on the fat to facilitate division. As the transverse mesocolon becomes tented up, it must be separated from the omentum with a combination of blunt dissection with graspers and sharp dissection with monopolar diathermy to allow it to drop down. As this is continued, the inner wall of the duodenal C-loop on 2nd part is reached with the right gastroepiploic pedicle still attached. The membrane between the duodenum and the pancreas is divided back toward the pylorus defining the lateral limit of number 6 lymph node dissection [1–3, 5–10].

Dissection of Number 6 Lymph Nodes

The position of the pylorus is determined anteriorly, and the dissection is commenced over the anterior surface of the pancreas to identify the right gastroepiploic vessels and dissect the surrounding lymph nodes. The right side assistant lifts the right gastroepiploic pedicle with perigastric fat near the pylorus ventrally to apply tension on the vessels. The root of the right gastroepiploic artery is usually found 2 cm below the pylorus in this configuration. The level of the head of the pancreas and the inferior border of the body are used for orientation during this dissection. As the plane anterior to the transverse mesocolon is followed superiorly toward the pancreas, the accessory right colic vein and gastrocolic trunk

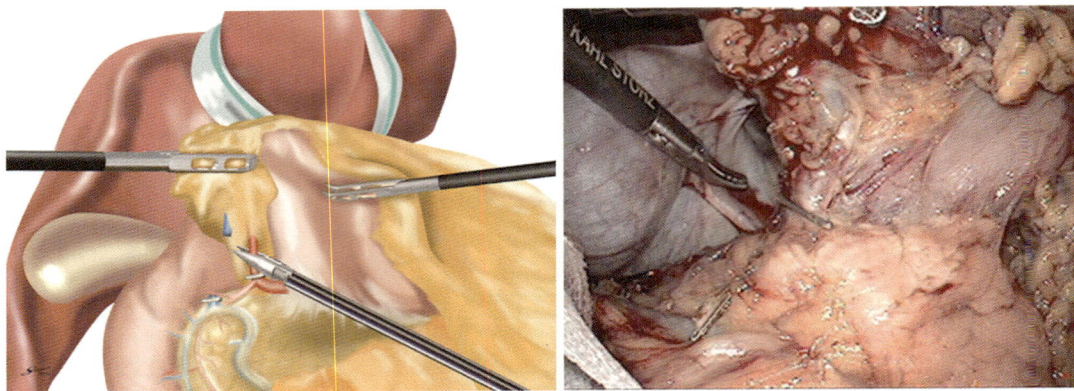

Fig. 24.12 Division of right gastroepiploic vessels (From Tanigawa [1] with permission)

can be seen within the mesenteric fat. Going over the anterior surface of the pancreas, the anterior superior pancreaticoduodenal vein comes into view and can be followed to its drainage into the right gastroepiploic vein. Once skeletonized, the right gastroepiploic vein is clipped above the anterior superior pancreaticoduodenal tributary, and the LigaSure V or Harmonic can be used to divide above the clip. The anterior surface of the pancreas can then be exposed further cranially in search of the artery. Care must be taken not to damage the pancreas as its head is tented up by the retraction on the artery. Energy devices in particular can cause thermal injury here and during dissection around the common hepatic and splenic arteries. Any damage can lead to postoperative inflammation. At our unit, we apply ice-cooled wet swabs on the surface of the pancreas during dissection in an attempt to minimize injury. As the fat is divided and the duodenal neck becomes mobilized laterally, small vessels and fibers running between the pancreas and duodenum require pre-coagulation with the LigaSure V or Marylands before division. Once exposed, the gastroduodenal artery on the pancreas can be followed to the origin of the right gastroepiploic artery. Approached from both sides, the artery can be dissected, clipped at its root, and divided above the clip (Fig. 24.12). The infrapyloric artery running to the pylorus can often be identified here and can either be clipped or coagulated. Once more space is created posterior to the duodenum, the remaining tissues connected to the

duodenum can be separated toward the pylorus. Further posterior mobilization along the gastroduodenal artery leads to the identification of the branching of the hepatic arteries defining the upper limit of the dissection from this approach. Several arterial branches to the lesser curve of the duodenum can also be opportunistically sealed and divided from this direction [1–3, 5–10].

Duodenal Transection

A gauze is packed behind the pylorus to help with mobilization of the lesser curve. The hepatoduodenal ligament is divided above the duodenal cap by incising the peritoneal layer with monopolar diathermy. In thin patients, the gauze may be visible through the transparent membrane, and the incision can be made in an avascular area. A wide window is created by dividing the vascular tissues along the lesser curve using the bipolar diathermy or coagulation devices. Once the duodenal neck is completely mobilized, the linear stapler is inserted for duodenal transection distal to the pylorus (Fig. 24.13).

Reinforcement of the Stapled Duodenal Stump

The staple line is buried with interrupted seromuscular 3/0 Vicryl. Once the corners are buried, 1–2 more sutures are usually enough to bury the middle portion of the staple line [3].

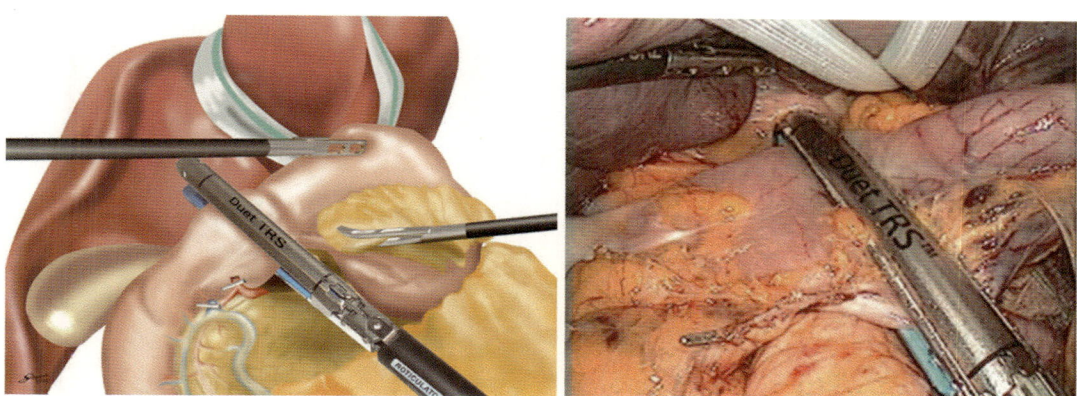

Fig. 24.13 Duodenal transection (From Tanigawa [1] with permission)

Division of the Right Gastric Artery and Dissection of Number 5 Lymph Nodes

The operator together with foot pedals shifts to the right side of the patient. The assistant stands in between the patient's legs and holds the camera with the left hand and an atraumatic grasper in the right hand. The peritoneal layer of the hepatoduodenal ligament is already divided and the common hepatic artery exposed from the dissection from below. The dissection can be continued toward the porta hepatis to expose the border of the hepatic artery proper with a combination of coagulation and sharp dissection. Large nerve fibers are present in this area and must be distinguished from lymphatics and small vessels. Inferiorly, the plane between the common hepatic artery and number 8a lymph nodes is separated cranially. The left side assistant retracts the right gastric pedicle in a 2–3 o'clock direction to facilitate dissection around its root. The retraction can, however, tent up the hepatic artery itself, so care must be taken not to divide this. The right gastric artery can also arise from the left hepatic artery. Anatomical variations are frequent here, and care must be taken not to cause any hepatic ischemia. Laterally, lymph nodes 12a and 5 are separated from the hepatic arteries, and the root of the right gastric artery is clipped before division (Fig. 24.14). The right gastric vein is also divided when encountered during this dissection [1–3, 5–10].

Division of the Lesser Omentum and the Peritoneum Overlying the Right Crus

The hepatogastric ligament forming the membranous proximal part of the lesser omentum is divided proximally toward the abdominal esophagus. The LigaSure and Harmonic are used to divide fatty layers, while membranes are divided by monopolar diathermy. In 15–20 % of cases, an accessory left hepatic artery runs from the lesser curve of stomach to the liver [11]. This artery needs to be dissected and its size and contribution to hepatic circulation estimated. In most cases, this artery can be divided. Once the upper limit near the hiatus is reached, the peritoneal membrane overlying the right crus of the diaphragm is divided to define the superior and right lateral limit of dissection of number 9 lymph nodes in front of the celiac trunk.

Dissection Above the Pancreas (Lymph Nodes 8a, 7, 11p, 11d, and 9)

The operator moves to the patient's right. The dissection is continued exposing the common hepatic artery toward the left gastric artery. The operator gently grasps the lymph nodes with a grasper or dissecting forceps in the left hand and continues separating the plane between the artery and lymph nodes using the monopolar diathermy in soft coagulation mode. This allows for

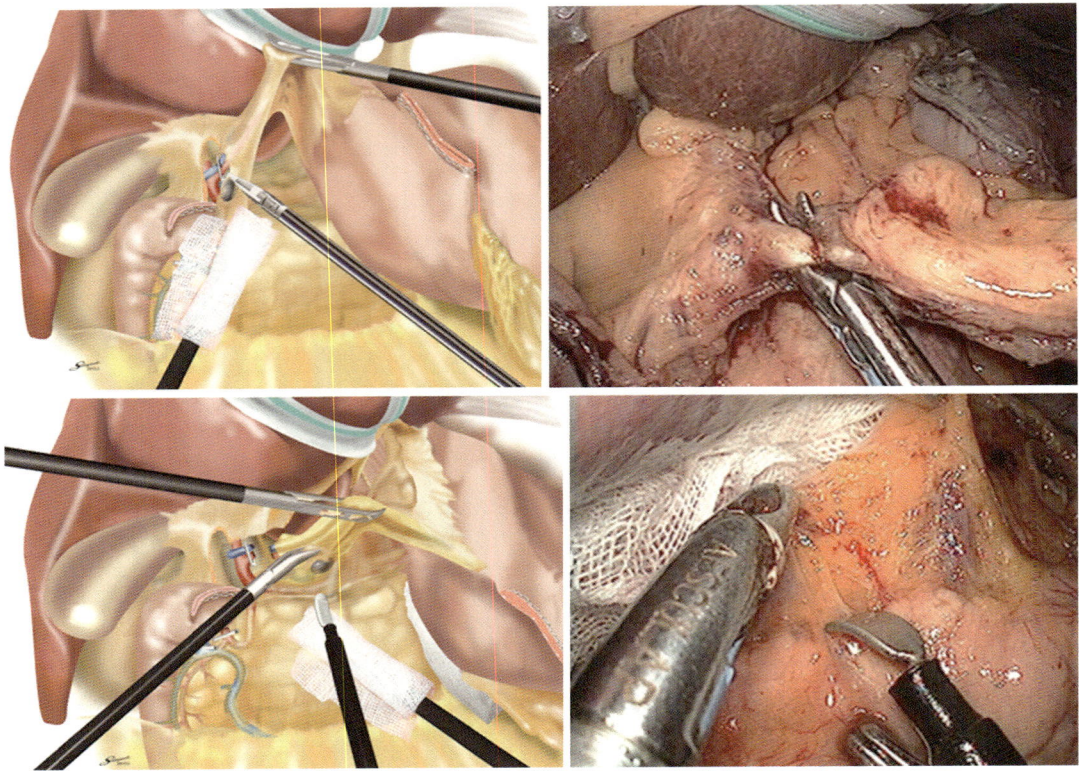

Fig. 24.14 Division of right gastric vessels (From Tanigawa [1] with permission)

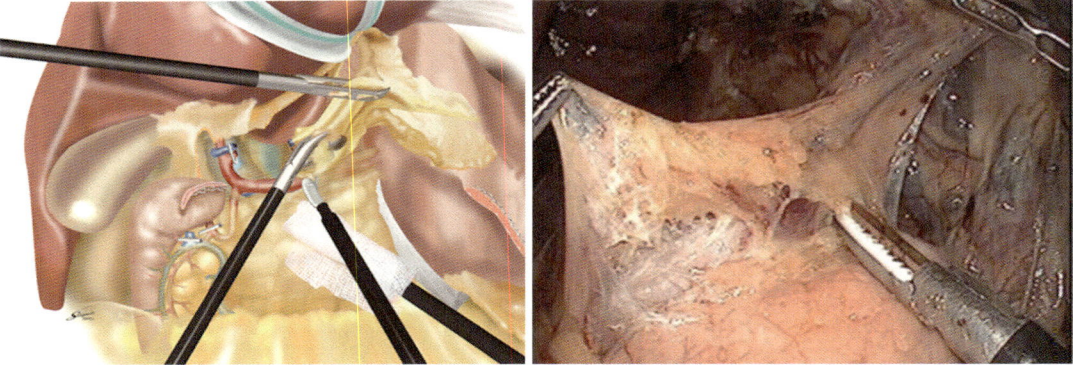

Fig. 24.15 Dissection of nodal tissue along the common hepatic artery (From Tanigawa [1] with permission)

hemostatic division of lymphatic tissues with a low risk of major vascular injury. The anterior surface of pancreas is pushed downward by the assistant to facilitate deeper dissection. Vessels running from the pancreas to the lymph nodes must be pre-coagulated with the soft coagulation diathermy or bipolar forceps (Marylands) before

sharp division with the cutting mode diathermy. Repetition of these gestures exposes the entire surface of the common hepatic artery to complete the inferior mobilization of number 8a lymph nodes (Fig. 24.15). The LigaSure can also be used for simultaneous coagulation and tissue division. The left gastric vein may be encountered

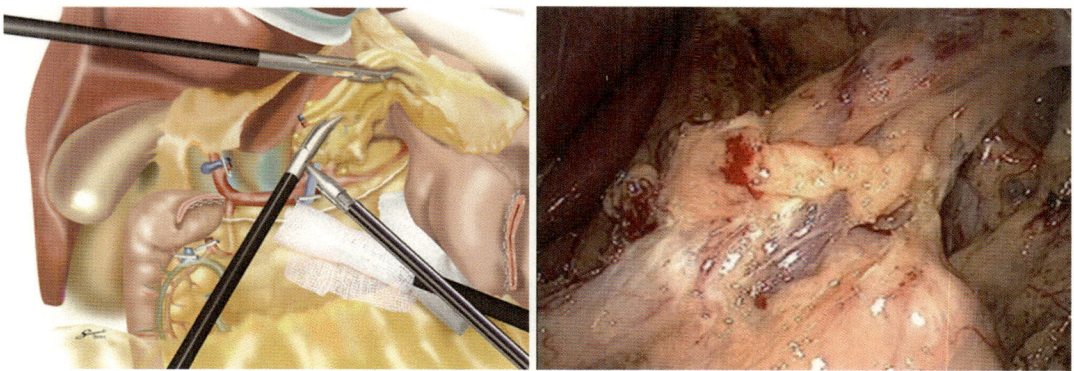

Fig. 24.16 Left gastric vein coursing anterior to the common hepatic artery (From Tanigawa [1] with permission)

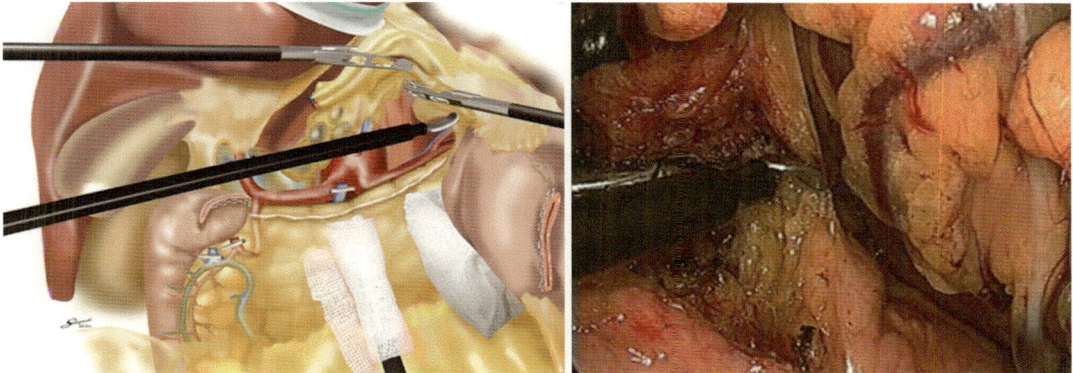

Fig. 24.17 Dissection of level 11p nodes along the splenic artery (From Tanigawa [1] with permission)

toward the pedicle. In cases where this vessel drains directly into the portal vein or into the junction between the portal vein and splenic vein, it runs posterior to the common hepatic artery, whereas in other cases where the vein drains into the splenic vein, it loops anterior to the common hepatic artery (Fig. 24.16). Rarely, the vein runs posterior to the splenic artery draining into the splenic vein. Once identified, the left gastric vein is clipped and divided.

The left gastric pedicle is grasped near the gastric wall and retracted ventrally with the operator's left-hand grasper. The dissection on the common hepatic artery is continued in front of the left gastric artery by dividing fibers running between the pancreas and the vessels. The dissecting forceps are used to create gaps in the lymphatic tissue then the LigaSure V or Harmonic is used to coagulate and cut simultaneously. The splenic artery is followed until the posterior gastric artery is reached. The splenic vein running posterior to the artery can occasionally be visualized during this part of the dissection. The loose space next to the left gastric pedicle can be opened and the lymphatic tissues divided laterally to dissect number 11p lymph nodes off the splenic artery (Fig. 24.17). Then, attachments to the left crus are divided to define the left lateral limit of the celiac lymph node dissection. Once tissues are separated from the crura on both sides, the posterior limit of number 9 dissection is defined. The root of the left gastric artery can then be dissected by dividing the fibrous nerve bundles around the vessel. The artery is then clipped and divided with number 7 lymph nodes on the side of the stomach (Fig. 24.18). A cut finger end of a surgical glove (Sensi-touch 8.0) is inserted into the abdomen through the 12 mm port, and the dissected lymph

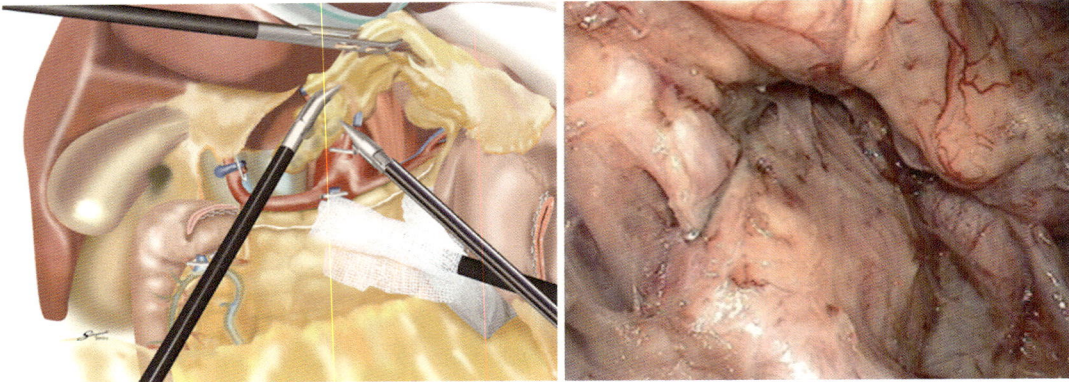

Fig. 24.18 Division of left gastric artery (From Tanigawa [1] with permission)

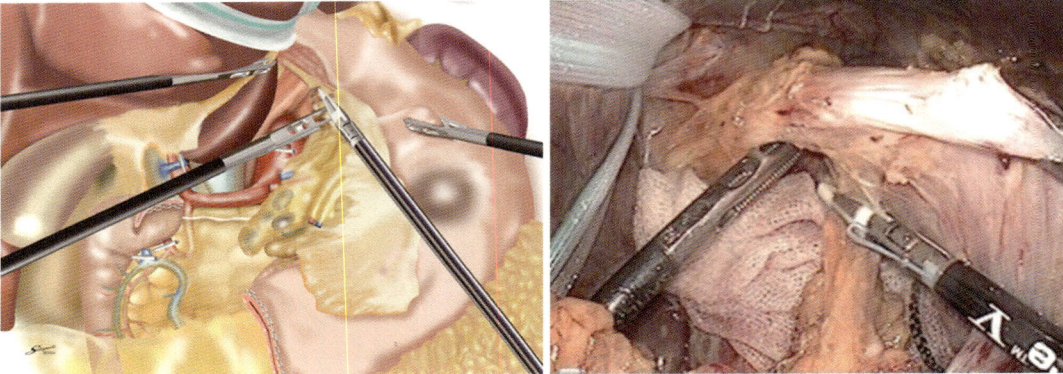

Fig. 24.19 Circumferential mobilization of gastroesophageal junction (From Tanigawa [1] with permission)

node is placed inside for retrieval from the abdominal cavity A [1–3, 5–10].

Hiatal Mobilization of the Abdominal Esophagus

Bearing in mind that the proximal transection will be on the esophagus, the anterior surface of the esophagus is approached from the right and freed from the diaphragm taking lymph nodes around the hiatus on the side of the stomach. The anterior vagus nerve running longitudinally on the anterior surface of the esophagus is divided distal to the origin of the hepatic branch preserving the nerve supply to the liver. As the dissection is continued posteriorly separating the esophagus from the right crus, the posterior vagus is divided leading to further lengthening of the abdominal part of the esophagus (Fig. 24.19). The Endo-Mini retractor is then passed behind and above the angle of His to confirm circumferential mobilization of the gastroesophageal junction [5, 6, 8, 12].

Insertion of Anvil and Esophageal Transection

The nasogastric tube is withdrawn in preparation for the insertion of the anvil of the circular stapler prior to esophageal transection and subsequent esophagojejunal anastomosis.

The authors have employed the hemi-double stapling technique at esophagojejunostomy,

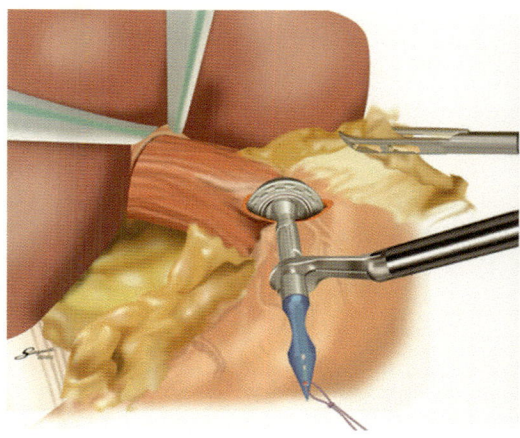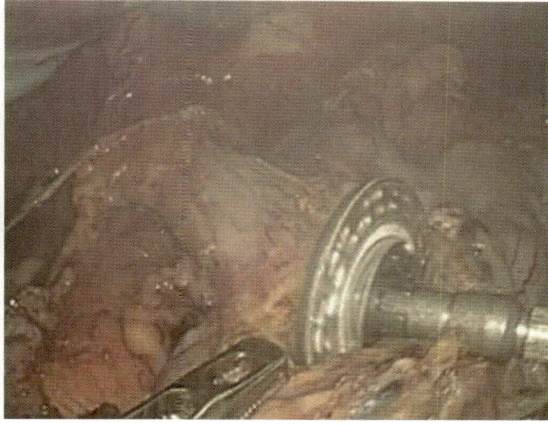

Fig. 24.20 Inserting the anvil through gastrotomy (From Tanigawa [1] with permission)

because it is simple without need of suturing techniques and the most familiar to every surgeon who has some experience of open gastrectomy. Insertion of the anvil is accomplished by two ways, one through gastrotomy which is made in the anterior wall of the fundus and another through the mouth by the use of OrVil Tilt-top.

Insertion of Anvil Through Gastrostomy (Video 24.1)

Using monopolar diathermy, a full-thickness gastrotomy is made on the lesser curve slightly anteriorly near the gastroesophageal junction to enter the lumen. The hole is extended longitudinally to about 3 cm enough for insertion of the 25 mm anvil. If the tumor is located on the proximal lesser curve, the entry hole is made anteriorly to avoid the tumor. A straight atraumatic grasper is inserted into the esophagus to confirm the direction of anvil insertion.

The anvil of a PCEAA 25 mm stapler is prepared outside the body by attaching a 2/0 Vicryl tie onto the center rod. As the Vicryl tie needs to be removed once the anvil is in position, it is tied loosely so that the tie can be easily cut laparoscopically. The length of the tie is left at 5 cm so that it can be identified once inside the body. The pneumoperitoneum is temporarily stopped, the umbilical port is removed, and the anvil is placed into the abdomen. The umbilical port is then reinserted and pneumoperitoneum reestablished. The center rod of the anvil is grasped with the anvil holder in the operator's right hand, and the anvil is inserted into the abdominal esophagus (Fig. 24.20). A rotating movement often facilitates insertion. The anvil is pushed in proximally so that there is adequate distal esophagus beyond the anvil rod for transection with the linear stapler. A grasper is used to palpate and confirm that the anvil rod is above the esophageal transection line. The Vicryl tie should still be within the transection line at this stage. The esophagus is then transected with the Echelon 60–3.5 blue inserted through the left lower 12 mm port (Fig. 24.21). Slight angulation of the staple line is appropriate when transection is complete (Fig. 24.22).

Once divided, the purple color of the Vicryl tie can be seen on the staple line. This is pulled so that the center rod abuts the staple line. While pulling on the Vicryl, the stapled line is incised with monopolar diathermy onto the center rod until the metal rod becomes visible and can be grasped and pulled out of the esophagus (Fig. 24.23). Once the anvil is in position, the Vicryl is cut and removed so that it does not get in the way when combining the anvil with the circular stapler.

Anvil Insertion Through Mouth

By the use of OrVil Tilt-top, the anvil is placed into the abdominal esophagus through the mouth by pulling down the tube, which is connected with the center rod (Fig. 24.24).

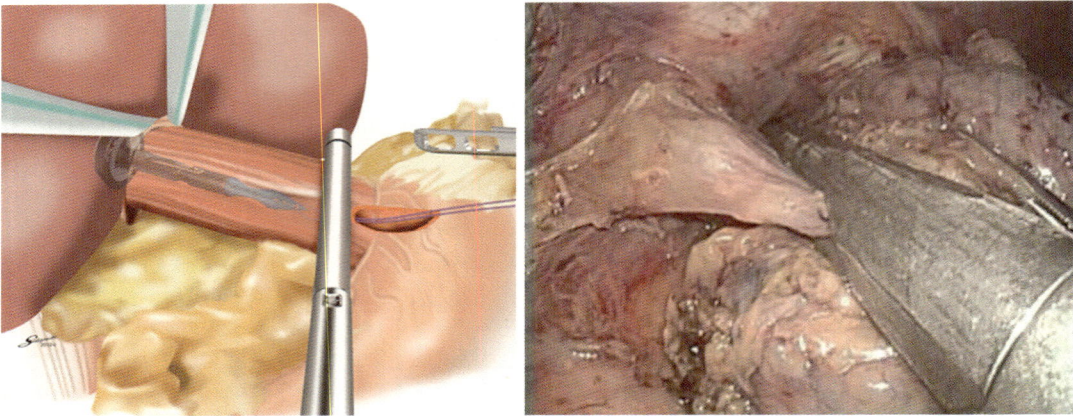

Fig. 24.21 Esophageal transection (From Tanigawa [1] with permission)

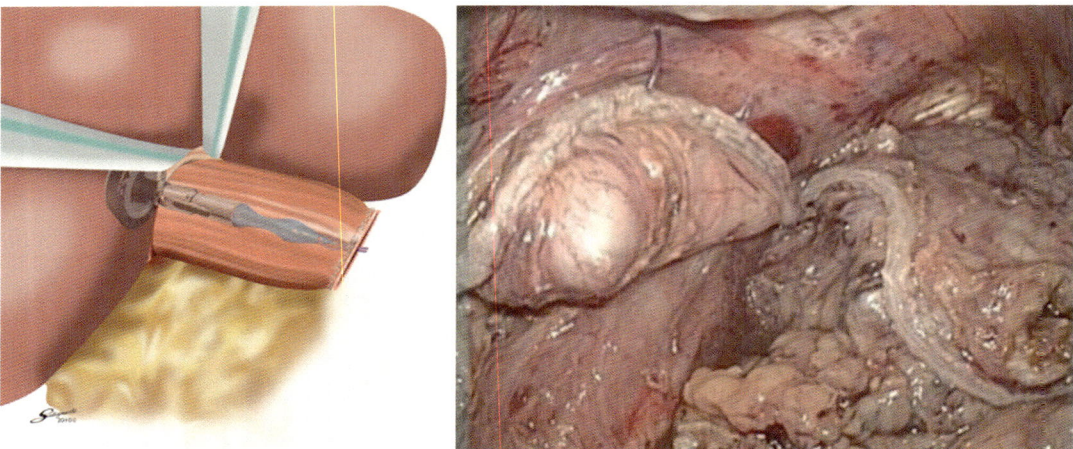

Fig. 24.22 Vicryl suture tied to the anvil identified post-esophageal transection (From Tanigawa [1] with permission)

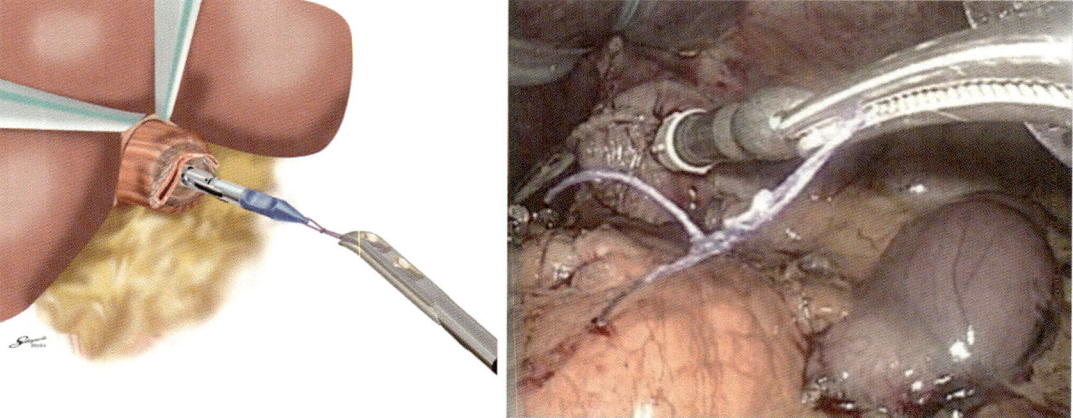

Fig. 24.23 Vicryl suture utilized to retrieve the anvil (From Tanigawa [1] with permission)

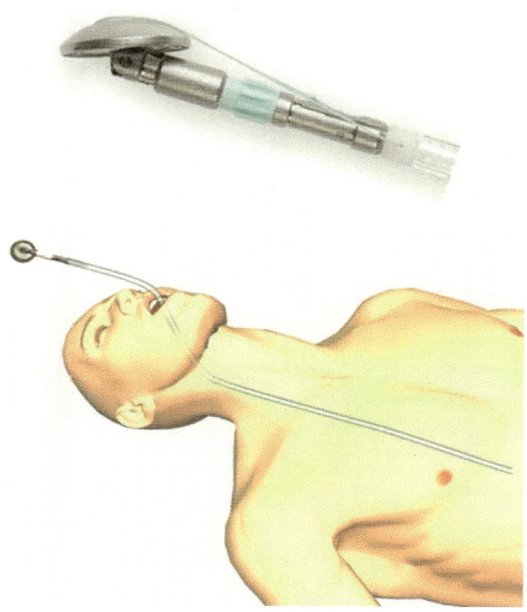

Fig. 24.24 Insertion of anvil through mouth (OrVil™) (From Tanigawa [1] with permission)

Marking of the Jejunum

The two assistants lift and spread the transverse mesocolon so that the operator can identify the ligament of Treitz. Using a 10 cm measuring tape, a distance of 20 cm is measured from the ligament of Treitz, and the bowel wall is marked with a dye-stained Endo-peanut. A metal clip is placed immediately distally to avoid confusion. The left side assistant grasps this part of the bowel while insufflation is stopped in preparation for the open part of the procedure.

Extension of the Umbilical Wound (Mini-laparotomy) and Specimen Retrieval (Video 24.2)

The umbilical port wound is extended to 4 cm superiorly using the diathermy onto the shaft of the port while it is still inserted. Once the wound is adequately large, the Lap Protector is inserted into the wound. Two towels are placed between the wound protector and the skin to prevent contamination. The specimen is removed through

the mini-laparotomy after which the marked jejunum is delivered outside [9, 13].

Division of the Jejunum

From the point on the jejunum marked with dye, the jejunal mesentery is divided for 10 cm distally using the LigaSure to coagulate vessels. This bowel becomes ischemic and is the sacrificed portion of jejunum. Another way of creating a gap in the jejunal mesentery without sacrificing the bowel is to cut into the mesentery toward its root. Once ready, the jejunum can be transected distal to the sacrifice jejunum using the Echelon 60–3.5 blue.

Insertion of the Anvil into the Jejunum at 20 cm from the Ligament of Treitz

To perform the jejunojejunostomy using the PCEEA 21 mm circular stapler, a purse-string applicator is placed on the healthy bowel just proximal to the sacrifice jejunum on the oral side. The redundant bowel is removed with the monopolar diathermy for external use, and a 2/0 Prolene with a straight needle on either end is used as the purse-string suture. Once in position, the needles are cut off, and the purse-string applicator is withdrawn. The anvil is then placed into the bowel lumen, and the purse-string is tightened around the center rod of the anvil.

Reinforcement of the Staple Line on the Divided Jejunum and Creation of the Enterotomy for Insertion of the Circular Stapler

The staple line on the divided distal jejunum of the alimentary limb is reinforced with interrupted seromuscular 3/0 Vicryl stitches. The last suture on the mesenteric edge of the stump is left long at 2 cm so that it can be grasped to maneuver the bowel intracorporeally during subsequent esophagojejunostomy.

After measuring 20 cm from the reinforced jejunal stump, a 25 mm enterotomy is made on the anti-mesenteric side of the jejunum. This is used to insert the circular stapler distally for the jejunojejunostomy and proximally for the esophagojejunostomy. Furthermore, this hole serves as the site where the subsequent gastrojejunostomy is created as part of double-tract reconstruction following proximal gastrectomy.

Extracorporeal Jejunojejunostomy (Using Circular Stapler)

The PCEEA 21 mm circular stapler is inserted into the enterotomy created. The shaft of the stapler is fed distally to a point 20 cm from the enterotomy. The center pin of the stapler is brought out to pierce the bowel wall here, and the stapler is connected to its corresponding anvil already secured in the biliopancreatic jejunum (on the side of the ligament of Treitz). The stapler is fired to create a stapled side-to-end jejunojejunostomy. Reinforcement of the staple line is not performed; however, any bleeding points are controlled with full-thickness hemostatic sutures across the staple line. The gap in the mesentery is closed with continuous 3/0 Vicryl to avoid internal herniation between the cut edges of the small bowel mesentery. The completed jejunojejunostomy is then pushed into the abdomen [3, 14].

Laparoscopic Esophagojejunostomy (Using Circular Stapler) (Video 24.3)

The end (2 cm) of the middle finger of a number 8 surgical glove is cut off, and the glove is fed over the shaft of the 25 mm PCEEA circular stapler through the finger hole. The head of the circular stapler is then fed into the enterotomy on the jejunum created earlier and passed proximally toward the stump. The center pin is brought out to pierce the bowel wall on the anti-mesenteric side near the stump. A window is made in the mesentery 2 cm away from the end to pass a cut rubber band through to the other side. The rubber band is pulled over the shaft and secured with a

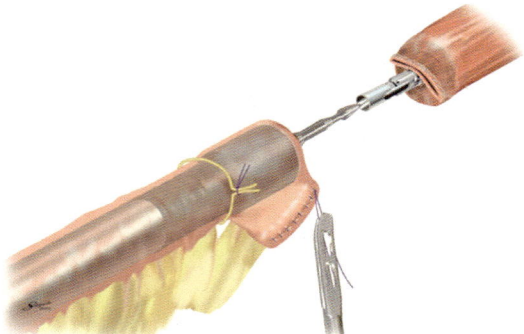

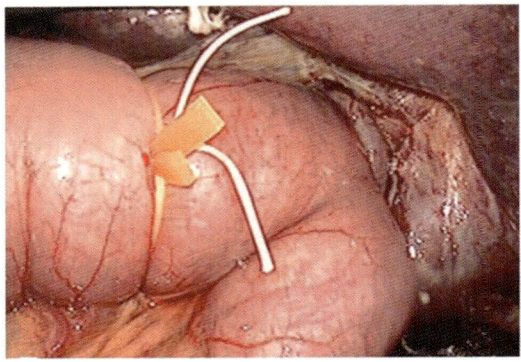

Fig. 24.25 Rubber band applied to the shaft of the stapler to stabilize for esophagojejunostomy (From Tanigawa [1] with permission)

heavy Vicryl tie so that the jejunum does not slip on the shaft during the anastomosis (Fig. 24.25). The whole apparatus including the jejunum connected to the stapler is inserted through the Lap Protector taking care not to cause any visceral damage inside the abdomen. The glove on the shaft is brought over the Lap Protector and fixed with three arterial clips to seal the gap for pneumoperitoneum. Insufflation is commenced through the left lower port through which the camera is also inserted. Using graspers, the center rods on the anvil and circular stapler are combined until securely clicked into position. The stapler is slowly closed ensuring that no tissues are caught in the anastomosis. The left-hand assistant helps by pulling on the Vicryl on the jejunal stump for retraction. Once closed and operators are satisfied, the circular stapler is fired. The rubber band is cut off and the stapler gently removed with some rotation so that it smoothly slips out from inside the bowel lumen (Fig. 24.26). Pneumoperitoneum is stopped again, and the

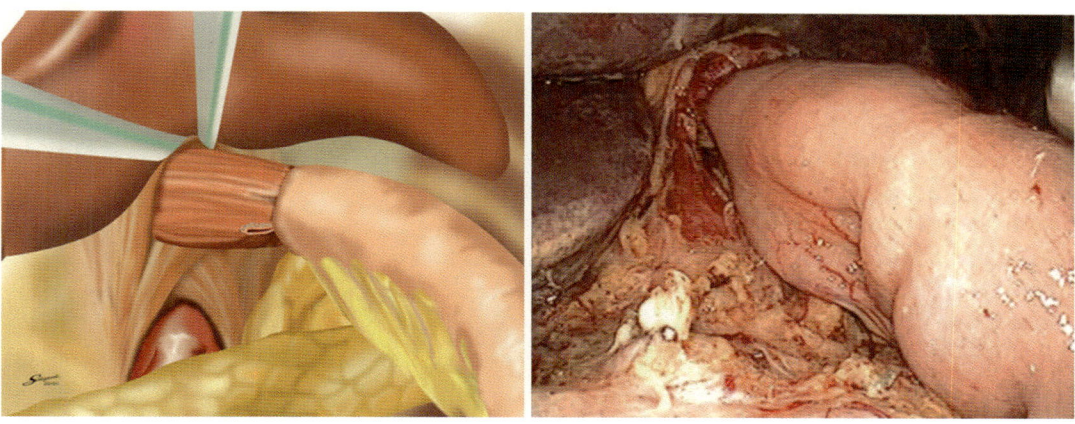

Fig. 24.26 Completed esophagojejunostomy (From Tanigawa [1] with permission)

glove is detached from the wound protector to completely free the stapler.

Another method for creation of the esophago-jejunostomy can be performed through division of the jejunum and insertion of the stapler through the end of the distal limb and advancing the head of the circular stapler distally toward healthy jejunum. By the use of a rubber band, the jejunal wall is fixed on the shaft so that the jejunum does not slip on the shaft during the anastomosis.

After pneumoperitoneum is established again, the shaft is introduced into the peritoneal cavity, and the center pin is brought out to pierce the bowel wall on the anti-mesenteric side. Using graspers, the center rods on the anvil and circular stapler are combined until securely clicked into position. The stapler is slowly closed ensuring that no tissues are caught in the anastomosis. After the circular stapler is fired, the rubber band is cut off and the stapler gently removed with some rotation so that it smoothly slips out from inside the bowel lumen.

Closure of the Jejunal Enterotomy (Used for Insertion of Circular Staplers) (Video 24.4)

The hole used for insertion of the circular stapler distally and proximally is closed using a two-layer Albert-Lembert technique (Fig. 24.27 depicts the completed anastomoses).

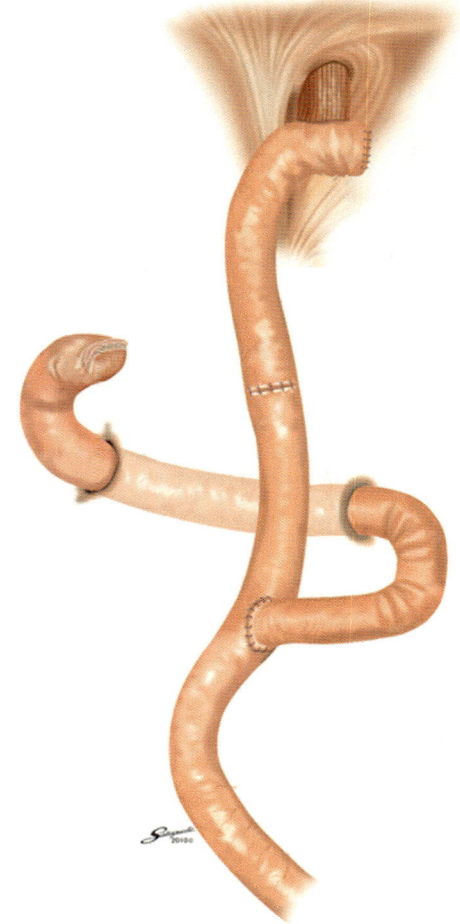

Fig. 24.27 Sketch depicting completed anastomoses (From Tanigawa [1] with permission)

Drain Insertion and Closure

A 10 mm flat-type Blake drain is inserted through the right lower port, passed between the peritoneum and abdominal wall and then into the space just distal to and behind the esophagojejunal anastomosis. The umbilical wound needs formal mass closure with 1 Vicryl. Skin closure is performed with interrupted 3/0 Vicryl subdermal stitches with buried knots. Steri-Strip tapes are used for accurate apposition of skin edges.

References

1. Tanigawa N. A manual for laparoscopic gastric resection. 1st ed. Osaka: Nagai Co, Ltd; 2009.
2. Shinohara H, Sonoda T, Niki M, Nomura E, Nishiguchi K, Tanigawa N. Laparoscopically-assisted pylorus-preserving gastrectomy with preservation of the vagus nerve. Eur J Surg. 2003;169:55–8.
3. Takaori K, Nomura E, Mabuchi H, Lee S, Agui T, Miyamoto Y, Iwamoto M, Watanabe H, Tanigawa N. A secure technique of intracorporeal Roux-Y reconstruction after laparoscopic distal gastrectomy. Am J Surg. 2005;189:178–83.
4. Lee SW, Bouras G, Nomura E, Yoshinaka R, Tokuhara T, Nitta T, Tsunemi S, Tanigawa N. Intracorporeal stapled anastomosis following laparoscopic segmental gastrectomy for gastric cancer: technical report and surgical outcomes. Surg Endosc. 2010;24: 1774–80.
5. Lee SW, Nomura E, Bouras G, Tokuhara T, Tsunemi S, Tanigawa N. Long-term oncological outcomes from laparoscopic gastrectomy for gastric cancer: a single-center experience of 601 consecutive resections. J Am Coll Surg. 2010;211:33–40.
6. Kim JJ, Song KY, Chin HM, Kim W, Jeon HM, Park CH, Park SM. Totally laparoscopic gastrectomy with various types of intracorporeal anastomosis using laparoscopic linear staplers: preliminary experience. Surg Endosc. 2008;22:436–42.
7. Japanese Gastric Cancer Association. Japanese classification of gastric carcinoma. 14th ed. Kanehara Co, Ltd; 2010.
8. Ikeda O, Sakaguchi Y, Aoki Y, Harimoto N, Taomoto J, Masuda T, Ohga T, Adachi E, Toh Y, Okamura T, Baba H. Advantages of totally laparoscopic distal gastrectomy over laparoscopically assisted distal gastrectomy for gastric cancer. Surg Endosc. 2009;23: 2374–9.
9. Nomura E, Isozaki H, Fujii K, Toyoda M, Niki M, Sako S, Mabuchi H, Nishiguchi K, Tanigawa N. Postoperative evaluation of function-preserving gastrectomy for early gastric cancer. Hepatogastroenterology. 2003;50:2246–50.
10. Bouras G, Lee SW, Nomura E, Tokuhara T, Tsunemi S, Tanigawa N. Comparative analysis of stration-specific lymph node yield in laparoscopic and open distal gastrectomy for early gastric cancer. Surg Laparosc Endosc Percutan Tech. 2011;21(6):424–8.
11. Lee SW, Shinohara H, Matsuki M, Okuda J, Nomura E, Mabuchi H, Nishiguchi K, Takaori K, Narabayashi I, Tangiawa N. Preoperative simulation of vascular anatomy by three –dimensional computed tomography imaging in laparoscopic gastric cancer surgery. J Am Coll Surg. 2003;197(6):927–36.
12. Tanigawa N, Nomura E, Lee SW, Kaminishi M, Sugiyama M, Aikou T, Kitajima M. Current state of gastric stump carcinoma in Japan: based on the results of a nationwide survey. World J Surg. 2010;34:1540–7.
13. Nomura E, Lee SW, Bouras G, Tokuhara T, Hayashi M, Hiramatsu M, Okuda J, Tanigawa N. Functional outcomes according to the size of the gastric remnant and type of reconstruction following laparoscopic distal gastrectomy for gastric cancer. Gastric Cancer. 2011; 14(3):279–84.
14. Lee SW, Nomura E, Tokuhara T, Kawai M, Matsuhashi N, Yokoyama K, Fujioka H, Hiramatsu M, Okuda J, Uchiyama K. Lapascopic technique and initial experience with knotless, unidirectional barbed suture closure for staple-conserving, delta-shaped gastroduodenostomy after distal gastrectomy. J Am Coll Surg. 2011; 213(6):e39–45.

Robotic Utilization in Gastric Cancer Surgery

Kaitlyn J. Kelly and Vivian E. Strong

Introduction

Utilization of minimally invasive techniques for gastric cancer surgery has increased in recent years. Laparoscopic distal gastrectomy for early-stage, distal gastric cancers is well established and is routinely practiced in the East where gastric cancer screening is routine. More than five randomized, prospective trials have confirmed improvements in short-term outcomes compared to open distal gastrectomy for patients with early-stage disease [1–6]. Laparoscopic resection of locally advanced and proximal gastric cancers, however, is not as well studied or widely performed. The two-dimensional view provided by the conventional laparoscope and limited range of motion of the instruments makes these complex resections challenging to perform

Electronic supplementary material Supplementary material is available in the online version of this chapter at 10.1007/978-3-319-09342-0_25. Videos can also be accessed at http://www.springerimages.com/videos/978-3-319-09341-3.

K.J. Kelly, MD
Department of Surgery,
University of California, San Diego,
3855 Health Sciences Drive,
La Jolla, CA 92093, USA
e-mail: k6kelly@ucsd.edu

V.E. Strong, MD (✉)
Department of Surgery,
Memorial Sloan-Kettering Cancer Center,
New York, NY, USA

laparoscopically. Controversy exists over the ability to perform an adequate lymphadenectomy laparoscopically in cases of locally advanced disease and over the safety of a laparoscopic esophagojejunal anastomosis in total gastrectomy.

The robotic surgery platform offers several technical advantages over laparoscopy. The camera provides a three-dimensional, magnified, high-definition view that is stable and is controlled by the primary surgeon. The articulated robotic instruments provide seven degrees of freedom and facilitate performance of difficult dissection and suturing. These advantages have led surgeons to investigate the use of the robotic platform for gastrectomy. Robot-assisted gastrectomy (RG) for gastric adenocarcinoma was first reported in 2003 [7, 8] and was first reported in the United States in 2007 [9]. Since that time, multiple retrospective series of RG for gastric adenocarcinoma have been published, almost all from the East [10–16]. The conclusions that can be drawn from these retrospective studies are limited due to great variability in inclusion criteria, surgeon experience, type of reconstruction performed, and the outcomes evaluated.

This chapter will describe the technical aspects of RG for gastric cancer and discuss considerations regarding the learning curve and patient selection. Additionally, the chapter will summarize current literature on RG for gastric cancer with a focus on outcomes and costs.

S.N. Hochwald, M. Kukar (eds.), *Minimally Invasive Foregut Surgery for Malignancy: Principles and Practice*,   261
DOI 10.1007/978-3-319-09342-0_25, © Springer International Publishing Switzerland 2015

Technical Aspects of Robotic Gastrectomy (Video 25.1)

Patient Positioning and Port Placement

RAG is performed with the patient in the supine position on a split-leg table. The patients' arms are tucked bilaterally with adequate padding of elbows and hands to avoid pressure points. The patient is secured to the table at the shoulders using foam blocks and heavy-duty adhesive tape applied circumferentially around the blocks and the table. Fixation is also applied at the hips with a safety belt and circumferentially at the knees. Footboards may also be applied at the feet as further means to avoid sliding during reverse Trendelenburg positioning. Once patient positioning is completed, it is important to place the patient in steep reverse Trendelenburg as a test to assure stability.

Port placement for RAG follows the same principles as for any robot-assisted procedure which include placement of the camera port at a distance of 15–20 cm from the target anatomy, placement of robot ports at least 8-cm apart from each other, and an assistant port at least 5 cm from adjacent robotic ports. While multiple variations of port placement have been described, the placement illustrated in Fig. 25.1 is recommended. Pneumoperitoneum is established with a Veress needle just off of the left costal margin. A 12-mm trocar is then placed in the midline above or below the umbilicus depending on the patient's body habitus but with a goal of port placement 15–20 cm from the target anatomy. In the majority of cases, the infraumbilical position is best. Two additional 8-mm da Vinci ports are then placed on the left side, at least 8 cm from each other and slightly off-set from the plane of the camera port. An additional 12-mm port is placed in the right mid-clavicular line, and an 8-mm robotic port is placed within it. A 5-mm assistant port is placed further laterally on the right side, approximately at the anterior axillary line.

At this point, the abdomen is explored for adhesions and for any evidence of peritoneal or

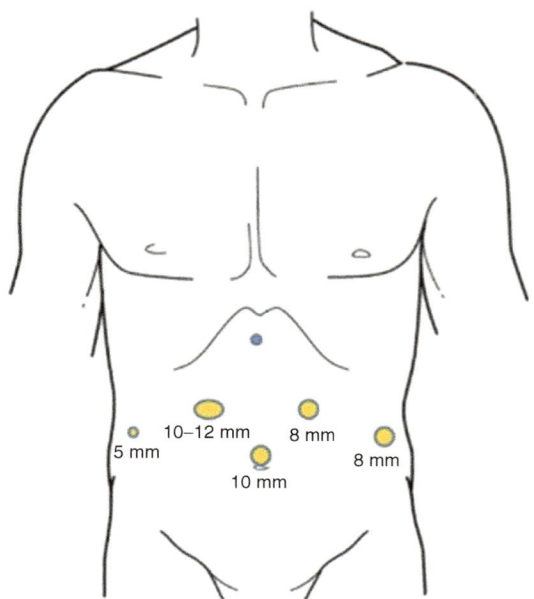

Fig. 25.1 Recommended port placement for robotic-assisted gastrectomy

extra-gastric disease. If a distal subtotal gastrectomy is to be performed and the lesion is not appreciable on the extraluminal surface, an endoscope is passed, and the lesion is localized. A silk stitch is placed laparoscopically to mark the level of transection of the stomach that will likely achieve a negative proximal margin. Once this is complete, the patient is placed in steep reverse Trendelenburg, and the robot is docked from directly over the patient's head. Arms 1 and 3 are attached to the left-sided ports, and arm 2 is attached to the right-sided port within the large 12-mm port. A fenestrated bipolar grasper is placed in arm 2, and a harmonic scalpel or monopolar scissor is placed in arm 1. A grasping forcep, preferably a Cardiere, is placed in arm 3.

Procedural Steps

The procedure commences by flipping the greater omentum cephalad and locating the transverse colon. The omentum is carefully taken off of the colon proceeding in the direction of the splenic flexure. With careful dissection, the omentum is separated from the transverse mesocolon, and the

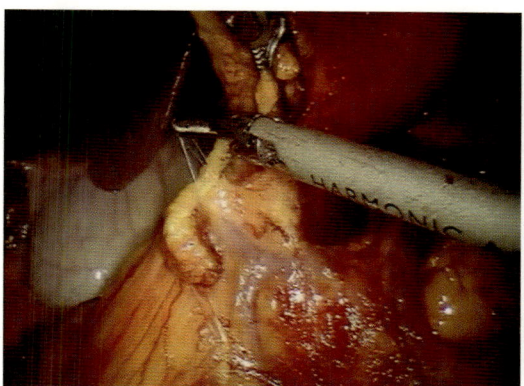

Fig. 25.2 Confluence of right gastroepiploic and right colic veins at anterior border of pancreas

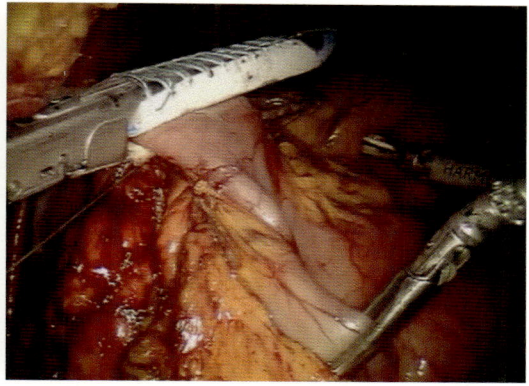

Fig. 25.3 Division of proximal duodenum just distal to pylorus

lesser sac is entered. Visualization of the posterior wall of the stomach confirms entry into the lesser sac. The posterior wall of the stomach is then grasped by the bedside assistant and is retracted anteriorly and to the patient's right side. The omentectomy is carried up toward the spleen and is stopped at the edge of the stomach just prior to reaching the short gastric vessels in a distal subtotal gastrectomy. For a total gastrectomy, the omentectomy is carried up to the esophageal hiatus, and the short gastric vessels are divided.

Once this is complete, the posterior wall of the stomach is grasped with the 3rd arm of the robot and is retracted toward the patient's left shoulder. The omentectomy then proceeds toward the hepatic flexure of the colon and is completed. The omentum can be placed in the left upper quadrant on the anterior wall of the stomach at this point. The posterior attachments between the stomach and pancreas are then divided sharply or with the harmonic scalpel in the direction of the pylorus. The right gastroepiploic vessels are identified and dissected circumferentially at the level of the anterior border of the pancreas (Fig. 25.2). The vessels are divided at their origin with a vascular load of a stapler or with clips. If the stapler is to be used, arm 2 of the robot together with its associated 8-mm port is removed from the larger 12-mm port, and the stapler is passed by the bedside assistant.

The pylorus is then identified by the vein of Mayo/white line, and attention is turned toward

the suprapyloric region. The gastrohepatic omentum is incised with hook monopolar cautery or a harmonic scalpel in arm 1. The right gastric artery is identified and is ligated at its take-off from the proper hepatic artery with the harmonic scalpel. The lymphatic tissue along the hepatic proper and common hepatic artery is swept medially toward the specimen, and a window is created at the level of the pylorus. The posterior aspect of the pylorus and proximal duodenum is elevated off of the retroperitoneum with a combination of blunt dissection and use of the harmonic scalpel. A blue load of the stapler with bioabsorbable reinforcement is then introduced, and the proximal duodenum is stapled and divided just distal to the pylorus (Fig. 25.3).

Once this is complete, the distal stomach can be retracted toward the patient's left shoulder utilizing robot arm 3. The lymph node dissection that was started previously is then continued along the common hepatic artery toward the celiac axis and proximal splenic artery. The left gastric artery is identified at the celiac axis and is divided at its base with a vascular load of the stapler. The gastrohepatic omentum is further incised up to the level of the esophageal hiatus with the harmonic scalpel. For distal subtotal gastrectomy, the level 1 and 2 lymph nodes are peeled down off of the proximal stomach down to the level where the stomach will be divided. For a total gastrectomy, the distal esophagus is divided with stapler (blue load).

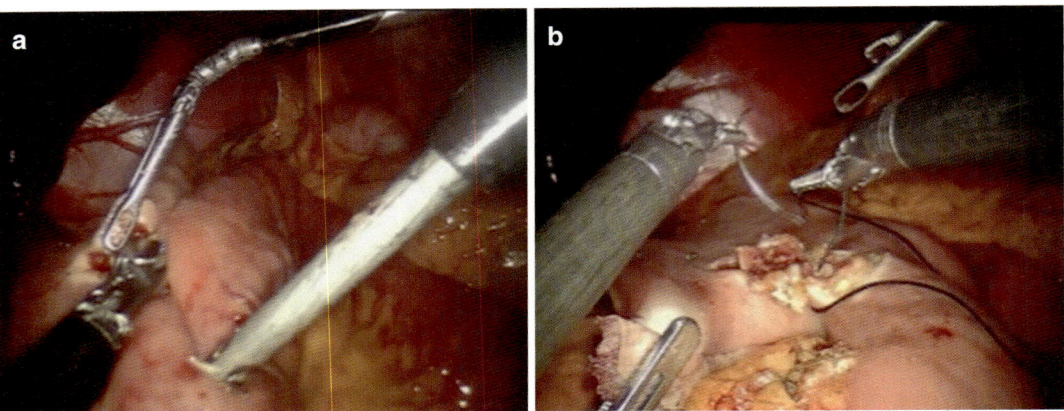

Fig. 25.4 (**a**) Creation of stapled side-to-side gastrojejunostomy. (**b**) Closure of gastroenterotomy

At this point, the specimen is placed in a specimen retrieval bag and is removed via the 12-mm port site in the right upper quadrant. The 12-mm port is then replaced, and the 8-mm robotic port attached to arm 2 is placed within it. Attention is then turned to the reconstruction.

For a distal subtotal gastrectomy in which no more than half of the stomach was removed, we prefer an antecolic, Billroth II reconstruction is preferred. If greater than half of the stomach is removed or if a total gastrectomy is performed, we prefer a Roux-Y reconstruction is preferred. The colon is elevated cephalad, and the ligament of Treitz is identified. A mobile piece of jejunum approximately 30-cm downstream is selected and is used for the reconstruction. For a Billroth II or Roux-Y reconstruction to a gastric remnant, a side-to-side stapled gastrojejunostomy is created with a 60-mm laparoscopic stapler. The remaining enterotomy is sutured closed with a running 3.0 silk stitch with needle drivers in robot arms 1 and 2 (Fig. 25.4). For an esophagojejunostomy, an end-to-side anastomosis is created with a circular stapler. To facilitate this, the Orvil of the stapler is passed transorally on a nasogastric tube which is then pulled through the distal esophagus. The tubing is then gently detached from the Orvil and is removed through the 12-mm right upper quadrant port. The stapler itself is inserted into the Roux limb after removing the staple line with the

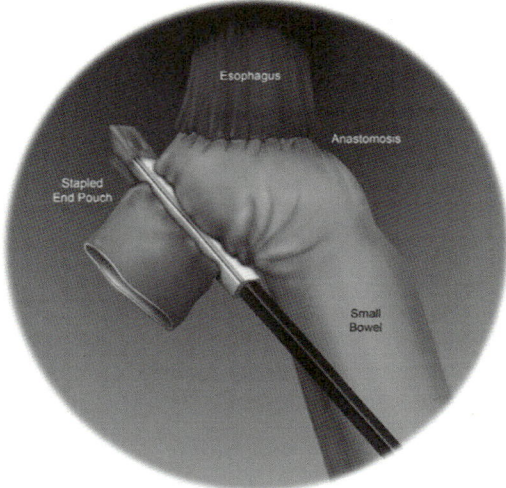

Fig. 25.5 Schematic diagram of stapled esophagojejunostomy following total gastrectomy

Harmonic scalpel. Once the anastomosis is created, the open end of the Roux limb is closed with a linear stapler (Fig. 25.5). All staplers are inserted via the right upper quadrant 12-mm incision by the bedside assistant. For Roux reconstruction, a side-to-side stapled jejunojejunostomy is created approximately 70-cm downstream from the proximal anastomosis, and the remaining enterotomy is sutured closed. Mesenteric defects are also sutured closed in a running fashion with 3.0 Vicryl.

The Learning Curve

It is hypothesized that the learning curve for RG is less than that for LG due to the ergonomic and technical advantages provided by the robotic platform. There is evidence suggesting that this is the case for surgeons already experienced with advanced laparoscopy, but the recommended number of procedures required for learning varies. Some authors have suggested 20 cases for learning RG by advanced laparoscopic surgeons [11, 17]. More recently, Kim et al. performed a comprehensive, multidimensional analysis of the learning curve for laparoscopic versus robotic distal gastrectomy [14]. With their more rigorous statistical analysis of stability in operating time and "surgical success," they found that 95 cases were required for learning RG, and 270 were required for LG. This was a retrospective analysis, however, and the surgeon had completed 177 LGs prior to the first robotic case. The number of robotic cases required might be greater for surgeons without prior laparoscopic experience.

There have been no studies to date prospectively evaluating learning curves from initial surgeon experience in RG versus LG. It has been suggested that experienced open surgeons can transition directly to the robotic platform without an intermediate laparoscopic step [18], but formal simulation training with the robotic platform with both dry and wet labs is a must. Furthermore, one should at least be familiar with laparoscopic exposure of relevant anatomy and with laparoscopic tissue handling while still having haptic feedback, which is lost with the robotic platform.

Patient Selection

For RG to be performed successfully, good patient selection is critical. This is especially true in a surgeon's initial experience. Ideal candidates for RG are patients with early-stage disease who have not received neoadjuvant therapy and those with normal BMI, distal tumors, and intestinal-type histology. As a surgeon's experience with the procedure increases, the incorporation of patients with more advanced disease, neoadjuvant treatment, proximal tumors, and higher BMI is reasonable. It may, in fact, be in these settings where the robotic platform is most advantageous over laparoscopy. It is in these scenarios where LG with D2 lymphadenectomy is most challenging.

We have noted an association between diffuse-type histology and microscopic proximal margin positivity (R1) in LG and therefore recommend selecting patients with intestinal-type histology in one's initial experience with minimally invasive gastrectomy (unpublished data). LG and RG are still feasible in patients with diffuse-type histology, but a frozen section of the proximal margin should be sent intraoperatively in all cases, and the surgeon should be comfortable with laparoscopic or robotic total gastrectomy or with conversion to an open procedure if necessary.

Perioperative Outcomes

Multiple retrospective series have been published evaluating perioperative outcomes following RG. Three of the largest studies, inclusive of patients reported in prior smaller studies, are summarized in Table 25.1 [10, 11, 15]. It is important to note that these studies contained a predominance of patients with T1–2, N0 disease. An association between decreased blood loss and RG has been shown, but no other measurable short-term outcomes have reliably been shown to be different between RG and LG. The study by Kim and colleagues was the largest and included 5,839 patients who underwent open ($n=4,542$), laparoscopic ($n=861$), or robotic ($n=436$) gastrectomy for gastric adenocarcinoma [15]. Patients in the open group had more advanced disease and proximal tumors than those in the LG and RG groups. The authors found no differences in overall perioperative morbidity or mortality among the groups, although interestingly, the types of complications did vary. The open

Table 25.1 Published studies comparing robotic and laparoscopic gastrectomy for cancer

Study	N	Op-time (min)[a]	Open conversion	Positive margin (R1/2)	Lymph nodes (N)	Length of stay (days)	EBL (mL)	Morbidity (%)	Mortality (%)
Kang et al. (2012) [11]									
RG	80	**202±52**[b]	NR	NR	NR	**10±12**	**93±85**	14	0
LG	282	**173±51**	NR	NR	NR	**8±4**	**173±51**	10	0
Kim et al. (2012) [15]									
RG	436	**226±54**	NR	1	40±15	8±14	85±160	10	0.5
LG	861	**176±63**	NR	2	38±14	8±9	112±229	9	0.3
Hyun et al. (2013) [10]									
RG	38	234±48	0	0	33±14	10±6	131±10	47.3	0
LG	83	220±61	0	0	33±13	12±10	130±18	38.5	0

RG robotic gastrectomy, *LG* laparoscopic gastrectomy, *NR* not reported
[a]Data expressed as means ± standard deviation
[b]Bolded variables were statistically significantly different

approach was associated with a greater incidence of postoperative bowel obstruction, ileus, and abscess formation. The minimally invasive approaches were associated with a greater incidence of anastomotic leak. In this study, complications were tracked out to 30 days postoperatively or to >30 days within the same hospitalization. Late complications were not reported, and conversion rates were not commented on.

One nonrandomized, prospective study of 150 patients undergoing RG (*N*=30) or LG (*N*=12) has been reported [17]. In this study, operative time was significantly longer with RG. There were no significant differences in margin status, number of lymph nodes retrieved, blood loss, length of stay, perioperative morbidity, or mortality. There were no conversions to open surgery in either group. This study evaluated CRP and IL-6 levels as markers of surgical stress and found them to be significantly lower with LG. Cost was significantly more with RG (approximately $4400 more per case).

The applicability of these studies to Western patients is limited given the high case volume of these surgeons, the very low overall morbidity reported, the exclusion of patients who received neoadjuvant therapy, and the predominance of patients with early-stage disease.

Finally, several meta-analyses of studies comparing LG and RG have recently been reported [19–21]. The most comprehensive of these included nine nonrandomized studies that compared the two procedures. One of these studies was from Italy, and the remaining eight were from China, Korea, or Japan. In the meta-analysis RG was again associated with decreased blood loss and increased operative time compared to LG. An association was also observed between RG and a shorter distal margin. There were no differences in any other short-term outcomes evaluated, including number of lymph nodes retrieved, proximal resection margin, rate of conversion to open surgery, overall morbidity, anastomotic leakage or stenosis, intestinal obstruction, time to first flatus, length of hospital stay, or perioperative mortality [21].

Long-Term Outcomes

Very limited data on long-term, oncologic outcomes of RG are available. Pugliese and colleagues reported 18 cases of RG including both early and advanced disease. At a median follow-up of 28 months, the 3-year overall survival was 78 %. Four patients (22 %) had recurrence within the follow-up period [22]. Decreased blood loss with RG over LG likely reflects the enhanced ability to perform a delicate lymphadenectomy near the celiac axis and major gastric vessels. Whether this advantage will translate into improvements in recurrence-free or disease-specific survival is not known. It was 15 years before the survival benefit of D2 lymphadenectomy in Western gastric cancer patients became apparent [23]. It may therefore be some time before a measureable difference in survival from a more precise lymphadenectomy emerges.

Cost

The cost of the robotic surgery platform is limiting in the current economy. In Korea, patients pay out of pocket for the extra costs of robotic-assisted procedures. In the United States, hospitals charge significantly more for robotic-assisted procedures than for open or laparoscopic surgeries to off-set the costs of the robots, instruments, and support. While the technical advantages of the robot definitely allow for better dissection and lymphadenectomy in some procedures, particularly gastrectomy, prostatectomy, and proctectomy, it is unknown whether the increased cost will continue to be justified in the absence of measurable clinical benefits over laparoscopy.

Summary

Utilization of the robot in gastrectomy for cancer allows for a more precise dissection and D2 lymphadenectomy than what can be achieved with standard laparoscopy. This advantage comes with significantly increased cost, however, and it is unclear whether it will translate into clinical benefits for patients. Further controlled, prospective studies inclusive of patients with advanced disease, neoadjuvant treatment, and higher BMI are needed to clarify the role of the robot in gastric cancer surgery. It may be in these settings, where laparoscopy is particularly challenging, where the robot may be most advantageous.

References

1. Hayashi H, Ochiai T, Shimada H, Gunji Y. Prospective randomized study of open versus laparoscopy-assisted distal gastrectomy with extraperigastric lymph node dissection for early gastric cancer. Surg Endosc. 2005;19:1172–6.
2. Huscher CG, Mingoli A, Sgarzini G, et al. Laparoscopic versus open subtotal gastrectomy for distal gastric cancer: five-year results of a randomized prospective trial. Ann Surg. 2005;241:232–7.
3. Kim HH, Hyung WJ, Cho GS, et al. Morbidity and mortality of laparoscopic gastrectomy versus open gastrectomy for gastric cancer: an interim report – a phase III multicenter, prospective, randomized Trial (KLASS Trial). Ann Surg. 2010;251:417–20.
4. Kim YW, Baik YH, Yun YH, et al. Improved quality of life outcomes after laparoscopy-assisted distal gastrectomy for early gastric cancer: results of a prospective randomized clinical trial. Ann Surg. 2008;248:721–7.
5. Lee JH, Han HS, Lee JH. A prospective randomized study comparing open vs laparoscopy-assisted distal gastrectomy in early gastric cancer: early results. Surg Endosc. 2005;19:168–73.
6. Kitano S, Shiraishi N, Fujii K, Yasuda K, Inomata M, Adachi Y. A randomized controlled trial comparing open vs laparoscopy-assisted distal gastrectomy for the treatment of early gastric cancer: an interim report. Surgery. 2002;131:S306–11.
7. Hashizume M, Sugimachi K. Robot-assisted gastric surgery. Surg Clin North Am. 2003;83:1429–44.
8. Giulianotti PC, Coratti A, Angelini M, et al. Robotics in general surgery: personal experience in a large community hospital. Arch Surg. 2003;138:777–84.
9. Anderson C, Ellenhorn J, Hellan M, Pigazzi A. Pilot series of robot-assisted laparoscopic subtotal gastrectomy with extended lymphadenectomy for gastric cancer. Surg Endosc. 2007;21:1662–6.
10. Hyun MH, Lee CH, Kwon YJ, et al. Robot versus laparoscopic gastrectomy for cancer by an experienced surgeon: comparisons of surgery, complications, and surgical stress. Ann Surg Oncol. 2013;20:1258–65.
11. Kang BH, Xuan Y, Hur H, Ahn CW, Cho YK, Han SU. Comparison of surgical outcomes between robotic and laparoscopic gastrectomy for gastric cancer: the learning curve of robotic surgery. J Gastric Cancer. 2012;12: 56–63.
12. Woo Y, Hyung WJ, Pak KH, et al. Robotic gastrectomy as an oncologically sound alternative to laparoscopic resections for the treatment of early-stage gastric cancers. Arch Surg. 2011;146:1086–92.
13. Song J, Oh SJ, Kang WH, Hyung WJ, Choi SH, Noh SH. Robot-assisted gastrectomy with lymph node dissection for gastric cancer: lessons learned from an initial 100 consecutive procedures. Ann Surg. 2009;249:927–32.
14. Kim HI, Park MS, Song KJ, Woo Y, Hyung WJ. Rapid and safe learning of robotic gastrectomy for gastric cancer: multidimensional analysis in a comparison with laparoscopic gastrectomy. Eur J Surg Oncol. 2013. Epub ahead of print.
15. Kim KM, An JY, Kim HI, Cheong JH, Hyung WJ, Noh SH. Major early complications following open, laparoscopic and robotic gastrectomy. Br J Surg. 2012; 99:1681–7.
16. Kim MC, Heo GU, Jung GJ. Robotic gastrectomy for gastric cancer: surgical techniques and clinical merits. Surg Endosc. 2010;24:610–5.
17. Park JY, Jo MJ, Nam BH, et al. Surgical stress after robot-assisted distal gastrectomy and its economic implications. Br J Surg. 2012;99:1554–61.

18. Coratti A, Annecchiarico M, Di Marino M, Gentile E, Coratti F, Giulianotti PC. Robot-assisted gastrectomy for gastric cancer: current status and technical considerations. World J Surg. 2013;37(12):2771–81.

19. Liao GX, Xie GZ, Li R, et al. Meta-analysis of outcomes compared between robotic and laparoscopic gastrectomy for gastric cancer. Asian Pac J Cancer Prev. 2013;14:4871–5.

20. Xiong B, Ma L, Zhang C. Robotic versus laparoscopic gastrectomy for gastric cancer: a meta-analysis of short outcomes. Surg Oncol. 2012;21:274–80.

21. Xiong J, Nunes QM, Tan C, et al. Comparison of short-term clinical outcomes between robotic and laparoscopic gastrectomy for gastric cancer: a meta-analysis of 2495 patients. J Laparoendosc Adv Surg Tech A. 2013;23(12):965–76.

22. Pugliese R, Maggioni D, Sansonna F, et al. Subtotal gastrectomy with D2 dissection by minimally invasive surgery for distal adenocarcinoma of the stomach: results and 5-year survival. Surg Endosc. 2010;24: 2594–602.

23. Songun I, Putter H, Kranenbarg EM, Sasako M, van de Velde CJ. Surgical treatment of gastric cancer: 15-year follow-up results of the randomised nationwide Dutch D1D2 trial. Lancet Oncol. 2010;11: 439–49.

Index

S.N. Hochwald, M. Kukar (eds.), *Minimally Invasive Foregut Surgery for Malignancy: Principles and Practice*,   269
DOI 10.1007/978-3-319-09342-0, © Springer International Publishing Switzerland 2015

Printed by Printforce, the Netherlands